YOGA & YOU

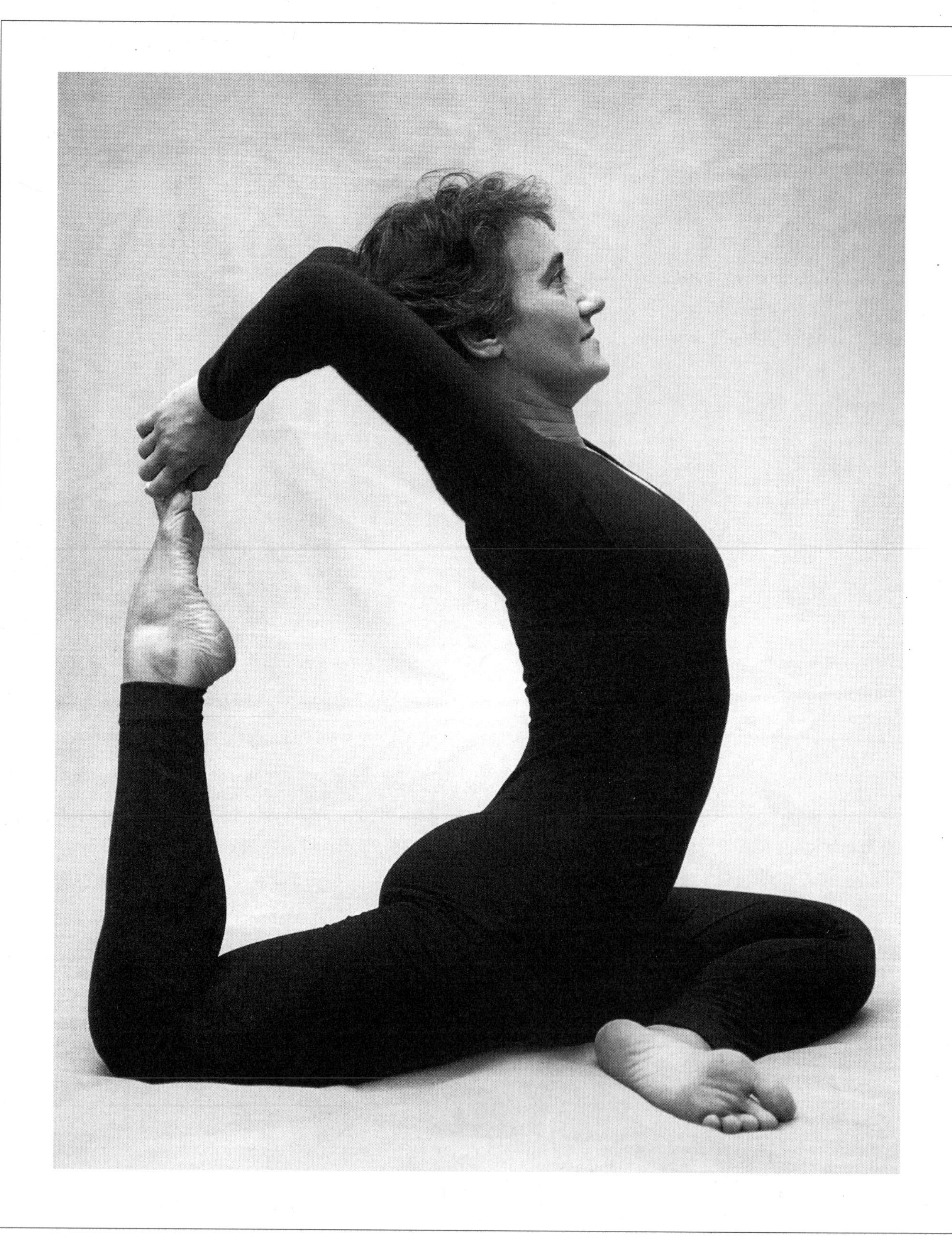

YOGA & YOU

Energizing and Relaxing Yoga for New and Experienced Students

ESTHER MYERS

RANDOM HOUSE OF CANADA
Toronto

Contents

Acknowledgements ix

Introduction 3

1. Yoga and its Roots 9

2. On the Way 21

3. Your Practice 31

4. From the Beginning: Basic Principles 45

5. Deep Relaxation: Letting Go 53

6. Pranayama: Attention to your Breath 59

7. Learning to Stand 81

8. Simple Stretches 87

9. Sun Salutation: The Wave 97

10. Standing Poses 109

11. Inverted Poses and Arm Balances 125

12. Backbends 159

13. Sitting Poses and Forward Bends 181

14. Sitting Twists 199

15. Suggested Practice Sequences 209

Suggested Reading 231

Glossary of Sanskrit Terms 235

Index 239

students, which I co-authored with Lynn Wylie. Lynn helped me to move from the idea of writing a practice book to the reality of putting something on paper. Danita Halldorson has inspired the discussion of yoga philosophy and its meaning today. My agent Lucinda Vardey, who is also a yoga teacher, encouraged me to write a book for people "on the path," those of you who are already committed to an on-going yoga practice. Sarah Davies, my editor, and the staff at Random House have been wonderfully supportive and patient.

Rick Pottruff and Rob Howard have been wonderfully generous with their time. Their talents have enhanced this book enormously.

I would also like to thank you, the reader. Whether you are starting yoga, returning to it, or wanting to expand and deepen your present practice, I hope that you will discover the joys, benefits, challenges and rewards of making yoga a part of your life, and that this book will be an aid and companion on your journey.

ESTHER MYERS
Toronto, 1996

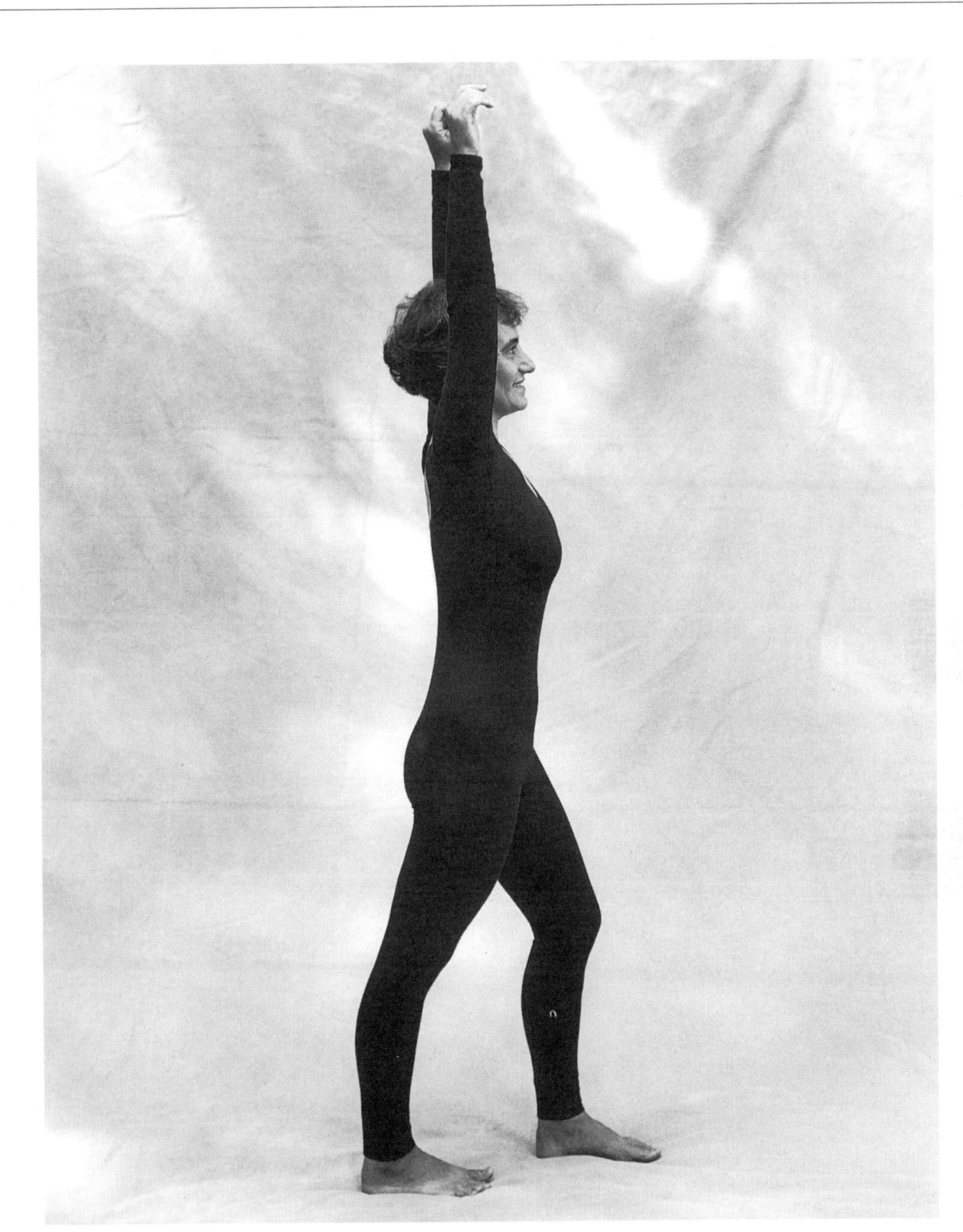

Warrior Pose I

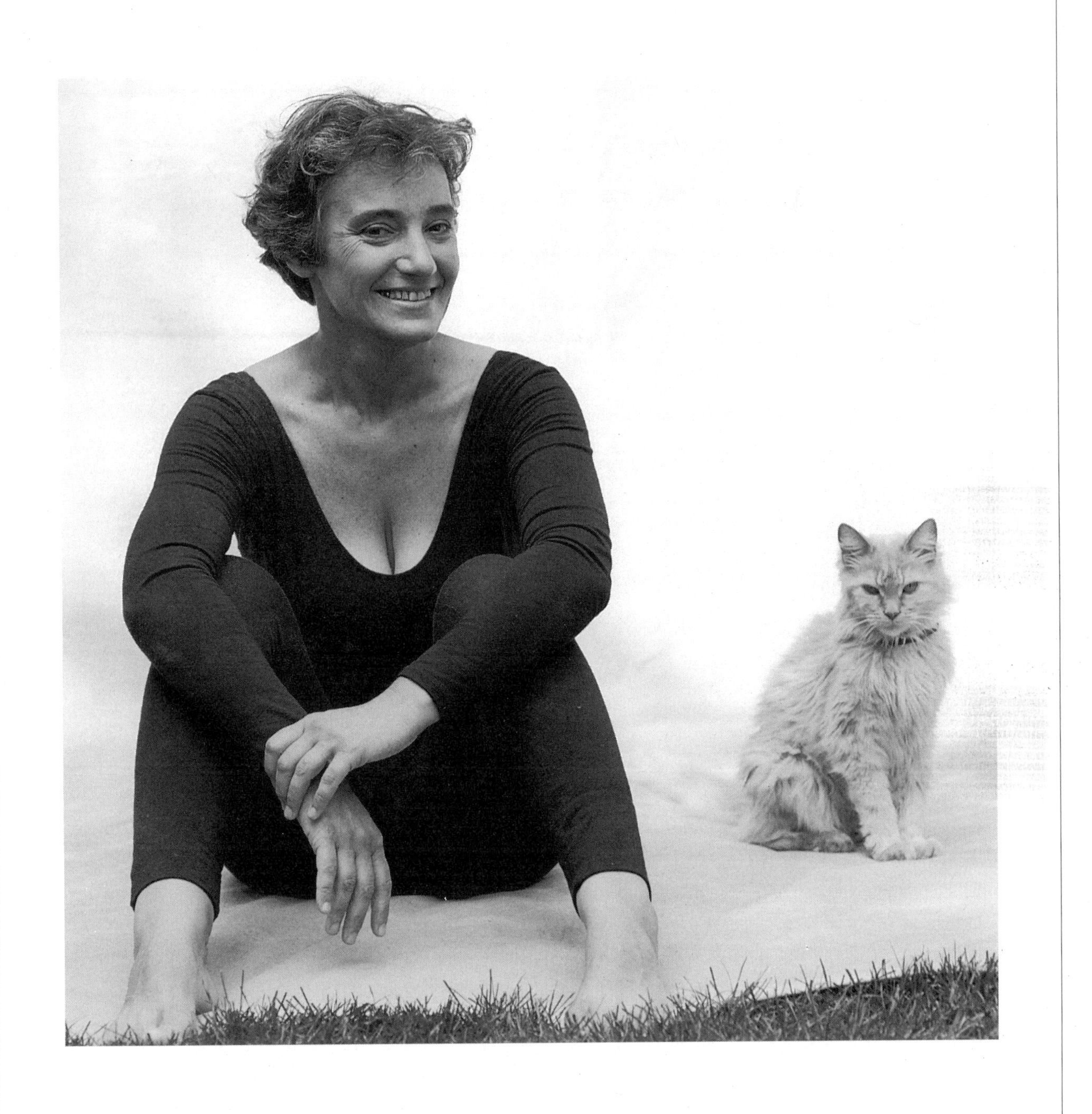

Introduction

I was introduced to Indian thought in high school when I read an essay by Rabindranath Tagore. He said that the East had a lot to learn from the West, *and* that the West could also learn from the East. At the time I was headed for a career in science and couldn't imagine what the West could possibly learn from the East. I've since discovered.

I began practising yoga in 1972, while I was living in London, England. I was part of an experimental community established under the auspices of the Philadelphia Association, a registered charity then under the chairmanship of psychiatrist R.D. Laing. The community's goal was to provide asylum, a place of refuge, to people who might otherwise be in mental hospitals, especially schizophrenics. It was a mixture of ex-patients, therapists, professionals-in-training and others, like me, who were simply interested in participating in this experiment. In the spirit of the sixties, we were attempting to strip away institutional roles and social façades. We wanted to create an environment in which people could be themselves — to heal and be healed in mind and spirit. I visited, lived and worked in the community and the network of friends surrounding it for about five years. When I left, I felt as though I had been through a mediaeval trial by ordeal. Having survived, I was both cleansed and healed. Much of what I have done and become since germinated there.

I was drawn to the community by the honesty, immediacy and rawness of the experience. We were asking questions about who we were, about the meaning and purpose of our lives. Much later I learned that these questions are central to yoga, and that the practice shows us a way to go inside to find the answers.

Arthur Balaskas was giving a free class in Iyengar yoga at the Archway community. I noticed that many people in the network were comfortable sitting on the floor. Since this was difficult for me and I thought that yoga might make it easier, I took the class. I was hooked instantly. A year and a half later, I began taking classes with Angela Farmer. When she decided to take a six-week holiday, I was faced with the prospect of six weeks without yoga, and in desperation started to practise on my own. I was helped by some simple sheets Angela had made up outlining a weekly practice. I hope that this book can guide you in the same way.

When Angela stopped teaching regular classes in London, I began classes with Mary Stewart (author of *Yoga for Children*, *Yoga over Fifty*, and others). The contrast between the two teachers couldn't have been greater. Angela is long, lithe, poetic and fluid; Mary is short, strong, a bundle of dynamic energy. With Mary, I became interested in training to teach. During my training, I studied with Mary, Angela and Diana Clifton, another senior Iyengar teacher. I was enriched by seeing the differences between these three women. I learned that we each practise and teach from who and where we are; that yoga frees us to be ourselves. At the same time, I could see the essence of the teaching being transmitted by each of them.

This zone, the zone of no-thing, of the silence of silences, is the source. We forget that we are all there all the time.

— R. D. LAING

I was on holiday in Toronto in the summer of 1975 when a casual acquaintance suggested that I come back and start a yoga school. Something inside me said "Yes." The following spring I moved back and began to teach. Iyengar yoga, a method of Hatha yoga developed by B.K.S. Iyengar, had not been taught in Toronto before, and I found myself teaching both novices and experienced teachers. It was quite overwhelming. It also showed me the contribution that Iyengar has made to yoga in the West. The combination of technical precision, strength, dynamic energy and the challenge to go beyond one's limits added a new dimension to the practice of many of my more experienced students.

In 1978, while I was in Italy studying with Dona Holleman, I met Vanda Scaravelli, author of *Awakening the Spine*. She had studied with B.K.S. Iyengar and also with T.K.V. Desikachar. After working with

them for a number of years, she branched out on her own. Trusting her body, and following the movement of her breath and her spine, she came to a "new world ... a world without aim and without competition, where the body can start to function naturally and happily, allowing expansion to take place in space."[1]

I got to know her daughter and son-in-law, who live quite close to my house in Toronto and had my first lesson with Vanda in 1984 when she was visiting them. She works one-on-one, and taught me almost entirely with her hands. I didn't really understand what she was doing, but again I felt a deep "Yes" inside. Her touch was absolutely right. My spine was starting to release, and her way of extension and elongation was a natural step for me. Even though I had not been looking for a teacher, I felt immediately that she was the person to take me further.

The following year, I attended a course at the Ramamani Iyengar Memorial Institute in India. Right from the beginning, it felt wrong. I realized that through my work with Vanda, I had moved away from Iyengar yoga and was now on a different path. It took me some time to integrate this "new way," and to learn to articulate and communicate it. I also had to let go of my identification with the Iyengar method. It was a difficult, painful and confusing period, internally and in the world of yoga politics. I ended up resigning from the Iyengar yoga association I had helped to create.

For the last ten years, Vanda has divided her time between Toronto and Florence, and I have had the privilege of working with her intensively over extended periods of time. I have been overwhelmed both by her teaching and by her love. I have never met anyone who accepted me so completely, and, at the same time, demanded so much of me. Much later I came to understand that love is the essence of this work, which begins and ends with loving acceptance of ourselves, our bodies, the earth and its energy. Vanda was seventy-six when I began to work with her. Her main concern was that her work be communicated to the world before she died. I hope that through my teaching and the writing of this book I have been able to contribute to the fulfillment of that wish. Vanda never wanted to name her work "The Scaravelli Method," because she believes that each us must carry on, looking inside and discovering for ourselves from within. I hope this book will give you the tools to discover your own way and the yoga that is right for you.

[1] Vanda Scaravelli, *Awakening the Spine*, p. 24.

As I look back over my years of practice and teaching, I find myself returning to my roots in the Philadelphia Association. I see my classes and practice, similar to the Archway community, as an "asylum" in the original sense, a quiet place in which it is possible to turn inward, breathe, reflect, release, heal and be healed.

I had just finished the first draft of this book when I was diagnosed with breast cancer. I had two operations, a biopsy/lumpectomy and a mastectomy. The shock of the diagnosis and surgery left me with very little energy or resources. I had to acknowledge the part of me that was too weak and frightened to even attempt to sit quietly. During this journey into darkness, yoga, the yoga community, friends, family and even strangers have provided an asylum for me: a place where I could collapse in exhaustion, reel in terror, be hurt, frightened, vulnerable and needy. The decision I made at the very beginning to tell students about my condition meant exposing myself publicly in a completely new way. The result has been a level of care and support that I could not have imagined or allowed in the past. In the process, I have realized that I have an extraordinary network of caring and supportive people around me, and I want to take this opportunity to thank them again.

What doesn't kill me makes me stronger.
— ALBERT CAMUS

It took eight months after the surgery for me to be ready to write. I decided to write about my experience because it felt right and true. This decision was confirmed for me at a recent fund-raising breakfast for breast cancer. I was reminded again of the sad and terrifying statistics. A number of speakers referred to the wall of silence that used to surround this disease, so that women went through their ordeals alone. If my writing serves to lessen one woman's anxiety, it will have served its purpose.

However, the issue here is not only my story and one disease. All of us at some point in our lives face illness, loss, fear and sometimes tragedy. At any time, something can pull the rug out from underneath us and shatter the framework of our lives. A friend wrote to me, "It is easy to say 'fear not' — not so easy to find that place of fearlessness in ourselves where we can really embrace what is and what comes." Yoga and meditation evolved to help us face suffering with equanimity and to find the quiet centre inside.

One of the goals of spiritual practice is to face our deaths with calm and dignity. Fear of death is one of the causes of pain and suffering. For most people, the word "cancer" is associated with death, and certainly the diagnosis confronted me with the possibility of a premature death. Through the terror, I have been able to clarify my

purpose, learned to live my life more fully and more passionately, and to value each day. My practice has gradually returned. I feel freer, lighter and more alive than before. At the same time, I am wounded, fragile and still frightened.

A student of mine who also had cancer said that for her cancer is a message to go deeper. She told me that when it comes right down to it you are alone. Through the months of uncertainty, surgery and recuperation, I felt surrounded by love, support, healing energy, light, prayers and compassion. As my student goes deeper into her practice, looking for the answer, I can now tell her, the answer is love.

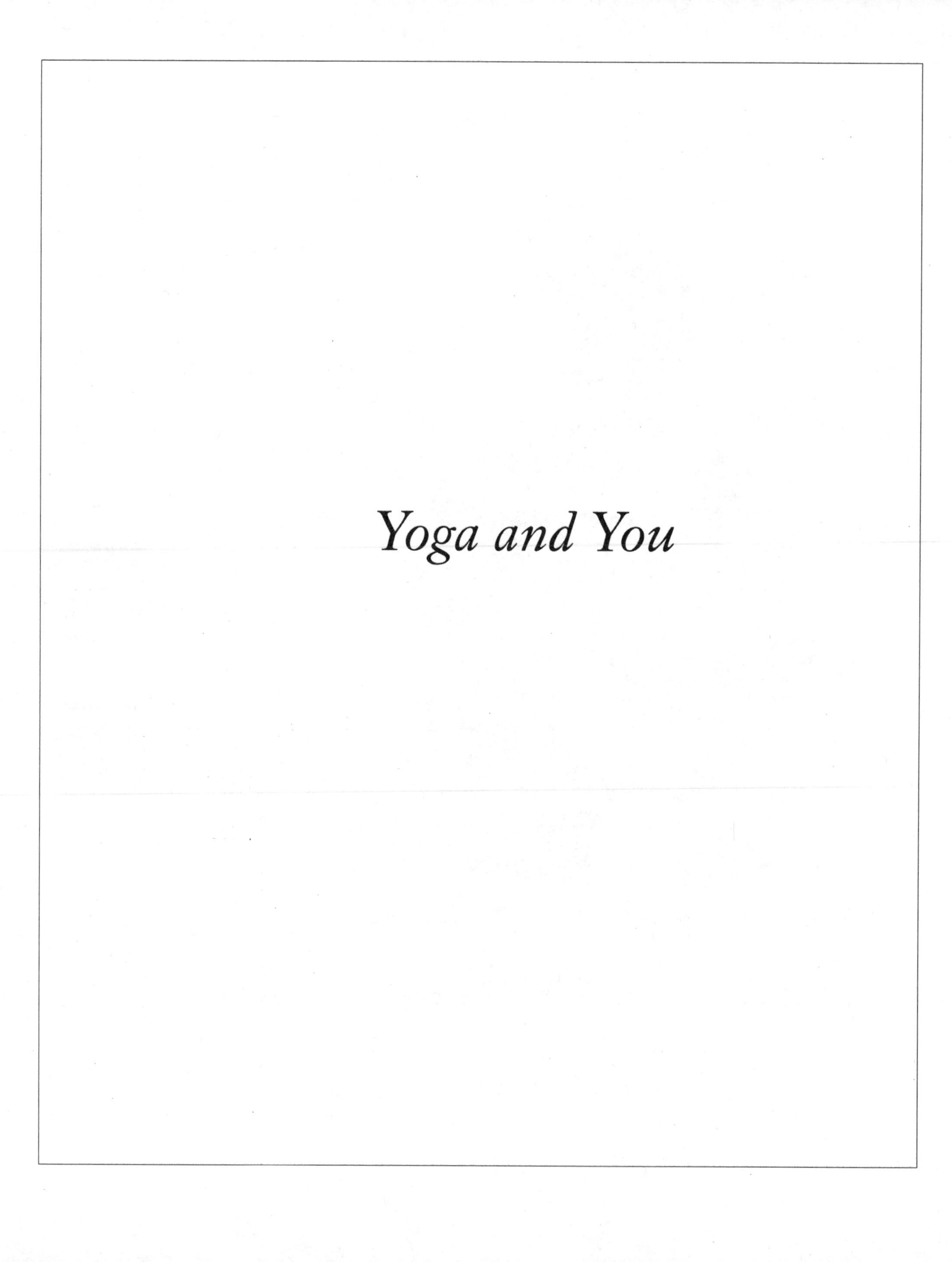

Yoga and You

CHAPTER I

Yoga and Its Roots

Yoga has its origins in the search for the spiritual and in primordial questions about the meaning of life. The awareness that yoga is a spiritual practice whose roots are ancient gives our journey continuity, richness and depth.

The word "yoga" comes from the Sanskrit root *yuj* meaning "to bind, join, attach and yoke, to direct and concentrate one's attention on, to use and apply." Yoga, in its original sense, is the joining or union of the individual self or soul with the higher Self—God. Yoga means mystical union, oneness with God, *and* the disciplines or practices that lead toward this union. It is related to religious concepts like communion, and modern psychological ideas of integration or wholeness. Through the practice of yoga, we yoke or harness ourselves to a discipline or a way of life that leads us toward harmony and balance. In the process, we integrate all aspects of our being—physical, emotional and spiritual—and discover our connections to the earth, the universe and each other.

Healing is a continual movement away from fragmentation toward wholeness and connection.

— DAWNA MARKOVA

Yoga developed from and within Indian philosophy and religion. It includes the idea of reincarnation, and considers our past actions (karma) both in this life and previous ones, as fundamental to our present physical, psychological and spiritual constitution. One of the purposes of yoga is to release us from the continuing cycle of death and rebirth, the result of the karma that we have accumulated. Our karma manifests as a combination of genetic predispositions and habits, patterns of behaviour and compulsions. Through practice, we can see how these reactions are triggered in us and how we can gradually weaken our tendency to repeat these patterns. However, the practice and benefits of yoga postures and breathing techniques do not require religious or spiritual beliefs and observances. On the contrary, we are taught that we must experience the practices personally in order to understand them. When I started yoga I found that it made me feel better, so I continued. Over the years, it has deepened and grown within me. Only in the last few years have yoga's traditional meaning and purpose become relevant and significant for me. It is certainly not necessary to believe in reincarnation to see the value in changing negative or dysfunctional patterns.

Classical texts

We do not know when or where yoga began. Archaeologists have unearthed seals showing figures seated in yoga postures that date from 2700 B.C., and the word "yoga" appears in the earliest Indian literature, the *Vedas* (3000–1200 B.C.). The *Bhagavad Gita* (Song of God) and Patanjali's *Yoga Sutras* are the most well known of the ancient texts on yoga. In very different ways, they each synthesize existing knowledge and practice.

The *Bhagavad Gita* is part of the epic *Mahabharata*, written around the time of the Buddha in the sixth century B.C. It is a philosophical poem, rich in imagery and symbolism. It brings together various meanings of the word yoga: equilibrium in success and failure, skill in action, the supreme secret of life, the producer of the greatest felicity, serenity, non-attachment and destroyer of pain.

> Some offer their outflowing breath into the breath that flows in; and the in-flowing breath into the breath that flows out; they aim at Pranayama, breath-harmony, and the flow of their breath is in peace.
>
> —*Bhagavad Gita*

We do not need to forsake the world or our responsibilities in order to find peace and enlightenment. Life in the world and spiritual practice can and should be cultivated simultaneously. The *Gita* is still used in India today as a guide for daily living. Mahatma Gandhi found both resource and solace in it.

Patanjali's *Yoga Sutras* (yoga threads), written somewhere between the second century B.C. and the fourth century A.D., were the first systematic descriptions of yoga philosophy and practice. Patanjali's method is sometimes referred to as Raja yoga, the royal path.

The four books consist of succinct aphorisms, distillations of the essence of yoga teaching as it had been passed down orally from ancient times. Patanjali defines yoga as "stilling of the restlessness of the mind." Quieting the mind is both the goal and the method of yoga. At the core of Patanjali's system is the "eight-fold path" (astanga yoga) which consists of **yamas, niyamas, asana, pranayama, pratyahara, dharana, dhyana** and **samadhi**.

The fundamentals of all yoga practice are the *yamas* and the *niyamas*: the ethical precepts of Patanjali's *Yoga Sutras*. As we shall see, these ethical principles, especially non-violence and non-greed, form the core of the practice of the postures. This attitude is in sharp contrast to the "no pain, no gain" philosophy of exercise and to the damage inflicted in sports today, where achievement, appearance and results have become the dominant values.

Yoga is the stilling of the restlessness of the mind.
— *Yoga Sutras*

Yamas

Yamas, restraints, are universal ethical principles. They govern social responsibilities and relationships with others. The five yamas are: non-violence, truth, non-stealing, chastity and non-greed.

According to Patanjali, yoga practice begins with non-violence in both thought and action. As we contemplate with horror the violence in the world today, this call to practise non-violence is more imperative than ever. The most obvious evidence of violence or aggression in our practice is injury. *Any* injury caused by practice is reason for concern. But even without an injury we need to watch for signs of force. Attention to our attitude in our yoga practice alerts us to ways that we are aggressive or hurtful in our lives, and gives us an opportunity to transform aggression through our practice.

Non-stealing and non-greed are very closely related to each other and to non-violence. Non-greed refers to having only what one needs, and non-stealing refers to both the act of stealing and the lusting after another's possessions. In terms of our asana practice we see these qualities in our competitiveness and aggression in the poses, pushing to do a pose that we aren't ready for or competing with ourselves and others. I have strained my knees a number of times because, as a yoga teacher, I thought I ought to be able to do Lotus Pose better. On one occasion this set me back nearly a year. We are all impatient with ourselves at some time. We need to remind ourselves over and over again that the practice is an on-going process of evolution, and that getting into the pose is not the goal. There is no value in achieving the position at the expense of your body, and no benefit in competing with yourself, other students or a picture in a book. But taking care of ourselves and respecting our bodies is not an easy lesson.

The precept of chastity shows that Patanjali has an ascetic approach to yoga practice. While very few students in the West make a commitment to chastity, this precept reminds us to conserve our energies and to pay attention to our contact with others, how we touch others and are touched by them.

Yoga calls us to be true to ourselves, as well as to be honest in word and deed. We need to be clear about who we are, and where we are. The body doesn't lie. The poses show us our strengths and weaknesses, our gifts and our limitations. They reflect our state of mind, and show us when we are centred and when we are disconnected or unstable. Practice brings to light the best and worst parts of ourselves that we have pushed aside or denied. We can learn to acknowledge difficult emotions like anger, despair, fear or sorrow, and find ways to work with and through them. Accepting your whole self is the essence of yoga. Yoga practice calls us to face ourselves with honesty and compassion.

These qualities which we develop in our practice radiate outwards into our lives. As Natalie Goldberg says in *Writing Down the Bones*, you can't be honest in your practice "and then step out of it, clamp down, go home 'be nice,' and not speak the truth. If you give yourself over to honesty in your practice, it will permeate your life." Notice, however, that truth follows non-violence. We must learn to speak and live the truth of who we are and what we believe in a way that does not do harm to others or ourselves.

Being true to yourself means being yourself. Liberation is the freedom not to conform. As the layers of expectations peel away, let the real you emerge and blossom. Funny, sad, silly, outrageous, angry, quiet, free.

Niyamas

Niyamas, disciplines, are concerned with the inner life, and relate directly to the committed practitioner. The niyamas are: purity, contentment, austerity, study and devotion to the Lord.

Most students today combine yoga with concern about their diet and eating habits. Some include periods of fasting and cleansing as part of their practice. These practices should be supervised by a qualified practitioner. Yoga is also being used in a variety of therapeutic contexts, a change from the ancient tradition when physical and mental health were prerequisites. The cleansing and purifying benefits of the poses and breathing practices help people who are working to overcome addictions, eating disorders and substance abuse. Students often find that as their yoga practice deepens they are able to stop or reduce smoking, drinking, over-eating, etc. Purity is a result of yoga practice.

Contentment is an active practice that goes beyond non-greed. Feelings of gratitude, abundance, joy and serenity need to be cultivated in an environment and culture that is constantly insisting on the need to have more, buy more and be more. We practice acceptance of our bodies and ourselves. Accepting our limitations and being willing to work with them often creates a release which allows us to move on. The practice is a way to help you move toward health, balance and stability.

The niyamas also include austerity, or *tapas*. The literal meaning of the word tapas is heat. It implies both psychic heat in the form of anger and aggression, and a burning fervour or zeal. Tapas stands as a counterbalance to contentment. It prevents us from allowing acceptance and contentment to slide into complacency. For me, tapas takes the form of anger and a strong drive to achieve. Most meditation books talk about observing your anger as a way to clear it, but I find that I need to express it in some way. I have used martial arts, journal writing, running and walking to do this. Karate provided a safe place and a structure for me to express my anger and to be centred in it. The dojo (way place) where karate is taught gave me a context where my anger and voice were encouraged and celebrated as expressions of spirit. Since I left martial arts (for a variety of personal reasons), I have worked to incorporate this kind of energy into my yoga. It is important to me that my yoga practice includes all of me — not just the quiet, peaceful, loving part. As a teacher, I feel that you can channel and express anger and rage in and through your practice if you want to, and that there are poses and techniques to help you do this.

In each pose, there is a place of balance. If we do less, we are not at our maximum; if we do more, we are forcing. Finding and staying on this edge is the middle way which balances and sustains contentment and challenge, self-acceptance and growth. Each of us needs to find our own balance of passive surrender and active practice, integrating these two extremes to become strong without effort and dynamic without force.

Study of sacred texts is not just intellectual knowledge, but a means for personal reflection and spiritual growth. Inspirational reading can nurture your spirit and counteract the images and messages of violence that surround us.

Devotion to the Lord is traditionally practised through prayer and mantras. Even without a formal devotional practice you can take a moment each day to be grateful for the gifts in your life

Asana

Asana now refers to all the yoga postures. In Patanjali's *Yoga Sutras*, it meant the place on which the yogi sits *and* the manner in which he sits there. All of the postures require a clear, conscious awareness of contact of our body with the ground. This connection between the posture and the ground, which we will be exploring throughout this book, is implied in the meaning of the word asana.

According to Patanjali, asana is both firm and relaxed. This is achieved through relaxation of effort, or by a mental state of balance. The idea that firm and stable posture could be achieved through relaxation of effort seems to be a contradiction. We need to learn how to find strength and stability without effort and stress.

> The tranquillity which is a pre-requisite for *samadhi* is a condition of extraordinary and habitual stability, and real stability cannot exist where there is strain.
>
> — I.K. TAIMNI

Steadiness of posture is also achieved by meditation on Ananta. In Hindu mythology, Ananta is the Chief of Serpents who upholds the globe of the earth and keeps it in orbit around the sun. He is the symbolic representation of the force of gravity. Through continuing to focus on this force, we bring ourselves into alignment with it. The combination of alignment with and surrender to gravity gives us the stability and ease described in the Sutras.

Pranayama

Pranayama, breathing practice, regulates and harmonizes the breath and its rhythm. Through breathing practices, prana or energy is contained and balanced. In B.K.S. Iyengar's classic book, *Light on Yoga*, he says "Prana is the breath of life of all beings in the universe. They are born through and live by it, and when they die their individual breath dissolves into the cosmic breath." Asana and pranayama are very closely linked and we always incorporate awareness of the breath into our practice of the poses.

Meditation

Pratyahara, withdrawal of the senses from the outer world, dharana, concentration, dhyana, contemplation or absorption/meditation and samadhi, ecstatic union, are the final stages of practice and are collectively known as *meditation*.

The word meditation (like the word yoga) refers to the goal of ecstatic union and the variety of practices used to reach this goal. In a very broad sense, meditation could be defined as a focusing of attention.

Attention to the breath is the foundation of most meditation systems, so pranayama is a form of meditation. Meditation techniques vary in the object or focus of attention. As Indian thought and practice travelled east through Tibet, China, Southeast Asia and Japan, the teachings and styles of practice were transformed by the various cultures they encountered. For example, in Vipassana (Insight Meditation) one observes the contents of the mind. Zen practice also includes focus on key questions, *koans*, like the famous "What is the sound of one hand clapping?" Mantra meditation uses sound or sacred phrases as a focus. Transcendental Meditation is the best known form of mantra meditation. Other types of meditation use the visualization of deities, mandalas or yantras (geometric forms). Chi Kung and Tibetan practices also visualize energy moving through the body.

> Meditation is a practice that can teach us to enter each moment with wisdom, lightness and a sense of humour.
>
> — JACK KORNFIELD

These practices are all now in the process of transformation and integration into our culture, and there are many different kinds of meditation practice to choose from today. They are all techniques for quieting the mind and focusing attention. The variety of practices, techniques and groups allows you to choose the one that feels right for you. Besides the differences in techniques, groups vary in the formality and ritual in their practice and in the understanding of the relation of the student to the master or teacher. It is very important that both the method and the teacher feel right to you.

Hatha Yoga

Meditation requires one to sit straight and still for long periods of time and to breathe easily and freely. Hatha yoga, the practice of the postures (asanas), was developed to give yogis the strength, energy and balance needed to sustain an intense meditation practice. Hatha is derived from two Sanskrit words: *Ha*—sun, and *Tha*—moon. Hatha yoga is a balance and integration of opposites: positive and negative, active and passive, left and right.

Because it is a physical practice, Hatha yoga is often seen as a lower practice than meditation, which focuses on the mind. This attitude can be re-enforced by Western spiritual teachings which emphasize transcending the body and sexuality and aspiring to something "higher." In my opinion, this splitting of body and spirit negates the essence of yoga — union and integration.

Hatha yoga is also a way of awakening *kundalini* (the energy dormant at the base of the spine), and opening the *chakras* (the energy centres located in the spine). The goal is to enable the energy to move freely to the highest, or crown, chakra. The awakening of this transforming energy has powerful repercussions on all levels. The poses establish the necessary foundation and clear the energy channels for this movement to take place in a safe and balanced way.

> This body is your home... You are filled with the source of all knowing... You are attuned to your body, and your body is attuned to the universe.
>
> — CHRISTINA BALDWIN

The primary text on Hatha yoga, the *Hatha Yoga Pradipika* says: "As Ananta, the Lord of Serpents, supports this whole Universe with its mountains and forests, so Kundalini is the main support of all the yoga practices." As we have seen, Ananta is a symbolic representation of the force of gravity. This verse connects kundalini with gravity, which is also an energy channelled through the spine. Our emphasis on alignment in the practice section is partly to prevent injuries and improve our functioning on the biomechanical level, but also to bring us into optimal alignment with this universal energy field. This energy is manifested in the wavelike movement that comes when the spine is released with the breath. Our spines move like a snake (which is all spine), so the classical image of kundalini as a serpent is both logical and appropriate.

There are many, many methods and styles of Hatha yoga. The practice of the postures, like meditation, is being transformed in coming to the West, as it is continuously being adapted for our bodies, needs and lifestyles. I cannot overemphasize the importance of finding the approach and teacher that are right for you.

I have always been drawn to the earthiness of asana practice. We see in babies a delight in movement and discovery of their bodies. Our aim is to re-discover this attunement, freedom and curiosity. While traditional Western spirituality has generally denied and denigrated the body, asana takes us into and through the body to something beyond— to integration, compassion, silence, spirit and love.

Yoga Today

Each teacher instructs from his own experiences and, as a result, there are innumerable forms of yoga practice. The most common types of yoga practised in the West today are **Hatha yoga** (the practice of yoga postures), **pranayama** (breathing techniques), and **meditation**. These three are the focus of this book. Other forms include **mantra** (repetition of a sacred syllable or phrase), **Jnana yoga** (study, self knowledge), **Karma yoga** (selfless service), **Bhakti yoga** (devotional practices), and **kriyas** (purification practices). Each of these categories has many variations and styles. The different aspects of yoga are like a hologram in which each part contains and reveals the whole. They are all aspects of yoga and alternative paths to the same goal.

The tradition of direct transmission from teacher to student and the on-going evolution of yoga continues today. Yoga is much more accessible than in the past especially with its appearance in books, magazines, videos, TV programs, etc. However, there are widely differing techniques and styles of practice, and sometimes conflicting viewpoints. It is important that you take the time to find the method and teacher that is right for you, and to assess intelligently and critically what is being taught.

As students today, we also need to look at the cultural roots of traditional teachings and reassess them in the light of our own contemporary values, needs, priorities and experiences. Since many yoga students in the West are women, their concerns need to be addressed and incorporated into yoga practice. We also need to find realistic ways of integrating yoga into our hectic lives.

Traditionally, disciples were men who turned to yoga in their later years when their children were grown and their responsibilities as a householder had been fulfilled. They studied under the direct supervision of a guru or teacher, who was seen as the embodiment of the Divine. Surrender to the guru was total, and his authority was not questioned. The guru/disciple relationship assumed that the aspirant was ready for the renunciation and devotion that total commitment to the spiritual life required, and the guru rejected students he did not think were ready.

Values like detachment from desires and surrender to the guru make sense as a counterbalance to the highly empowered position of the typical Indian male. But we are now living in a society where isolation, alienation and impersonal detachment are the norm. It seems far more important for us to give weight to the values of relatedness, interconnectedness, support and integration.

We also need to look at how these teachings relate to women who are deeply conditioned to put others first, and often have difficulty acknowledging their own needs, feelings and priorities. They often need encouragement and support to stand on their own two feet, to find their ground and stand firm in who they are and what they believe. They need to learn to take care of themselves, to find their own authority, financial resources and sense of self. Women students are seeking to find a sense of inner worth, self-esteem, empowerment and creativity. The ability to accept, free and enjoy their bodies needs to be cultivated in the face of the predominant cultural stereotypes of beauty and desirability. At the same time, men are making an increasing effort to free themselves from the macho stereotype, and the body armouring that goes with it. Rather than learning detachment from their feelings and desires, they are finding ways of acknowledging and expressing them without sacrificing their masculinity and strength.

Today many students are looking for physical and psychological healing. The whole notion of surrendering the will becomes problematic for people who are deeply scarred and wounded, or survivors of abuse. Unfortunately, an increasing range of abusive relationships is being exposed in the yoga and meditation communities. We are now seeing gurus and spiritual teachers who are physically, emotionally, financially or sexually abusive. Some are involved in drug and alcohol abuse. Do not assume that everything a teacher says and does is beyond question or sacrifice yourself in your devotion to a teacher or group. As much as we recognize the benefits of yoga and the related disciplines, it is essential that we practise discrimination and continually examine the practice or teaching to be sure that it is right and beneficial for us at the moment. This is entirely in keeping with the early yoga teachings that warn us not to accept anything we do not know to be true from our own experience.

As our bodies release and our minds clear, memories, feelings and conflicts that have been repressed often surface. Spiritual teachers are often ill-equipped to deal with the issues and feelings that arise. These feelings need to be addressed with clarity and skill. Increasing numbers of therapists and students involved in spiritual practices are becoming aware of the need to integrate psychological awareness with spiritual practice. Later, we will look at some of the ways you can work with these feelings in your practice.

Through spiritual practice, we become more open, sensitive and attuned. Sometimes we need to learn to protect ourselves from the vulnerability that this opening creates, or to ground ourselves more deeply as energy is freed. Some people are also gifted with psychic abilities and clear intuition, which can be developed or increased through yoga. Possession of these powers does not make one "spiritual." In fact, the *Yoga Sutras* refer to them as a distraction, which can become an obstacle to enlightenment. Yoga is first and foremost about wholeness and integration, stillness, and interconnectedness. Increased awareness needs to go hand in hand with the wisdom and discretion to use these abilities responsibly and with care.

Yoga and holistic approaches to healing offer us many opportunities for self-care and empowerment. When this recognition is taken to an extreme, we are told that we are totally responsible for our health, mental and physical, as well as our emotional and even financial well-being. The issue was brought home very strongly when I was diagnosed with cancer. One person told me that I didn't have to have it if I didn't want to. There were various explanations for my illness: genetic predisposition, my mind, the stress of difficulties in a relationship, the stress of moving my studio, the fear of cancer, emotions I had "taken in" from my mother, etc. I don't know what caused my cancer. The best response I received was: "You never know what life has in store for you."

I found it completely counter-productive to dwell on why I had cancer, and much more useful to focus on my immediate situation, the decisions that had to be made and what I could do to promote my own healing. Yoga is a tremendous resource and I am very grateful to have it as an ally. But it does not offer us any guarantees.

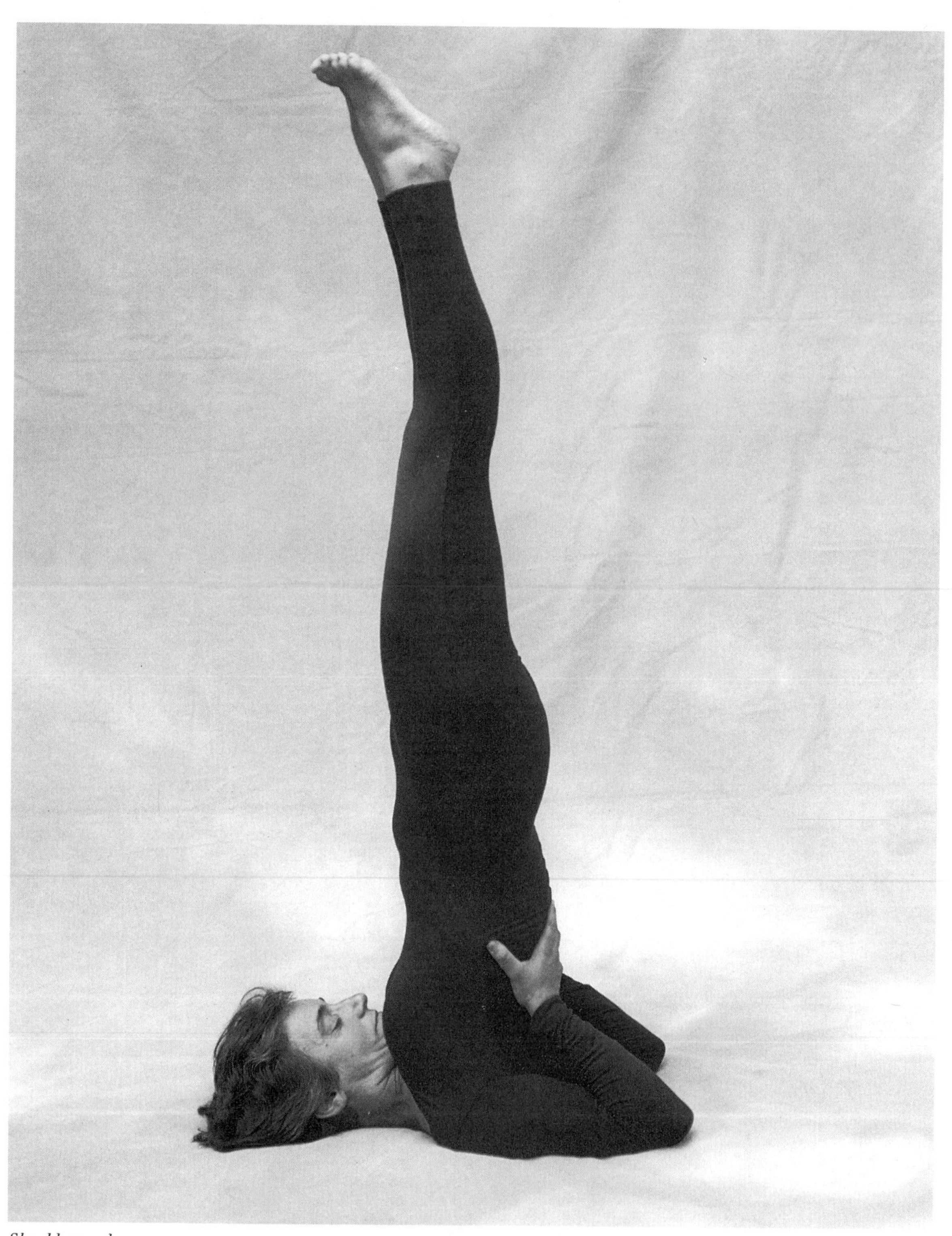

Shoulderstand

CHAPTER 2

On the Way

MOST PEOPLE start yoga for flexibility and relaxation, as a way of slowing down and unwinding, as well as getting some gentle exercise. Many people use yoga to complement a fitness programme, or to heal a sports-related injury. As the pace and pressures of our lives increase, we are desperate for ways to touch something quieter and slower, more whole and healing. There is a prevalent need for meaning beyond oneself and one's material pursuits.

Yoga today is accessible to people who do not accept or are not interested in spiritual practice. Some find a sacred space grows within them, and others are happy simply to stretch and relax. Each of us comes to yoga in our own time and in our own way. Its meaning for us and its place in our lives is unique and changes over time. Beginners' reasons for wanting to do yoga are usually much clearer than those of more experienced students and teachers for whom yoga is simply a part of their lives. Yoga is much more acceptable today than in the past and many people who did yoga ten or fifteen years ago are returning to it now.

"To twist, stretch, and move around, is pleasant and enjoyable, a body holiday."

—VANDA SCARAVELLI

Asana practice, the practice of the yoga postures, is visible and tangible. Giving oneself over to gravity and the breath teaches us the meaning of surrender in a way that is direct, concrete and immediate.

Mystics teach us that the way to achieve spiritual awareness is to look within. The gradual deepening of the exhalation provides a direction and becomes our guide. It is like having a flashlight in a dark tunnel. Through our breathing practice, we touch the unlimited capacity for depth within us. From this depth we receive the inhalation, allowing ourselves to be "inspired."

Stress Management

Since so many people start yoga for relaxation or stress reduction, it is worthwhile to take a little time to understand what stress is and how it affects us.

Stress is the body's automatic reaction to perceived danger. The nervous system directs the body to prepare for action. Blood pressure, blood volume and heart rate go up as blood is directed from the digestive system into the large muscles. The digestive, reproductive, immune and healing systems are inhibited. Breathing becomes quick and agitated. When we decide that our situation is no longer dangerous, we can return to normal in three minutes. This is the relaxation response. Stress-related problems arise when we remain in this heightened "fight or flight" state over a long period of time.

Our bodies react to our thoughts. Thinking about a tense situation will generate a physical reaction that is similar to being in one. This can work both negatively and positively. Replaying mental tapes of tense situations creates tension; images of peace and quiet are relaxing. This is the basis for imagery and visualization techniques for healing, improving skills and general functioning. Conversely, when we change or transform a physical response, our thoughts and emotions are affected. For example: as mental activity is reflected in eye movement, letting our eyes become passive quietens the thinking mind; dropping our shoulders lessens the feeling of being burdened. The poses all work toward a shift in both our bodies and our states of mind.

From the point of view of yoga practice, the key element of the relaxation response is the shift in our breathing, which becomes slower, smoother and more regular as we calm down. The breath is central because we can be conscious of it and affect it through our practice.

Shifting our attention to our breath facilitates the relaxation response. When we practise pranayama, our systems get the message that this is "down time" and there is a deep exhalation that says "Now I can stop. Thank you." This shift is accompanied by an internal or sometimes vocal sigh. Saying "Ha" or sighing also helps us unwind. Implicit in the relationship between breathing and stress is the connection between our breathing and our state of mind.

When the energy that has been held in tension is freed through the postures, we start to see how we take stress into our bodies. During a difficult day at work you may notice your shoulders tighten or feel your jaw clench. With increased awareness, that comes from your practice, you can release the tension as it arises.

Our work with the body inevitably brings in our emotions as well. The fight/flight analysis of stress fails to address the tension that goes into suppressing legitimate and valid emotions. We have all had the experience of maintaining a façade in a social or business situation where it would be inappropriate to express what we are actually feeling. While this may be inevitable occasionally, if we maintain this façade constantly, keeping up a false image, then our bodies lock into a pattern of holding or with-holding. As our bodies release, we re-connect with our true feelings, needs and aspirations.

Stress management strategies may call on us to adapt to untenable situations, and learn to "manage" the stress better. But we also need to consider the deeper causes of stress and burnout. We need to have meaning and purpose in our lives. As Sam Keen says in his book, *Fire in the Belly*,"When we spend the majority of our time doing work that gives us a paycheck but no sense of meaning we inevitably get bored and depressed. When the requirements of our work do not match our creative potential we rust out." Living under constant stress and pressure in an environment that is like a war zone depletes energy and deadens the spirit. You may find that managing your stress is simply a temporary solution and that real healing means leaving the battlefield.

As we become clearer and quieter, we develop a better perspective on ourselves and our lives. Although it takes time and courage, many people find that through yoga practice they are able to make major changes in their lives toward a happier, more peaceful and harmonious way of living.

Ups, Downs, Plateaus and Changes

Yoga books often praise the benefits of yoga without addressing the difficulties, trials and tribulations, dangers and risks. However, like everything else in life, yoga practice has its ups and downs.

You may finish your practice feeling pure and peaceful yet explode at the first person to walk into the room. Or just when you think everything is going well, a pulled muscle sets you back six months. Sometimes it seems like your practice is going nowhere and you wonder why you bother at all. Feelings of despair can be the prelude to a breakthrough, or they can indicate the need for serious change in your lifestyle or approach. At the same time, the practice gives us access to a quiet centre in which we can integrate these changes. It takes time to learn to stand tall and free, to grow and blossom.

Classical teachings outline obstacles to practice such as sickness, doubt, illusion and despair. Even the positive attributes of enlightenment can present difficulties. Tibetans say that one of the faults that prevents us from full self-realization is the idea that enlightenment is too wonderful for us to accommodate. I am always encouraged when I read these texts. They remind me that many people have taken this path before and have encountered these roadblocks.

In the same way our bodies easily let go of impurities in the breathing process, emotional and mental toxins can also be released in a natural way.

— NANCY ROSE EXETER

It can be disconcerting to discover just how difficult it is to follow the first instruction of yoga and meditation practice: "Pay attention to your breathing." Focusing on our breathing makes us immediately aware of our mental chatter. This chatter is incessant and draining and often negative, anxious, angry and controlling. You will discover your own way to respond to this chatter. The practice reveals our thoughts and feelings while giving us the security and courage to face and accept them. Through this process of integration, yoga leads us toward wholeness. With time and attention to your breath, you will find that the internal static and noise gradually die down. Underneath the "chatter" lies a layer of deeper insight. Through practice we can reach these deeper layers. Solutions to problems come to us; the practice creates a quiet space that opens us to insight and intuition. Mary Stewart describes this process in her book *Yoga*, "It is as if the water of a lake becomes still and clear so that you begin to see things lying long submerged on the bottom. In the choppy weather of everyday living many things lie forgotten; when you change the pattern of your thoughts and become quiet they can emerge and demand your attention."

There are hundreds of ways to avoid practice. The plants suddenly need watering, and there's nothing like Headstand for revealing the dust under the furniture. Consistent practice takes commitment and discipline, tempered by compassion and self acceptance and finding the way that is right for you.

When we are extremely stressed, it sometimes seems as if our whole practice is dissipated in distraction. At times like this, remind yourself that the practice itself is valuable. The *Bhagavad Gita* instructs us to work without regard to success or failure. A regular practice trains us to centre and release. The effort to focus your attention will have benefits in your day-to-day life, even at times when the practice itself seems impossible.

Learning to stay with your practice through these stressful times also means that your practice will be there for you when you need it. Yoga is not always a blissful experience, nor an escape. It is a resource that you can build within that has the capacity to guide you through good times and bad.

There are many ways to deal with thoughts and feelings that arise during your practice. Some people use activities like a brisk walk, journal writing, enjoying music or art, but our focus here is to look at ways that you can use yoga practice to move through emotional blocks.

Our approach is to remain with your breath, following the feelings either until they are resolved or until some insight is reached. As you do this, observe the effects of your thoughts and feelings on your body and breath. Another option when you are feeling overwhelmed by emotion is to do the poses that you find the most grounding and stabilizing. Breathing, standing poses and inversions are commonly used for this purpose. You can also use breathing or asana practice to express the emotion. For example, relaxation poses, Child's Pose and sitting forward bends have a surrendering quality through which sadness can be released.

Yoga is calming and centring, but it is also a vehicle for expressing and clearing strong energy and emotions, especially when you are experienced and can do the poses well. You can release anger and rage through Rapid Abdominal Breathing, which you can do either sitting or in the poses. Sun Salutations, Handstands and backbends are vigorous and energetic poses through which you can channel intense energy. (Just be careful to protect your lower back.) Shaking your arms vigorously between the standing poses frees up the shoulder girdle and shakes off pent-up anger and frustration. These actions will not resolve the issues, but will clear some of the turmoil so you can deal with them more effectively. If you find that the feelings that arise are consistently overwhelming or disturbing to you or those around you, you may want to consult a counsellor or therapist. Continuing your practice through this period will provide you with an inner resource.

At the same time, it is important to have compassion and respect for your resistance and denial. This has been a very hard lesson for me to learn. Immediately after the mastectomy, I felt quite disconnected from my body and feelings. I decided that this was fine and that I would

When we make friends with our changes, we don't become weaker, but stronger. We don't need to correct our moods or interfere with them. The moon reminds us to resonate and become whole with all of our moods.

— ADELHEID OHLIG

have plenty of time to get in touch with my feelings later. This denial enabled me to focus my energy on healing, and I am sure helped in my recovery. For years I had pushed myself and my students to confront fears and resistance. I have since gained a greater respect for resistance and denial.

In addition to resistance to negative emotions, we also have resistance to positive states of mind. I have found myself asking questions like: What terrible things would happen if I were secure, relaxed and peaceful? What right do I have to be happy? To exist? Would I really be me without my anxieties, anger, frustration, insecurities and rage? Where would my friends be if I became strong and dynamic?

Give yourself permission to be happy. For most of us, it takes lots of practice!

Yoga opens us up to love, compassion, caring and creativity. It inspires us to look inside, to face our deepest fears and find the essence of our being that lies beyond the veils of fear and illusion. We gradually come to a place of peace from which the still small voice within can be heard. The experience of stillness, even for a moment, touches a power and resource of infinite love, and energy.

Body Image

The pressure to conform to an external body image is intense and pervasive. We are surrounded by images of how we should look. What's attractive, what's sexy, what's young, what sells. Millions of dollars are spent by women and men trying to look like pictures in a magazine. In some ways I think it is wonderful that movie stars are now making yoga videos, and that the image of yoga in the media is changing. Yoga is now much more recognized and acceptable than when I began. But we must remember that the goal of yoga is integration and inner peace. I teach people of all shapes and sizes, most of whom will never look like Raquel Welch, Jane Fonda or Ali McGraw.

When we practice yoga, we free our bodies to breathe and release, and in the process they are re-aligned softened, lengthened and toned. What emerges is the body of someone who is allowing themselves to be and to blossom. The sign of the practice taking hold is a budding clarity, fullness and radiance that is unmistakable.

> *Practice transforms us.... We become more beautiful, our faces change and our walk gains in elasticity. Our way of standing is steady and poised, our legs are firmer, and our toes and feet spread out, giving us more stability. Our chests expand, the muscles of the*

abdomen start to work, the head is lighter on the neck (like the corolla of a flower on its stem moving easily with flexibility while the wind blows). To watch these enchanting changes is amazing.

A different life begins and the body expresses a happiness never felt before. These are not just words, it actually happens.

— VANDA SCARAVELLI

The dominant cultural and medical message is also that our posture and flexibility inevitably deteriorate with age. This deterioration is not necessary. I want to emphasize how much your body can improve over time. Chronic patterns of stress and tension can be relieved and postural problems can be reversed. Your bunions, knocked knees, sway-back, or hunched shoulders can all change for the better. There is no reason to believe that at age thirty-five or forty we start an inevitable downhill slide. As you become more familiar with the poses, you will find out which ones help you the most. Hundreds of poses have evolved to help us reach various parts of our bodies. You will gradually discover which ones do the most to release that stiff hip or free that tight shoulder. You *can* improve.

Energy is eternal delight,
and is from the body.

— WILLIAM BLAKE

Improved posture frees energy, relieves aches and pains, promotes and radiates ease and self-confidence. As your posture and body change, so will your self-image. For example, as your shoulders open and spine lengthens, you come face to face with the parts of yourself that have assumed a withdrawn, frightened or victimized stance. Changes in the body affect self image, body language and the image and attitude you project.

When our bodies release, suppressed emotions come to the surface, sometimes as feelings, sometimes as memories. Do not try to deny what you are feeling. Our bodies can only be truly free when we are willing to recognize and accept emotions that have been buried. Work with your emotions with the same attitude that you are developing toward your body—allowing/accepting, observing/releasing. The purpose of the practice is to create a safe, secure and stable environment within, where thoughts and feelings can arise and be accepted.

While I was writing the first draft of this book, I was struggling with my own issues of body image. I had put on nearly fifteen pounds and was feeling heavy and sluggish. I had always had a fast metabolism and had been able to eat as much as I wanted without thinking about it. It took me three years to realize that something fundamental in my metabolism had changed with menopause. Simply, I was not as lean and taut as I had been. I tried to accept that the changes came with a softer, more feminine approach to yoga and to my life, but the fact was that I hated my body, and I did not feel like myself at all.

I tried to love my body as it was, but couldn't. Then I got more upset with myself for being so judgemental. When I was able to listen to the message in my judgement, I started to accept the change in my metabolism, started swimming to get more exercise and found that I loved it.

At the same time, my yoga practice was plagued with minor injuries. It seemed as if every time I tried to stretch and move, I simply pulled another muscle or strained another joint. While I was writing about the acceptance of one's body and not trying to conform to an outer image, I was going through a period of intense frustration. Faced with a mastectomy, I was forced to confront issues of sexuality and body image underlying my self hatred. My mother had lost both breasts, and it was my father who was able to reassure me that I would be no less a woman without one breast.

My practice improved. The weight disappeared, not only from anxiety, but also from letting go, and my practice felt freer and clearer than it had in a very long time. I was able to change my diet, instantly dropping dairy products, caffeine and fats.

I rarely use a prosthesis since I find it uncomfortable, but mainly wear loose fitting clothing. I feel that I have a choice between being uncomfortable and feeling self-conscious, and am choosing the latter. I don't think there is only one right answer as to how we should look or what feels right. A student of mine who had a mastectomy six months before I did, told me that since the surgery she has learned to love her body in a new way. I feel the same way.

I am still grappling with issues of sexuality, and the integration of strength, dynamic energy and passive surrender. I see this struggle as part of the redefinition of roles and relationships that is taking place today, generating a transformation in our understanding of masculinity and femininity. This new understanding, which is being explored and articulated through emerging women's and men's consciousness groups, also needs to be reflected in our body awareness, structure, tone and self-image.

A Note to Encourage Men

Men face added difficulties when considering yoga. People often think that yoga is about flexibility, and flexibility is considerably more challenging for men. Yoga is often seen as flaky and effeminate, making it even harder for men to consider. If they do go to a yoga class, they find that the vast majority of students are women. As one of my students said, he feels as if he was invading a women's retreat.

Because men are naturally less flexible than women, the sitting poses and forward bends can be difficult and frustrating. However, men do have certain advantages in yoga. The poses requiring stability and balance often come much more easily to them. Remember: flexibility will come with practice, and is certainly not a prerequisite.

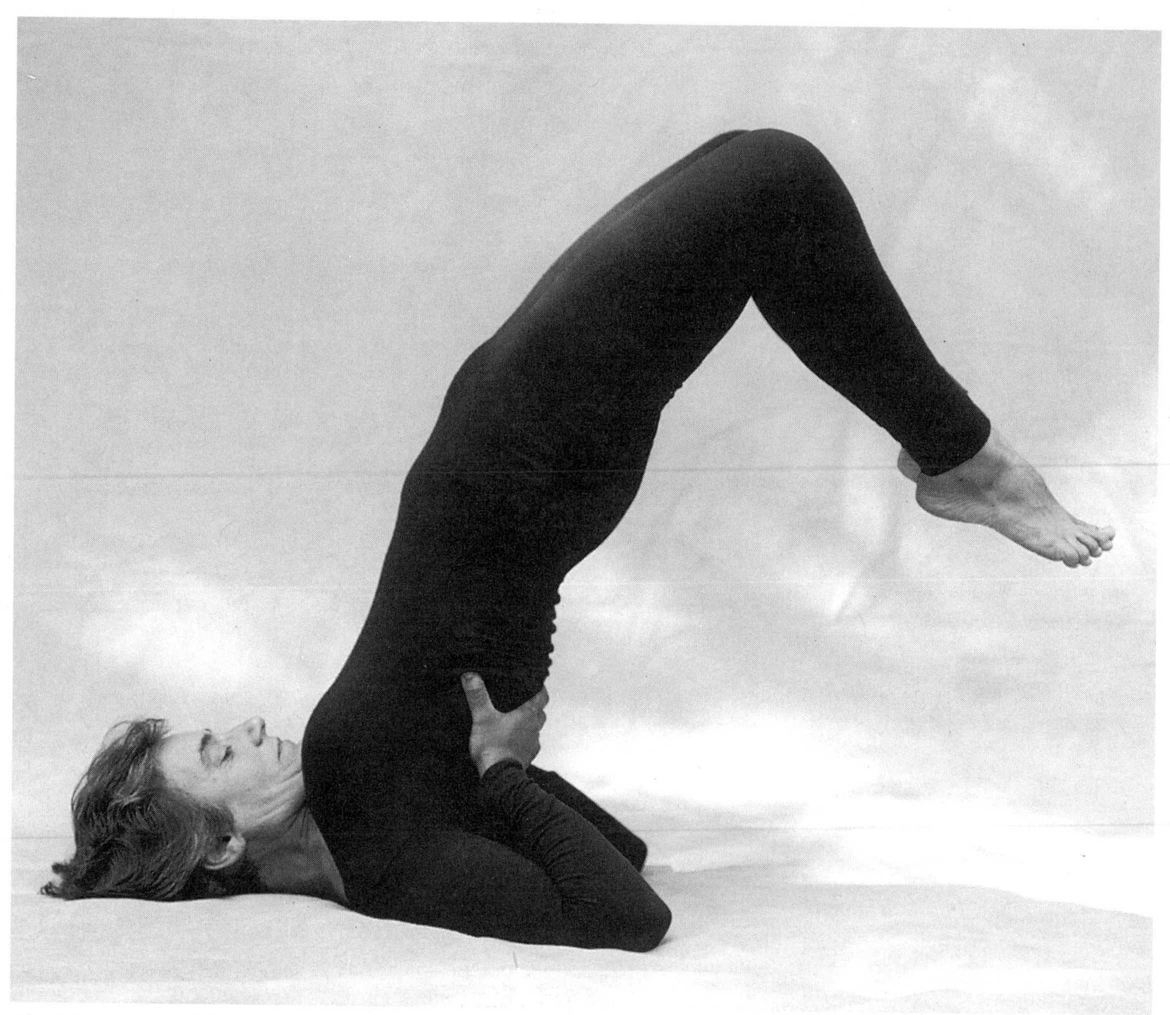

Shoulderstand into Bridge Pose

CHAPTER 3

Your Practice

Caution: If you have any concerns about your health or fitness, consult your doctor, qualified health practitioner or a yoga teacher before undertaking a yoga practice.

YOGA IS NON-COMPETITIVE and can be practised by anyone of any age or level of fitness. It does not require special equipment and can be practised anywhere. You can find the ground and focus your breath under any circumstances. Your yoga practice is always with you.

The sequence of poses in this book have been arranged to follow the basic principles outlined in Chapter 4. The book starts with deep relaxation, passively following your breath, feeling the support of the floor underneath you, and letting your body release to gravity. We then move on to upright positions, sitting and standing, to establish an understanding of gravity, breath and the support of the spine. The simple stretches and Sun Salutation teach the movement of the spine with the breath, and the wave. These principles are then incorporated into the other poses.

Basic instructions are given for each pose. Variations for many of the poses and guidelines for going deeper in the postures are also included. A series of graduated practice sequences at the end of the book will help you get started or develop your practice.

Guidelines

- *Practise on an empty or nearly empty stomach.*
- *Wear loose comfortable clothing.*
  You should be barefoot for the active poses (standing poses, backbends, inversions). If you are at the office, take off your shoes and loosen your clothing as much as possible.
- *Take time to breathe.*
  Awareness of the breath is at the core of yoga and meditation. If you don't have time to do anything else, take a few minutes (sitting or lying down) to focus your attention on your breathing.
- *Practise regularly.*
  It is better to do small amounts often than occasional intensive bursts.
- *Pay attention to your body.*
  Do not force or push your body into a pose. You will know when you have had enough or when you are ready to move on.
- *Start with the poses that you like the most.*
  Your practice will be enjoyable and beneficial. If you enjoy your practice, you are more likely to continue practising regularly. The poses highlight particular movements in the joints or specific muscle groups. As your repertoire of poses increases, you will discover the poses you need to free the parts of your body that need attention. Use the ones that are most beneficial for you. At the same time, be aware of balancing your practice.
- *Adjust your practice to your schedule and biorhythms.*
  Some people feel too stiff to practise in the morning, others prefer it. Some people find it soothing to do yoga in the evening, others find it wakes them up and affects their sleep. Try to practise at the same time each day so that your body becomes familiar with the rhythm. However, if your schedule is variable, you will have to work around that. For instance, my practice times are different on days when I teach than on those when I don't.
- *Be aware of the effect of the poses on your mood and energy.*
  Different types of poses have different moods or energies. Standing poses, Sun Salutation and backbends are strong,

stimulating poses that were traditionally done early in the day. Doing them in the evening may keep you awake. Inversions and forward bends are restorative poses that can be done in the evening.

- *Set aside a place to practise.*
  Having a place to practise helps to focus your attention and bring you to a quieter state. Simply being there will help you focus. Even a corner of a room can be your yoga place.

- *Incorporate bits of practice throughout the day.*
  There are many ways that you can do this. For example:
  Whenever you feel tense, exhale and drop your shoulders.
  When you are walking, be conscious of the contact of your feet with the ground, and focus your attention on your breathing.
  When you are standing for a long time, be aware of your breath and relax your shoulders.
  Be aware of your spine as you walk, stand or sit.
  Take little yoga breaks during the day. Current recommendations from professionals such as physiotherapists are 5–10 minutes every hour.

"In the beginning you have to make room for yoga in your daily life, and give it the place it deserves. But after some time yoga itself will pull you up by the hair and make you do it."
—VANDA SCARAVELLI

Finding the Time

Lack of time is one of the key issues facing us today. We seem to spend most of our lives trying to catch up. Fitting in a yoga class or practice can seem like just one more thing to do, another obligation, another responsibility. But we need time to "undo" or unwind. When my students start to become quiet, their first reaction is often, "I feel like I ought to be *doing* something." Yoga practice gives us time set aside from these pressures, in which we can come back to ourselves, become a little clearer and quieter. It is a resource which can enhance everything else that you do.

Taking this time may seem like an indulgence that is hard to justify. Learning to take time for ourselves and to be kind to ourselves takes practice. It may be painful at first, and surprisingly difficult, but do persist. You and everyone around you will reap the benefits. Turning inward provides a resource and clarity which enhances all other aspects of our lives. The practice of accepting ourselves leads to concern and compassion for others. Being able to return to an inner source and draw from it can give us the strength to carry on in trying and difficult situations.

The mastectomy left me so exhausted that I quickly learned a lot about setting priorities and valuing my time and energy. As a result, I have become more committed to my practice. Less and less gets in the way. The phone calls can wait and so can the chores. I still constantly ask myself the question: "Is this what I want to be doing right now?" and I strive to eliminate anything in my life for which the answer to that question is "No."

The value of an on-going practice cannot be over-estimated. Start with a realistic assessment of how much time you have for yoga. Even 5 or 10 minutes a day makes yoga a part of your daily life. Regular short practices are more beneficial than occasional long ones. With time, your practice will naturally grow. If your practice slips, don't punish yourself. Breathe and start again. Even spending time in your practice place will help you focus.

The voice that says: "Only 5 minutes a day won't make any difference" is wrong. Even when you can only manage a few minutes, those few minutes will keep you in touch with the thread of yoga. One of my students, a working mother with two young children, sets one pose a day as her bottom line; another, after the birth of her third child, did five rounds of Rapid Abdominal Breathing as a daily minimum. I have had students make significant improvement by practising 15 minutes a day.

As yoga germinates and takes root in your life, you will find the rhythm and level of practice that is right for you. There is a multitude of ways you can approach and use your yoga practice. I have students who have been coming to class once a week for years, but rarely practice, and others whose lives have been transformed through their practice.

Starting to Practise

If you are just beginning to practise, start with poses that you like and feel immediate benefit from. You might be able to convince yourself for a while that you are doing yoga because it is good for you, but in the long run the only reason to continue is because you love it. As your practice grows, include more poses.

With time you may want to try more difficult and challenging poses. Approach them with the same attitude that you have developed through the basics. When you are working on a pose you find difficult, you are much more likely to push and struggle. This creates tension that will block you and will actually prevent you from doing the pose.

Take time, breathe and go as far as your body is ready. Eventually, these poses will come with ease, and the distinction between beginning and advanced poses will dissolve. Have faith that you will progress. Your faith will build slowly over time as you start to improve.

Finding Support for your Practice

Yoga is solitary by nature. Being able to share your experience with others will help sustain you over time. After a recent talk on yoga philosophy at my studio, one of the students commented that it was nice to simply be in a group where these topics are discussed and "normalized."

Find a yoga class that suits you. Shop around. Classes vary enormously in energy, pacing, intensity and focus. Both the style and the teacher should feel right for you. The teacher is both a role model and a "product" of the practice. Trust your intuition; if it doesn't feel right, keep looking.

In selecting a class, consider the following questions:

- *Does the space feel comfortable?*
- *Do you enjoy being there? Do you leave feeling better?*
- *Do you want to learn from this teacher?*
- *Is the teacher at ease and relaxed in his or her own body and in the class?*
- *Is the class well-organized? Are the poses clearly explained?*
- *How big is the class? Is there personal contact and correction?*
- *Are there adaptations for your particular needs?*
- *Are the time, location, and price of the class appropriate? If not, is the class so good you want to go anyhow?*
- *Can you make up missed classes?*
- *Do you feel safe in the area, especially if the classes are at night?*

If you can't find a class, try to find a friend to practise with occasionally, someone you can talk to about your practice or others involved in similar kinds of activities. Read books on yoga or spiritual practice, or start a journal.

One of the reasons I decided to teach was to create a context to support my practice. I was teaching Iyengar yoga, which had not been taught in Toronto before, so I had to look outside the yoga community for resources. Over the years, I have been involved in the martial arts, various forms of bodywork and psychotherapy. I have travelled to the United States, Europe and India for yoga classes. These have all nourished and enriched my practice.

There is always the risk of dabbling in so many different techniques that you never penetrate deeply in any of them. Once you have found an approach that is right, wait until you are established in it before you branch out. Ultimately, you are the only one who can decide what combination of activities and practices is realistic and right for you.

How to Structure and Balance your Practice

While it is important to start with poses that you enjoy and derive immediate benefit from, you also need to consider the overall balance of your practice. Make a list of the poses you enjoy and practise them regularly. See what you need to add to create a more rounded practice. A balanced practice includes all of the major types of movement—upright, forward, backwards, sideways, twisting and inverted.

Shape your practice like a bell curve: start gently, peak in the middle and cool down at the end.

- *Start your practice with easy warm-up poses.*
  Begin your practice with poses that centre you and prepare your body for more intense postures that follow. Take longer to warm up when you are unusually tense, recovering from an illness, when there has been a break in your practise, or when you are affected by external factors like allergies or the weather.
- *Build up to the core poses of your practice that day.*
- *Follow intense postures with counterbalancing poses.*
- *End with quiet relaxation poses.*
  These include Deep Relaxation, Little Boat and Child's Pose, long forward bends or breathing.

Consider both the risks and the benefits of the poses. Counterbalancing postures offers us a way to protect ourselves physically and emotionally. For example, if you do backbends incorrectly you might compress your lower back. Forward bends stretch the lower back. They are also cooling, introverted and passive, in contrast to the backbends which are opening, energizing and extroverted.

Keep these basic guidelines in mind as you practise:

- *Try to do a breathing practice every day.*
  I can't emphasize enough how valuable a breathing practice is.
- *Practise forward bends after backbends.*
- *Do sitting twists after forward bends.*
  The spine is already lengthened, and there is less likely to be compression in the twist.
- *Shoulderstand follows Headstand.*
  Shoulderstand is a more basic pose than Headstand, but it is also a more intense stretch on the neck. It releases compression in the neck and upper back that may be caused by the Headstand.
- *After a long series of forward bends or Crow Pose variations, you may want to do some gentle pelvic tilts or Cobra preparation to stabilize your spine, if it feels overstretched.*

For your practice to deepen, you need regular, longer practices (at least 45 minutes to an hour). You should include an extended breathing practice, preceded and/or followed by a long relaxation at least once a week. As your breath deepens, its movement will permeate through your postures, opening, deepening and altering them profoundly. Take time to let this happen.

As your practice develops, you may want to spend more time on a particular type of pose or movement. In that case, balance your practice over a longer period of time, perhaps a week or ten days. For example, you might spend one day doing backbends with only one short forward bend afterwards. Another day could be devoted to forward bends, etc. You should still end your practise with at least one counterbalancing pose.

As your body changes, you may find that you need to go "back to square one" periodically as you integrate this "new body" into the postures. This sometimes means that you can no longer do poses that you were able to do before, which is disconcerting and frustrating. For example, people with very stiff upper backs can often do Headstand easily because they are building on a solid foundation. As their upper backs become freer and more flexible, the pose may lose stability and collapse for a while. When that happens they need to go back to re-establishing the foundation in their arms, and learn to do the pose with extension and lightness instead of rigidity.

Look at the pattern of your practice over a few weeks or months and see which poses you focus on and which you avoid. It can be quite helpful to keep a journal of your practice to see which areas you are drawn to, and to record any insights that you may have during your practice. You will probably find that you go through phases where you focus on a particular movement or type of pose for an extended period of time. Follow your body and its needs. At the same time, be aware of maintaining an overall balance in your practice. If there is a pose or type of pose that you consistently avoid, try doing it briefly at the beginning of your practice and then go on to something else. I find this helps to minimize the guilt and the feeling of a huge block which must be overcome.

The rhythm of your practice will vary. There will be times when you want a strong, active dynamic practice; others when you are slow and quiet. Your practice is an opportunity to re-connect with, honour and respect your own biorhythms.

Sometimes we need to be very gentle and accepting and at other times we need to challenge ourselves to go deeper and further. If you have a lot of drive, you may need to learn to temper it somewhat. I learned that through a series of minor injuries which forced me to slow down. If you are naturally slow and passive, you may need to give yourself a bit of a push occasionally.

When I was convalescing from surgery, Vanda was adamant that I should rest and not push myself. At the same time, a Chinese doctor gave me a Chi Kung walking meditation for cancer and told me to walk for an hour a day—even if I was tired and my knee or shoulder hurt. At the time, I thought he was out of his mind. But walking helped me to rebuild my energy.

It seemed to me that they were both right. I needed lots of R and R, *and* ways to re-energize. Your practice may alternate between high energy phases and times of very gentle practice, or you may find a steady rhythm that suits you. The rhythm and structure of your practice is constantly changing and evolving, as your practice matures and your life changes. Follow these changes and go with them, to make your practice truly your own.

Alignment and Technique

The poses were developed to improve posture, promote health, and increase vitality and energy. We need to be aware of the benefits of

Caution: Doing yoga incorrectly can cause damage over a long period of time if the underlying imbalances are not corrected.

yoga, but we also need to be aware of the risks. It is essential that yoga poses are correctly aligned because of the intensity of the positions.

When we build a house we need to be sure that the ground underneath it is solid and the foundation is strong, stable and balanced. We expect the floors to be level, and the windows and doors to be square. Otherwise, there will be cracks and distortions and the house might even collapse. It is exactly the same with our bodies. We look for a secure and stable foundation, and for alignment and elongation of the spine.

Alignment and technique are essential components of asana practice. Correct alignment prevents injury, promotes healing of existing injuries, reduces stress on the tissues and joints, and improves our overall function and feeling of well-being. Concern for technique does not in any way undermine the spiritual dimension of our practice. Great musicians and dancers have flawless technique. The tremendous sense of repose that we see in statues of the Buddha comes in part from the ease of his posture. Technique alone is not spirit, but provides a vehicle through which spirit and creativity can manifest and express themselves.

A picture placed in just the right position on the wall is satisfying, whereas if it's not in balance with whatever else is in the room, it is not quite right and it doesn't satisfy.

— NANCY ROSE EXETER

Alignment allows the body to integrate and elongate. Energy which was used to compensate for imbalances is freed as our muscles and joints come into better balance. Organs occupy space, and their arrangement and function can also be affected by tension, injury, and psychological states. Internal organs function better when they have sufficient space and appropriate support from the musculoskeletal system. The more precise our alignment, the greater our sense of ease and balance. Gravity becomes our ally instead of our enemy.

As you go on in yoga, correct alignment becomes more and more important. For example, a slight tilt in your neck becomes serious if you are doing Headstand regularly. While the feeling of release and extension is usually clear, it is almost impossible to know if you are straight in a pose. We are so used to our own posture that our inner feelings will often tell us we are straight when we are crooked and vice versa. Even if you are aware of your structural imbalances, you will almost always feel strange or crooked when straightened. You should check your poses in a mirror regularly and, if possible, have someone look at them from time to time. Be particularly careful with backbends and inverted poses.

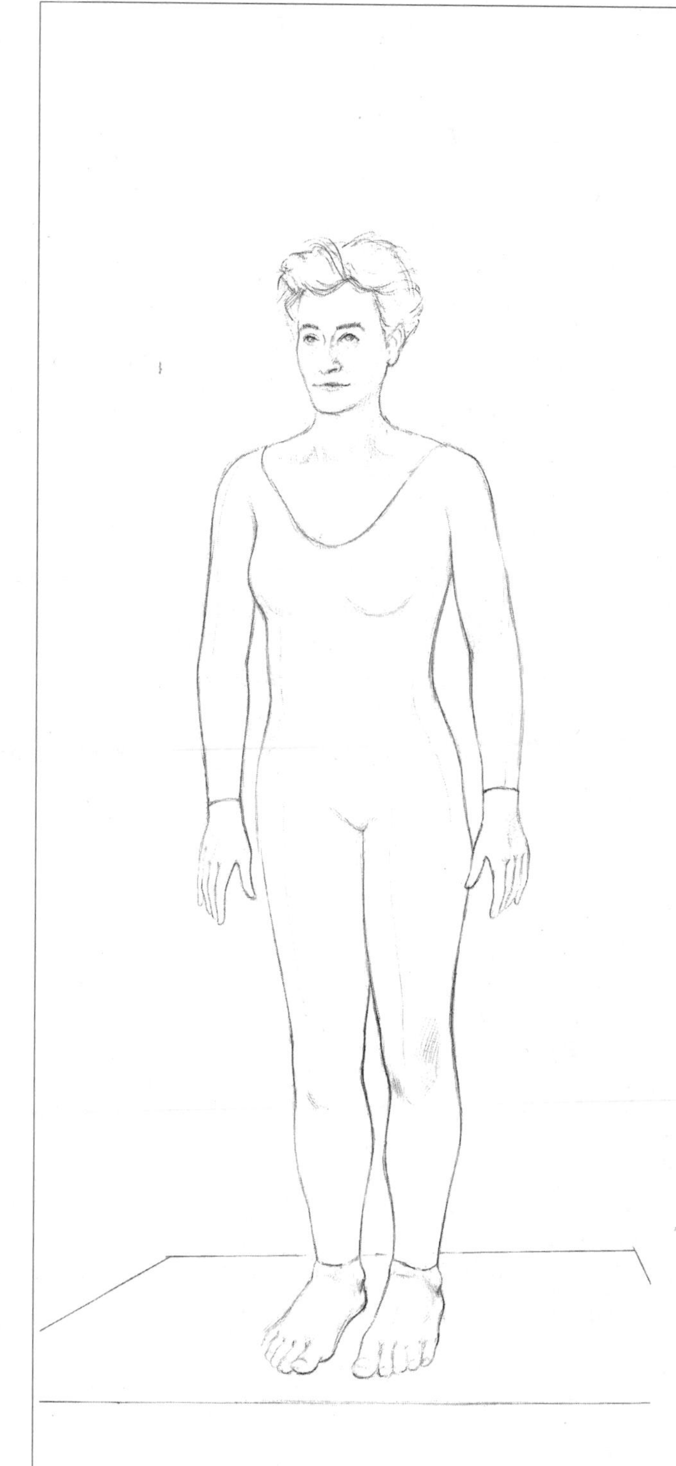

We often avoid giving kind attention to areas that are problematic, because of the negative feelings associated with them. Perhaps you "hate" your hips, or fear a recurring injury, or become frustrated when you can't do a pose. Our practice highlights the ways that we punish ourselves. Trusting the process weakens the "inner critic," enabling us to focus our attention on a tension area and gradually release it. Areas that are out of proportion reveal body blocks. As your body comes into greater balance, these areas will tone and lengthen.

What Is Ideal Alignment?

Understanding your goal while observing the alignment of your poses is essential. There is no clear image of a balanced body in our culture. Ancient Egyptian art shows a much better understanding of structure. Take some time to look at some books on Egyptian art and you will notice the extension and ease in the illustrated bodies — even though the artistic style is very formal.

There are common patterns of imbalance, and general rules or guidelines for correction are included in the instructions for the poses. For example, we focus on the outer edges of the feet in standing poses because many people have weak arches. If your arches are too high, then you need to let them relax and drop. You must pay careful attention to your own body, and determine what is appropriate for you. Begin by getting a general impression, then move on to more detail.

Aligning the foundation of the pose creates a horizontal base for the spine. The line of the spine is fundamental to our practice. When the spine is vertical, ankles, hips, shoulders and ears are in a line, and the back of the head balances over the back of the pelvis. You can use the edge of a doorway as a guideline when you are standing straight, sitting, or in Headstand. The back of your head and the back of your pelvis should touch the doorway. When you are standing or in Headstand, the curve at the back of your waist should be minimal. When you are sitting, the back of your waist should touch the doorway, as the lumbar curve disappears.

Focus on the base of your body in contact with the ground. The base needs to be stable, secure and aligned. When you stand, shift your weight until your pelvis is horizontal to provide a balanced foundation for your spine. (Most people stand with more weight on the dominant side. If you are right-handed, shift your weight to the left, and vice versa.) Similarly, when you are in symmetrical sitting poses, your pelvis should be horizontal. If you do Dog Pose or a Standing Forward Bend with your back to a mirror, you can see whether your sitting bones are horizontal.

The line of your shoulders, shoulder blades or collarbones will establish the base for inverted poses. Adjust the position of your arms to balance your shoulders. In Handstand, Elbow Balance and Headstand, you can use a mirror. There is no way to be absolutely sure about the alignment of your head and neck in Shoulderstand by yourself. The best advice I can offer is to place your chin in line with the notch between your collarbones. If possible, ask someone to look at your poses. It is very easy to miss your own imbalances.

Always remember that correct alignment is a goal or an ideal. Never force your body into a position that it is not ready for, even if it's a "correct" position.

Pain and Injuries

It is important to distinguish between the pain or discomfort of a muscle stretching and a warning pain that indicates strain or stress. Any pain in your back during or after your practice is cause for concern. Necks, lower backs and knees are particularly vulnerable to injury. Treat them with care. When in doubt, err on the side of caution. If problems persist, consult a doctor or a professional bodyworker such as a physiotherapist, chiropractor or massage therapist.

> In every injury, there is the potential gift of healing.
>
> — DAWNA MARKOVA

Injuries are a reflection of structural imbalance. Even when the injury is caused by an accident, weaker areas are the most likely to be injured. In order to truly heal, you will need to find the source of the

- Injured knees are usually reflections of weak feet and/or stiffness and imbalance in the pelvis.
- Neck, shoulder, elbow and wrist problems are related to stiffness in the upper back.
- The neck and lower back balance each other. Problems in one are often mirrored in the other.

problem and work to bring your entire body into alignment. As you balance your body as a whole, problems will gradually be alleviated. In line with our basic principles, work from your spine outward to your limbs. The injured area can also be a symptom of tension or imbalance elsewhere.

As your body changes, you will find that you are most vulnerable to injury in times of transition. As a stiff area becomes more flexible, it can be overstretched or slip out of alignment. Old injuries can recur, as the area is opened up, very often just when you have made a huge breakthrough. It is intensely frustrating to work through this kind of setback.

If you are injured, you need to allow time for recuperation. The first seven to ten days are considered the classical "RICE" stage — rest, ice, compression, elevation. During this period you can continue your breathing practice. No matter how injured or ill you are, you can always focus on your breath. This focus will bring you back to a quiet centre, which is both soothing and healing. You can also do postures that do not involve the injured area. For example, if you have a sprained ankle, you can benefit tremendously from leg stretches or inversions.

As the injury heals, start to work the injured area, but go easy until healing is complete. Soft tissue injuries can take six months to a year to heal. After the tissue is healed, your task will be to restore full function and undo any imbalances caused by compensation for the injury.

There is always tension, compression and misalignment around an injured or diseased area, no matter how long ago the injury occurred. Compensation patterns will remain until you consciously work on changing them. Release, elongation and structural balance are essential, but the transition must be gradual enough that the condition is not exacerbated. This is a matter of trial and error. Be patient. It is a very slow process, but the rewards are great freedom and balance.

Repetitive Stress Injuries

Repetitive Stress Injuries (RSI) are soft tissue injuries that come from repeating the same action over and over. If you are performing the same movement daily, try to counterbalance it in your practice. Years ago, I taught a flute payer who had developed a scoliosis (curve in her spine) from spending so much time turning to one side. Her yoga practice helped her to stay relatively balanced and pain free.

Computer-related injuries are now becoming more common. They generally start from the middle of the back and then move through the shoulders and down the arms. By the time the problem has reached the arms or wrists it can be quite serious. If you are working at a computer all day, remember to breathe and keep the principles of alignment in mind. Find the support in your pelvis, just as you do in your yoga practice. Take at least 5–10 minute stretch breaks every hour. Regular practice of Shoulderstand, backbends and sitting twists will also help keep your upper back, arms and shoulders free and supple.

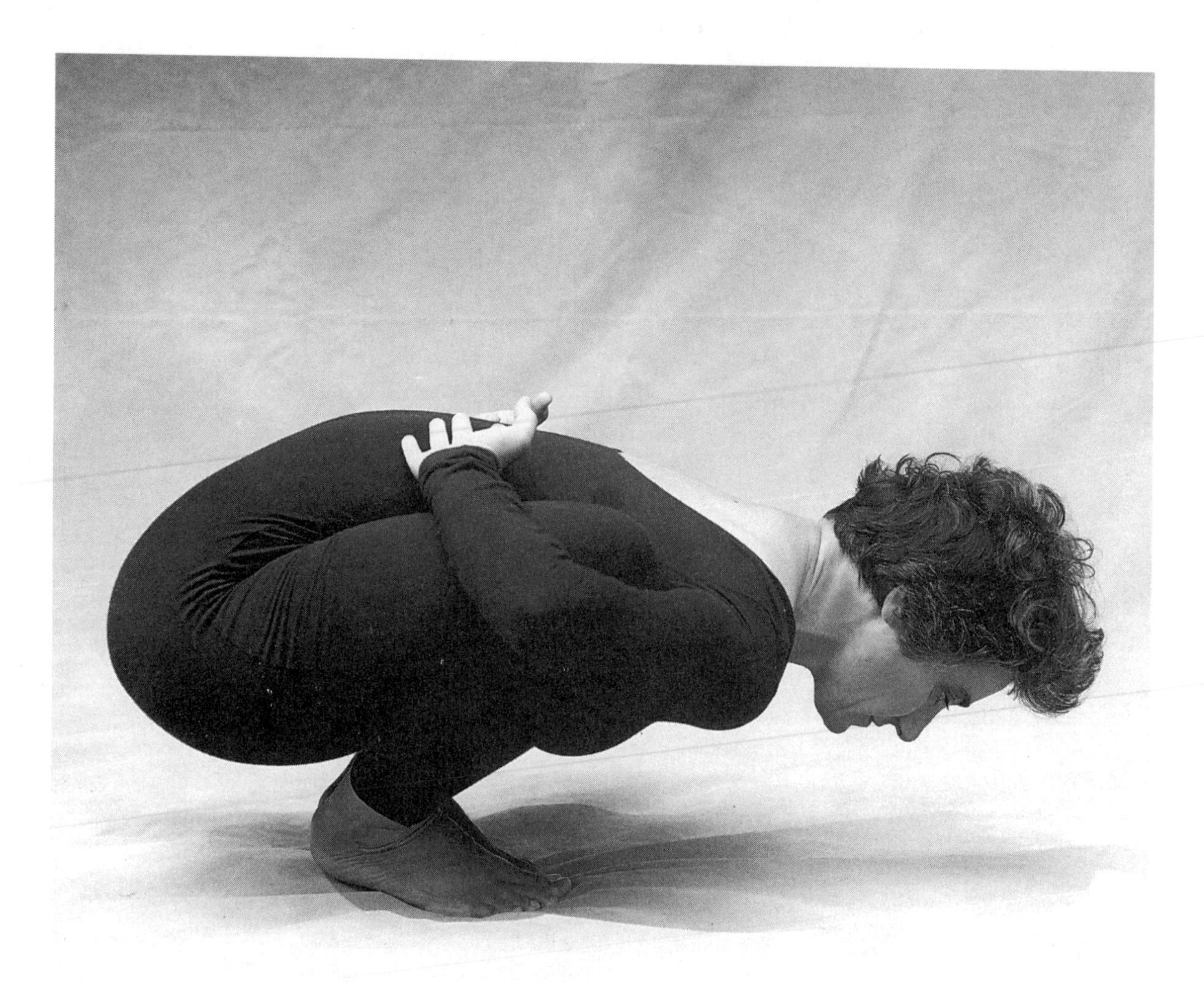

Garland Pose

CHAPTER 4

From the Beginning: Basic Principles

THE YOGA DESCRIBED in this book was developed by Vanda Scaravelli, author of *Awakening the Spine*. She studied with B.K.S. Iyengar and T.K.V. Desikachar, but after working with them for a number of years branched out on her own. Trusting her own body, and following the movement of her breath and her spine, she came to a "new world... a world without aim and without competition, where the body can start to function naturally and happily, allowing expansion to take place in space."

One of the beauties of Vanda's approach is its simplicity. The principles remain the same throughout practice, regardless of your level. The approach to the advanced poses is the same as to the most basic.

As I mentioned earlier, the word asana, which has come to mean pose, originally referred to the ground on which the yogi sat. In our practice, we remind ourselves over and over again that the earth is supporting us and drawing us to her. Our breath is always with us, and we can turn to it whenever we are lost, disoriented or confused.

Each time we practice, we begin again with an acceptance of our bodies and ourselves. We give ourselves time and quiet attention, and allow our bodies to release and unwind naturally. From this acceptance and a willingness to work *with* our bodies rather than against them, we find happiness, security, serenity and balance within and through our bodies. This process gradually takes us deeper and deeper, opening up infinite possibilities.

First we should notice that we are already supported every moment. There is the earth below our feet and there is the air, filling our lungs and emptying them. We should begin from this when we need support.
—NATALIE GOLDBERG

This book begins with Deep Relaxation Pose to help you develop an awareness of the breath and the contact of your body with the ground, and the support it provides. This will enable you to give yourself time to bring your attention into your body. As you relax, you will feel your muscles become passive and the weight of your body drop to the ground.

Begin each pose the same way. Focus on your breath. Be conscious of the support of the ground, and feel gravity as an active force anchoring you and pulling you toward the centre of the earth.

Breath

Breath is the gift of life: one we rarely take the time to appreciate. Breathing practice is our time for quiet attention to ourselves and to the miracle of our lives.

"God formed man from the dust of the ground, and breathed into his nostrils the breath of life; and man became a living being."

— GENESIS 2:7

Even if you don't have time for anything else, take a few minutes each day to stop and focus on your breath. Incorporating a daily breathing practice into your routine builds a tremendous resource for bringing yourself back to centre when you are stressed, upset or disturbed. The ability to sit easily and quietly even for a few minutes frees you from tensions which drain your energy. Bringing your attention to your body and your breath brings you into the present moment.

The exhalation especially releases tension and facilitates dropping and weightedness ("gravitating"). With time and practice, the mind becomes calmer and a steadier, quieter focus emerges. While thoughts and images continue, we are able to see and feel them with greater clarity, and gain perspective on them. The rhythm of the breath becomes slower and more even, and the body more relaxed and passive. In this state of passive receptivity, the inhalation comes freely and easily, without effort or force.

At first, there is a release of day-to-day stresses and tensions. Gradually, more deeply held patterns of fear, defense and resistance can surface and a powerful transformation begins. Out of the experience of quiet security come ease, freedom, joy and spontaneity. An inner light and beauty shine forth.

Once you are familiar with following your breath, incorporate awareness of your breathing into your practice of the poses. Co-ordination of breath and movement has a cumulative effect on all effort and action.

Focus on your breath, especially your exhalation, to release your body and allow the tension to drop. Allow the tension to flow out with your out-breath. Remain passive as you inhale, letting your body open to receive the breath. Active movement comes with the exhalation. As your breathing deepens, the release that takes place in the postures is correspondingly deeper and more powerful. Even strong demanding poses like Headstand and Crow have within them this rhythm of relaxation and action.

Approach the advanced poses just as you would the most basic. In theory, this makes perfect sense. However, in practice, when we encounter a pose we find difficult, the immediate impulse is to push and struggle. Notice when and how you do this. Come back to your breath, and start again. When you encounter stiffness, pain or fear, continue to breathe and give your body time to release. With time, you will find the release that allows you to go further. This requires patience and faith. We all have a strong tendency to push and force the position or to give up in despair. Staying quiet and focused on your breath is a valuable and beneficial practice, whether you can "do" the pose or not.

Gravity and the Ground

Because gravity is with us all the time, we rarely stop to think about what it is or how it affects us. But as Brian Swimme and Thomas Berry say in their book *The Universe Story*, gravity "is not an independent power that acts.... Always and everywhere, it is the universe that holds all things together and is the primary activating power in every activity."

Be conscious of the support of the ground underneath you. Think of gravity as an active force anchoring you and pulling you toward the centre of the earth. Gravity is acting on you. It does not take any effort for you to be on the ground. Your yoga mat rests there easily. Connecting with gravity means stopping, relaxing, not trying, doing nothing, letting go, undoing.

> Every organ, every limb is one with a force in the universe.
>
> — *Talking with Angels*

Once you are familiar with the feeling of releasing with gravity when your body is completely supported, learn to feel the ground underneath you when you are sitting or standing. When you are upright, you can also work with gravity. Learn to work with gravity by focusing attention on the part of your body in contact with the floor. Each pose has a foundation or anchoring point. Take time to find it and to experience it. Can you actually feel your feet on the floor?

While it is obvious psychologically that when we feel more secure we are more at ease and function better, this same logic is rarely applied to the body. We find, however, that when we clearly feel a stable base on the ground, we relax. Having a secure physical foundation also helps us to feel more at ease emotionally. In standing poses, for example, this can be expressed or experienced as "knowing where you stand," "holding your ground," or "standing on your own two feet."

Think of your body as a plant with roots growing from the back of your waist down into the ground. Your spine is the stem of the plant and your head is the flower. The lotus flower is a classical image, with its roots in the mud, its long stem and the flower floating on the water. Finding this base takes time. When I first started lessons with Vanda, she had me stand straight and told me to "grow the roots." Then she went away for twenty minutes. By the time she came back, I was beginning to feel rooted. There is really no substitute for this time. Your practice will be very slow for a while as you learn to find the earth beneath you and to let it support you. The anchoring points vary depending on the pose: the heels in standing poses, sitting bones in the sitting poses. In inverted poses the roots are in the arms and the feet are the "flower." If you are confused in a pose and don't know where to start or what to do, come back to the foundation, follow your breath and wait.

Aligning ourselves with gravity involves both feeling and technique. Correct alignment in the poses is essential to prevent injury and for gravity to truly support us. As you align yourself with gravity, you will find increasing strength emerging from this surrender.

Undoing

Muscles that are relaxed are longer, softer and fuller than tense ones. We are all familiar with the hard knots that form when we are stressed or injured. The opposite experience is less familiar. In your practice, cultivate the experience of undoing the tensions and untying the knots. This means that your muscles will lengthen and there will be more space and freedom in your joints. We do not collapse under the weight of time, but are gradually able to grow longer and lighter.

Release happens. It is not something you can manufacture or create. It comes spontaneously, as a gift. The aim of our practice is to create conditions which are conducive to release. But it requires both trust and security. In order to surrender you need patience and an open-ended sense of time: time to unwind, and to return to the natural rhythm of your breath. You will gradually find your basic rhythms. Learn to go with the day-to-day variations. Even if you only have a very short time to practice, don't rush. This is your breathing space and your time.

I learned this lesson again after my mastectomy. The recovery from the surgery took much longer than I had anticipated. My energy was extremely limited, much more limited than I could have imagined or predicted. I had no choice but to listen to my body and to respect its needs and its limits. I couldn't stretch because any stretch anywhere pulled on the scar. I could however, wait, breathe, unwind and let go. Through absolute necessity, I was forced to practice what I preach and to follow my body.

Walking helped me get moving when my yoga practice was limited to breathing, forward bends and passive stretches. Over a period of months, the areas of holding and blockage gradually receded. Five months after the operation, I began to believe that the practice I had yearned for would return. I learned again to trust this process.

The release of the body, and especially of the spine, comes as a result of surrender and openness. It is something that we can neither control nor predict, nor do we know where it will take us. Therefore, each release, however small, is a move into the unknown. At times this process is supportive and confirming, at others it is frightening and overwhelming. Coming back to our breathing again and again, re-establishing once more a sense of contact with the ground, can help build the security and faith that we need to move through difficult transitions.

Each release carries a new risk and opens up with it a new fear. When I began to understand the implications of this method, I was terrified. I took a good friend to lunch and asked him: "If I really let go, what's going to happen? Where will it take me?" I will be eternally grateful for his answer: "It will take you home."

Spine

Particular attention is given to the release of the spine. The spine is the structural, nervous and energy core of the body. It is an axis around which we can orient and through which we can ground. When we connect to our spines we are connected to the core of who we are, where we stand, and what we believe and value.

As you find your spine and let it support you, the need to support yourself through muscular tensions will decrease. As the spine releases,

A value is a spindle that aligns everything as if it were a spine running through one's life… Centring brings us back to that spindle again and again.

— DAWNA MARKOVA

it lengthens. This release divides the body at the waist. The lower half is pulled into the ground like the roots of a plant, and the upper half is released toward the sky like the growing stem. While grounding gives a sense of where we are, the elongation of the spine gives a sense of direction, where we are going.

"Movement is the song of the body.... This song, if you care to listen to it, is beauty. We could say that it is part of nature. We sing when we are happy and the body goes with it like waves in the sea."
—VANDA SCARAVELLI

The Wave

The segmented and curved structure of the spine gives the release a wavelike quality. This wave radiates out from the spine and is transmitted through the entire body, gradually freeing areas that are blocked, stiff and tense. The multiplicity of poses give us a variety of forms through which this movement is explored and developed. In poses like Child's Pose and the Standing Forward Bend it is relatively easy to feel the release and lengthening of the spine. They are good poses to practice to get a sense of the movement. Sun Salutation is a dynamic expression of the wave, especially in the Dip/Eight Parts Pose illustrated below.

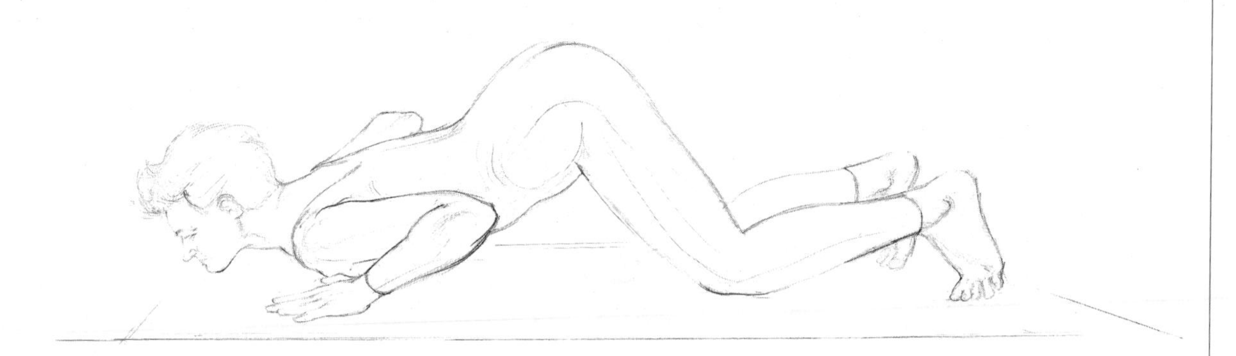

You can learn to "catch the wave" like a surfer, re-enforcing its action and giving the poses a strong and dynamic energy. Doing Rapid Abdominal Breathing in the poses is one way to get a sense of this dynamic quality. Actively extending as you feel the wave of the breath take hold is another. For example: in the standing poses, as you come to the end of the exhalation, actively extend your back leg by pressing the heel into the floor and stretching your knee. Then relax, as you inhale. This gives the poses a pulse or rhythm that alternates relaxation with dynamic extension. As a result of this action, your legs will become stronger and more pliant, your shoulders light and free. The extension of the thoracic spine frees the chest, expanding your breathing capacity and creating space around your heart. It takes time and practice to get the feeling of this rhythm. If your pose feels strained in any way, come back to passive attention to your breath and your roots.

Your poses will become strong and vibrant without effort or strain and your muscles toned through release and extension. This is hard to imagine at first. We are so conditioned to believe that strength comes from effort, and by building muscles. Instead we can begin by building a secure foundation, and gradually find strength from the support of the spine, the inner core of the body, and the ease that comes from a balanced structure. A graceful fluidity emerges similar to the movement of animals. Our bodies express confidence, energy, freedom and joy.

I finally discovered the source of all movement, the unity from which all diversities are born.

— ISADORA DUNCAN

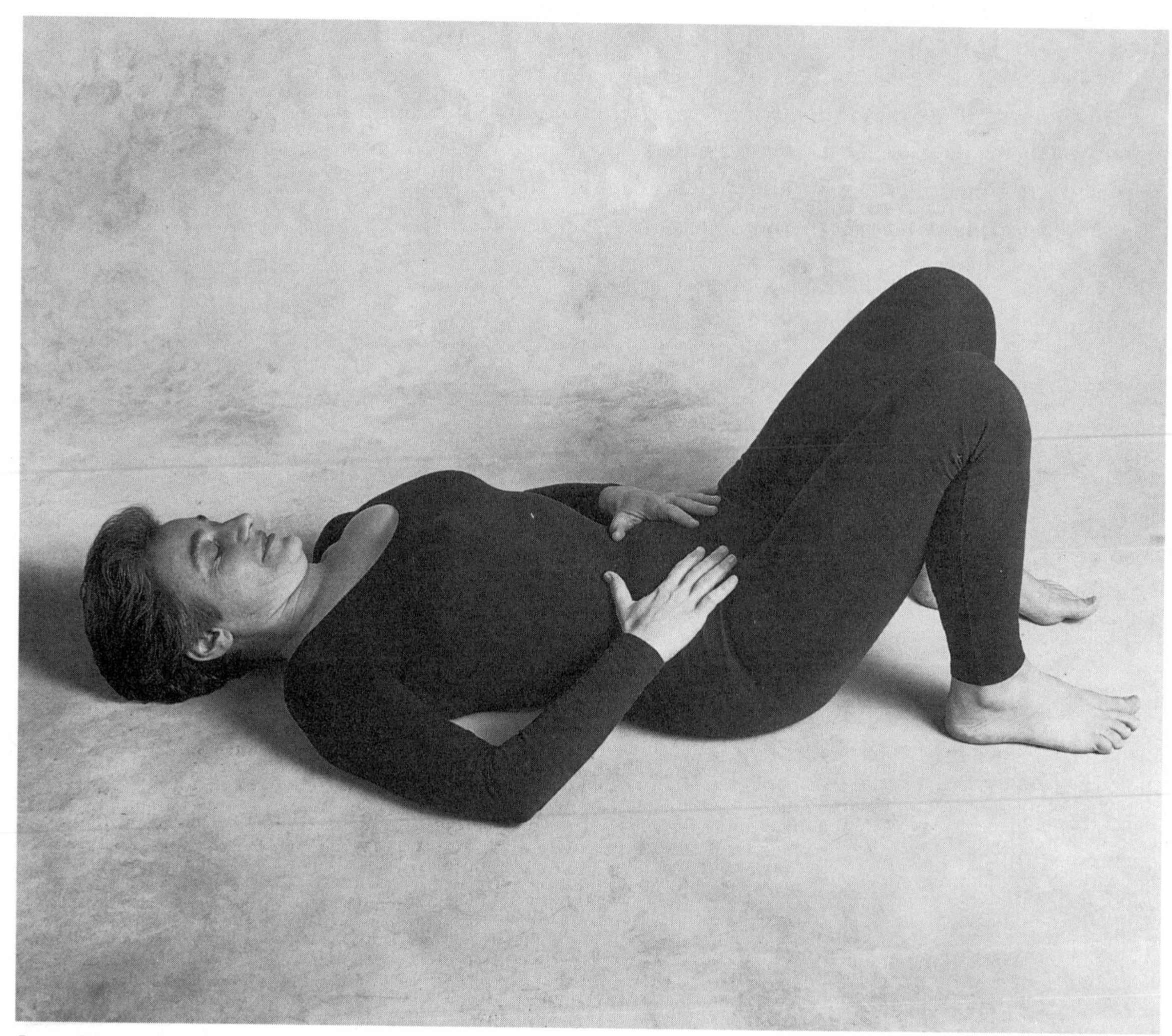

Lying Release Pose

CHAPTER 5

Deep Relaxation: Letting Go

WE ARE ALL FAMILIAR with the way that our bodies harden and tense when we are under stress, but we are less accustomed to the experience of easing and undoing. Deep Relaxation (Corpse Pose) teaches us quietness and surrender, and gives us an experience of being completely supported. We can see and feel our breath and become aware of the power of our attention. We discover the release that takes place spontaneously in our bodies when we are still and attentive.

Notice that your muscles soften and lengthen as they relax, and that this relaxation can radiate through your body. As you relax, you will feel heavier and more in contact with the floor. These sensations increase with time. You may think that eventually you will reach a point of complete relaxation from which there is no further release. In fact, the quieter you become and the longer you practise, the more you will be able to go on releasing further and further with your breath.

Deep Relaxation brings you into contact with the back of your body and gives you the experience of being completely supported from the back. Passive breathing, which you learn in Deep Relaxation, is the foundation of all of the poses. If your breathing is strained or stressed at any time, it is telling you that there is strain or undue force in the pose.

Deep Relaxation is an orientation to your entire practice. It is not simply a way of resting or a counterbalance to more active poses. It brings you to the passive release which is at the core of the work. It is a benchmark that shows us what it means to release with gravity, what a passive breath feels like. We see in Deep Relaxation that our bodies do release spontaneously and without effort on our part. Deep Relaxation shows us that something really can and does happen when we become quiet and surrender. There is a tremendous simplicity, integration and wholeness to the pose.

Little Boat, and Child's Pose in Chapter 8 will take you a step further in the process of easing rather than straining into the poses. Experienced students can also use the Standing Forward Bend (p. 111), and the Sitting Forward Bend (p. 190) to learn more about the release of the spine with gravity and the breath. As you learn to carry the ease of Deep Relaxation through into other poses, even strenuous or difficult ones, the distinction between easy and difficult dissolves. You will find ways of doing advanced poses with less and less effort.

Deep Relaxation (Corpse Pose, Savasana)

- Lie on your back with your legs straight and your arms at your side, palms up.

In addition to being comfortable, you must also be lying straight. Deep Relaxation is an excellent opportunity to observe your alignment. Lift your head and check to see if your spine is straight, your hips bones are level with each other and your legs are hip-width apart. Your arms should be equal distances from the sides of your body.

To relax your neck, reach behind the back of your head and feel the muscles just under the rim of your skull. Gently massage them, then stretch the back of your neck away from your shoulders. As the back of your neck releases, your chin will drop. Centre your chin in line with the notch between your collarbones, as you let your head rest back.

As your lower back releases, imagine that your heels are being gently stretched away from the back of your waist.

If your upper back is stiff, place a folded towel or blanket behind your head to keep the back of your neck long.

If you have lower back problems, you will probably prefer to put a pillow or rolled blanket under your knees, or to do Lying Release Pose.

Lying Release Pose

- Lie on the floor with your knees bent, arms at your sides, palms up.

Sink down into the floor with your exhalation to release and lengthen your lower back. You can also rest your hands on your belly to follow your breath.

Variations

- Lie with your legs resting against a wall or on the seat of a chair. These positions improve circulation in your legs and support your lower back.

How to Practise

Deep Relaxation Pose is difficult precisely because the position is so simple. Your eyes are closed and it is easy to be distracted. Concentration takes practice, and many people give up too soon. Like anything else worthwhile, you will need time, focus and commitment to come to a state of quiet balance. And it takes many years of practice to be able to sustain it. But the value of this practice is inestimable. There are a number of simple techniques that you can use to help your concentration.

- *Talk yourself through the relaxation.*
  Start from your head and work down to your feet. Finish with a passive focus on the movement of your belly as you breathe. You may find a relaxation tape helpful.
- *Mentally say "inhaling" while you are inhaling, and "exhaling" while you are exhaling.*
- *Count your breaths: inhale one, exhale two, inhale three.*
  When you get to ten or lose the count, start again.
- *Place your hands on your chest or belly, wherever you can feel your breath.*
  As you become quiet, slowly move your hands lower until you can feel your breathing in the area between your pubic bone and your navel.
- *Start with your hands on your lower abdomen, and wait for your breath to drop.*

- *Cover your eyes with a small towel or wrap a scarf or tensor bandage loosely around your head.*
  Relaxing your eyes is soothing and helpful. Try using eye bags filled with rice or flax seed or eye masks like the ones people use to help them sleep on airplanes.

You can start your practice with relaxation in order to give yourself time to shift your attention from your day-to-day concerns inward to your body and your breath. Quiet attention to your breath clears your mind, and your nervous system shifts to the passive relaxation response.

It is also important to take time to be quiet after doing the poses so that you can integrate your practice, physically and mentally. Observe the cumulative effects and benefits of your practice. Seeing these positive changes give you encouragement, direction and purpose. If your practice has gone well, you will be more in contact with the floor, and you will be able to feel continuing release without effort or intervention. Your mind will be quieter and your attention more focused. Gradually, you will find a place of inner quiet. The final relaxation also gives you time to make the transition back to the "outer" world.

We all go through periods of more intense stress when even a moment of quiet attention is elusive. However, if you are consistently tense and distracted at the end of your practice, you should think about why, and determine what changes you need to make. You may be forcing your breathing or pushing yourself in the poses, creating tension rather than releasing it. You may find that you need more time to practise, or that you need to make some other changes in your life to reduce the stress.

While most people love Deep Relaxation Pose, some people are frightened or threatened by the passivity and stillness. If it is a very difficult pose for you, and you keep finding reasons to avoid it, try sitting in one of the simple sitting poses, Child's Pose or Little Boat, instead.

On the other hand, some people fall asleep during the relaxation. You may fall asleep because you are tired, or because you cannot separate relaxation and sleep. At times, sleep is a form of resistance to the awareness that comes with deep and conscious relaxation.

When you are used to lying quietly, lengthen the period of relaxation from time to time. This deepens the experience and prepares you for more advanced breathing techniques. It is beneficial when you are tired, ill or burnt out. A long Deep Relaxation Pose is cooling and you may want to cover yourself before you start. You may also want to lie on a folded blanket, so that your back can relax more easily.

As we discussed in the Introduction, both Deep Relaxation Pose and pranayama (breathing practice) bring one's attention to the mind and emotions. As you become quieter, you can observe your thoughts and feelings, which may have been pushed aside or repressed. Knowing that feelings may surface will reduce your guilt or confusion if it happens. You may sometimes burst into tears or have powerful dreams after a deep relaxation or breathing practice, but this is all part of the process, and is often a sign of opening or progress.

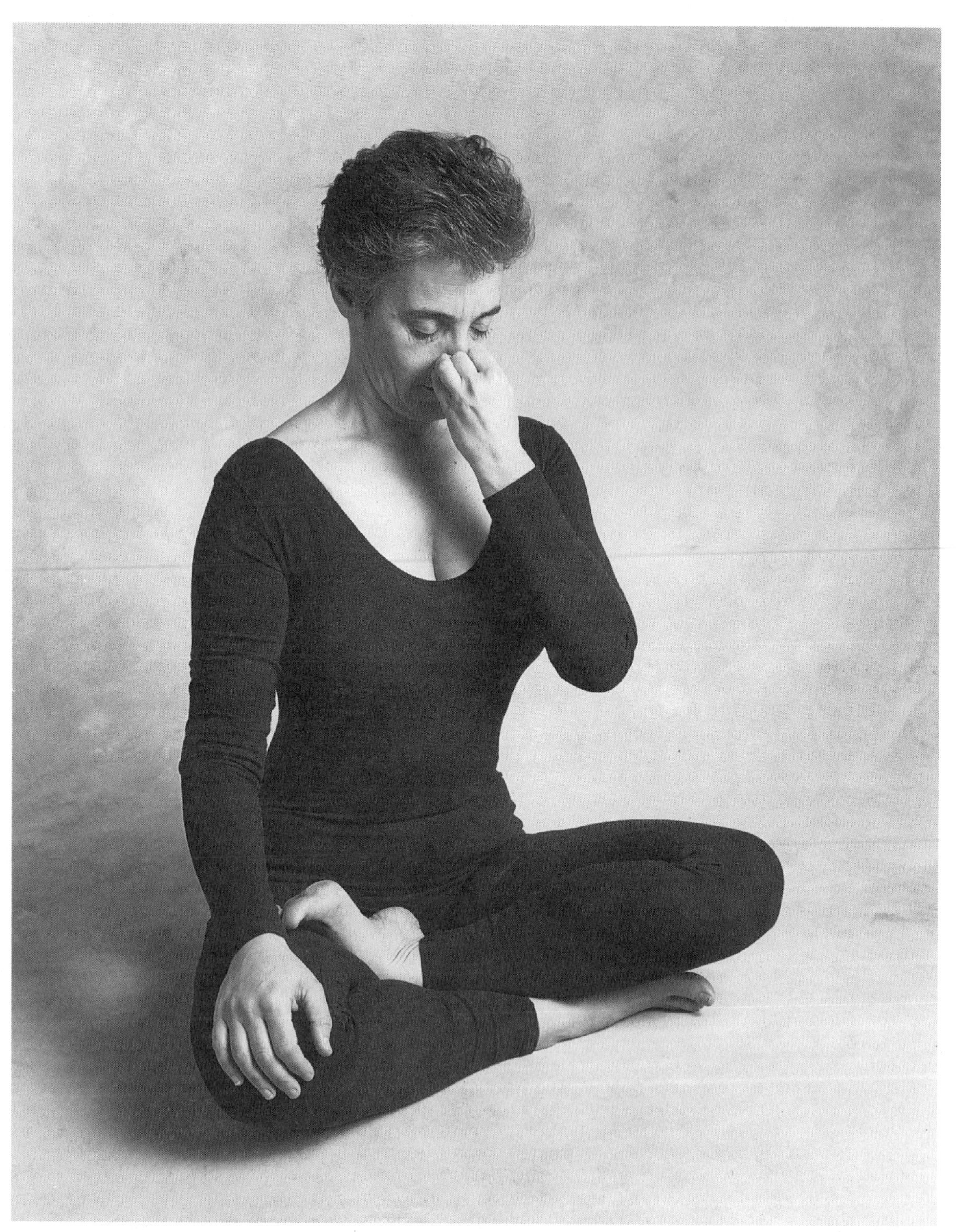

Alternate Nostril Breathing

CHAPTER 6

Pranayama: Attention to your Breath

PRANAYAMA MEANS the mastery and containing of prana, the universal energy. We achieve this mastery through breathing practices which progressively deepen, balance and harmonize the breath.

As I mentioned in the Introduction, attention to and awareness of our breath is central to the practice of yoga. In many languages the words for breath and spirit are the same. Awareness of our breathing gives life to the postures, and builds the bridge between body and spirit.

And just as stress can affect our entire body, so can the relaxation that comes with deep and quiet breathing. The increased expiration of carbon dioxide and improved oxygen intake give us energy and improve metabolic function by cleansing and detoxifying our bodies. The cardiovascular system benefits from greater ease in breathing. The overall benefits of a regular breathing practice—physically, emotionally, mentally and spiritually—cannot be over-estimated.

I enter each living creature and dwell within as the life-giving breath.

— *Bhagavad Gita*

Guidelines

Always respect your natural breathing pattern and rhythm, as everyone's breathing is different. Your breathing will naturally become slower, smoother and deeper as you become quieter. Do not try to make your breath slower or force your breath in any way. Let it slow down on its own, and find its own rhythm.

Our breathing is directly connected to our nervous system, so you will begin to feel the effects of your breathing practice immediately. As you practise deep breathing and the different breathing techniques, be aware of any signs of stress or tension. These include:

- *Strain in the eyes, forehead or throat*
- *A forced sound in the throat as you breathe*
- *Gasping for the inhalation*
- *Pushing to deepen the breath*
- *Hyperventilation or light-headedness*
- *Feeling tense, "hyper" or light-headed after the practice*
- *More emotional release than you can handle*

If you feel any stress from your breathing practice, come back to passive breathing and take more time to become quiet and grounded. Use less effort. Watch carefully to find the cause of the stress in your posture or practice.

Lying Down

If you are a beginner, start your breathing practice lying down. You can relax more easily, and your spine will be straight and supported. You can practise any of the breathing techniques in this position. Use the techniques described for Deep Relaxation to bring your attention to your breath.

Even if you are an experienced student, you may want to lie down when you are too tired or sick to sit comfortably. If necessary, you can do a breathing practice in bed.

- Start in Lying Release Pose, and follow your breathing.
- Let the exhalation drop lower and lower into your body.
- As you exhale, let the back of your waist relax toward the floor.
- Remain passive as you inhale.

Sitting

When you are able to sit comfortably and can follow your breath, try sitting for your breathing practice. In the long run, you will be able to breathe more deeply sitting than lying down. It is easier to concentrate, and the practice is more powerful. And there is a wonderful reciprocal relationship between deep breathing and posture.

When we are upright, gravity supports the base of the pose and anchors the spine. The upper body is then light and free, which is essential for deep breathing as any tension in the diaphragm or upper body limits the movement of the breath. Deep breathing supports the spine, which will lengthen and become stronger from your breathing practice, improving your posture.

There are many poses which can be used for pranayama. Lotus Pose is the classical position because it is secure and grounded. If you can do Lotus easily, you will find it easier to sit straight. However, for most Western people it takes years of practice to be able to sit in Lotus comfortably for extended periods of time.

You can sit in any of the simple sitting poses described in Chapter 13. Use the one(s) you find most comfortable, and feel free to try different postures for variety. When your knees are on the floor, the base of your pose is a triangle, a strong and stable structure. Be sure to alternate your legs in any of the cross-legged positions.

- Focus on the contact of your pelvis and legs with the floor.
- Feel the back of your pelvis and your legs being pulled down toward the centre of the earth as you exhale.
- Feel your spine rooted in your pelvis.
- Let your upper body relax.
- Drop your arms and your shoulders.
- Release the back of your head away from the back of your shoulders, so that your chin drops.
- Let your eyes remain passive and rest back, just as they did when you were lying down.
- Relax your forehead and your eyebrows.
- Let your jaw release and the muscles of your face become passive.
- Watch the movement of your belly as you breathe.

Following Your Breath

The simplest breathing practice, which we also use in the poses, is attention to your breath. Learn to simply watch your breath, without trying to adjust or control it.

- Watch your breathing, noting the rhythm, the "texture" and the sound of your breath.
- Be aware of the places that you can feel easy, free, relaxed movement.
- Notice the areas that feel tense or blocked. Imagine what it would be like if they were also relaxed and free.
- Notice what happens as you pay attention. Be aware of the power of your attention and the changes that result simply from watching.
- As you exhale, allow the back of your pelvis be pulled into the floor and your knees to drop.
- Pay attention to the release of your spine as your legs and pelvis drop.
- Let your shoulders relax and your arms remain passive, especially as you inhale.
- Be aware of the base of your spine rooted in your pelvis and let your upper body be light and free.
- Let the inhalation come to you.
- Remain dropped and rooted to the floor as you inhale.

As you pay attention to your breathing, let your eyes remain passive and rest back, as you did when you were lying down. This shift of awareness will also help to bring the back of your head in line with the back of your pelvis. Relax your eyebrows and let your forehead broaden. When you are sitting, be aware of the tendency to tighten your eyebrows and forehead as you watch your breath.

When you begin to follow your breathing, you will probably be busy and distracted. Your breathing rhythm will reflect this, and be erratic and jagged. Take time to come to your breath, and to let your attention and your breath settle.

Be aware of the polarities of the breathing cycle: the end of your exhalation and the end of your inhalation. Feel that gravity is pulling your exhalation down. Eventually, you will be able to feel your breath moving all the way down to your sitting bones. Your hips will be free and relaxed and you will be able to sit with your pelvis upright. In this position, the back of your waist will be supported by the action of your breathing. The security of this foundation allows your upper body to relax. Your head will balance easily over your pelvis; your upper back, arms and shoulders will be relaxed and free. In the classical framework of energy and chakras (see p. 16), following the breath will gradually connect you to the bottom of your tailbone, the root or first chakra, representing stability and security.

As you become quieter, your breathing naturally becomes slower and steadier. You may find a natural pause at the end of your exhalation. In this very quiet moment, let yourself drop further within.

As your exhalation deepens, your inhalation becomes fuller as a result. The inhalation follows naturally at the end of the exhalation. There is no need to "take" a deep breath. Wait. Allow the inhalation to come to you. Trust that it will. Open yourself to receive it. This is an example of non-greed and non-grasping (see p. 11) in practice. There is no limit to the potential depth and fullness of your breath. Your exhalation may be deeper than you thought possible; your inhalation can expand beyond your expectations.

As always, this physical experience of greater depth has corresponding emotional and spiritual aspects. The feeling of being pulled down with gravity will also draw you inward to the roots of your thoughts and feelings. It is important not to close off your thoughts or deny your feelings. Many of the tensions in our bodies have been caused by this denial. Allow yourself to feel your feelings.

The quieter you become the more clearly you will see your innermost thoughts. One of the goals of meditation is to see things as they are, free of expectations, preconceptions and projections. When you can keep your attention steady on your breathing, then you will have glimpses of this clarity.

Time in the wilderness, surrounded by quiet and the sounds of nature has helped me to be patient with myself as I breathe. In the country, I am often surrounded by silence while I am still noisy and distracted inside. This silence provides an inspiration for my breathing practice in the city. With time, I can find a quiet space around my thoughts, while my thoughts continue. Touching moments of true quietness are a rare and precious gift.

Breathing Practices

Complete Yoga Breath

Complete Yoga Breath is the term is used to describe movement of the breath which includes the belly, the diaphragm and the chest. It is the basis of all of the breathing techniques discussed here.

Extended Exhalation

When you are comfortable following your breath, you can begin to deepen your exhalation. Consciously, deepening your breath is an extension of the passive breathing that you have already been practising. The exhalation is primary because it is the vehicle for release or letting go. A deep exhalation creates the conditions for a deep, passive inhalation. When we are able to let go we create the opening which allows us to receive breath, to be inspired.

- Start by watching the movement of your belly as you breathe.
- When your breath is quiet and relaxed, gently draw your abdominal muscle further back as you come to the end of your exhalation.
- As you exhale, "touch" the back of your waist with your breath, let the back of your pelvis drop and your spine lengthen.
- As your pelvis drops, let your knees drop also.
- The movement of your abdomen back also supports your spine. As your pelvis drops, your upper body is supported and lifts upward.
- Remain completely passive as you inhale.

This movement should be smooth and even, a reinforcement of the natural and passive movement of the breath. You will feel as though your abdomen has been sucked back, as if gravity becomes stronger at the end of your exhalation and pulls you further into the floor. The abdominal wall remains smooth and wide. It is like pushing a child on a swing; you intensify the swinging motion which is already taking place, adding energy and momentum. It is much more a question of rhythm and timing than of strength.

Extending your exhalation massages your abdominal organs and strengthens your stomach muscles. Internal tensions can be released.

As your belly becomes softer and more elastic, imagine that your abdominal wall could move right back to your spine, so that the front of your spine is being massaged with each exhalation. As the back of your waist releases and lengthens, the movement is transmitted down through your legs. When you feel your head and neck start to adjust themselves, you will know that the release has also transmitted itself through the length of your spine. Distinguish clearly between your spine, which is supporting you, and your arms and shoulders, which are not. As your spine lengthens, the back of your head lifts and your shoulders drop.

Do not force your breath or create tension. If there is any tension or anxiety at the end of your exhalation, then you have pushed your breath too far. Relax and come back to a passive breath. At first, allow at least three passive breaths between the extended exhalations. Any strain will show in the quality of these breaths. As you become more comfortable with the technique, you can extend every other breath, and then every breath.

When you are comfortable with this technique, you can incorporate it into your poses to give them more power and depth.

Ujjayi

Ujjayi means "to pronounce loudly." A sound is created by narrowing the breathing passage in the throat, which makes the breath loud and forceful. The students I have seen practising this type of breathing seem to me to be creating stress in their necks and throats. Since many people already have too much tension in their necks, throats, jaws and shoulders, I do not recommend this type of practice. I think it would be very difficult to narrow your throat in this way and still remain relaxed.

Stronger Breaths

The following three techniques, Ha, Lion and Rapid Abdominal Breathing, are all useful when you have pent up energy or emotion and you want a strong technique for discharging it. Once you are comfortable with these techniques, you can use them in the postures to give your practice more dynamic energy and emotional release.

Ha

- As you exhale, say "Haaaa..."

Saying "Ha" with the exhalation gives added release to the breath. Said loudly, it discharges emotional stress; said more quietly it has a quality of relief and unwinding. It is particularly effective in releasing tension in the neck, throat and jaw.

In the beginning, you may be shy about vocalizing. I have done it in the shower, in a car with the windows closed, or with the vacuum cleaner on.

Lion (Simhasana)

Lion breath is another technique for discharging pent up energy and negative emotions. It is also very effective for releasing tension in the neck and throat. It can be quite helpful when you have a sore throat.

- As you exhale, stick out your tongue as far as you can, and try to touch the tip of your tongue to the bottom of your chin.
- At the same time make a loud noise, like a child imitating a lion's roar.
- Inhale passively.
- Continue for as long as you want. When your feel ready, return to passive breathing.

Rapid Abdominal Breathing (Kapalabhati)

The word *Kapalabhati* is derived from two words meaning "to clean the skull" or "shining skull." It is intended to clear the nostrils, the ears and the other air ducts in the head.

Rapid Abdominal Breathing is warming and stimulating as well as an energetic massage of the internal organs. Particularly effective for toning the abdominal muscle, it develops strength and tone without the shortening and contraction of sit-ups. The back of the waist is lengthened, and the pelvis firmly grounded. At the same time, the upper back is released upward, giving you a direct experience of the two-way movement of the spine.

You can start Rapid Abdominal Breathing when you are comfortable with the Extended Exhalation. It is like a controlled sneeze. To learn it, say "Ha" quickly and loudly and watch the movement of your stomach.

- ✦ Pull your stomach muscle back sharply to expel the air through your nose.
- ✦ Relax and let the inhalation follow automatically when your abdomen is released.
- ✦ Begin with 5–10 breaths.
- ✦ When your rhythm is steady, increase to 20–30 breaths per round, about one breath per second.
- ✦ Make the last exhalation in the series stronger and slower, to connect with the following slow inhalation.
- ✦ Take at least one complete slow breath between the rounds.

You can continue repeating the series of breaths for as long as you want. Eventually you can go up to 120 breaths per minute. When it is done correctly, Rapid Abdominal Breathing leaves you feeling clear and grounded, and your breath is smooth and even.

The impulse of Rapid Abdominal Breathing should radiate through your entire body and break up patterns of holding or tension. Be sure that you are not holding your head and neck.

This technique is faster and more dynamic than in passive breathing, but the basic mechanics remain the same: the abdomen fills with the inhalation and moves back on the exhalation. If you find yourself reversing the movement, go back to simple breathing, wait and try again.

Do not push *down* on your diaphragm. Move the abdominal muscle back. Dropping of the hips is a result, not an action.

Incorporating Rapid Abdominal Breathing into the poses makes your practice more dynamic, and helps you to move in poses where you feel stuck. Be sure that you are not creating any stress in the pose with the stronger breathing.

- ✦ Caution: Rapid Abdominal Breathing should be avoided by people with eye or ear problems, high or low blood pressure or emphysema. It does, however, benefit people with asthma, since it helps empty the lungs, allowing better inhalation. Start with very light movements.

- ✦ This technique should not be practised during the first trimester of pregnancy or toward the end of term. In the middle trimester, experienced students can practise light Rapid Abdominal Breathing.

- ✦ If you hyperventilate or begin to feel light-headed, you are practising incorrectly and should stop.

breath. You can gradually increase the length of the pauses, and the number of sections in the breath.

Interval breathing helps you to lengthen your breath, and prepares you for the longer pauses in breathing retention.

Square Breath (Sama Vrtti Pranayama)

In this technique, you pause at the end of the inhalation and at the end of the exhalation. The length of all of the sections of the breath are the same. Unless you are very comfortable with long pauses, the breaths themselves will be very short. Soften and drop during the pauses so there is no holding or tension.

This breath is very stabilizing.

- Take a few normal breaths to establish an easy, steady rhythm.
- Then pause after the inhalation and after the exhalation: exhale, pause, inhale, pause.
- Gradually increase the length of the pauses until all four parts of the breath are of equal length.
- Continue with this pattern for as long as you are comfortable and then return to normal breathing.

Retention (Kumbhaka)

Retention techniques involve more extended pauses at the end of the exhalation (exhalation retention) and the end of the inhalation (inhalation retention). Retention creates a moment of stillness within the breath, when even the action of breathing stops.

- Take a few normal breaths to establish an easy, steady rhythm.
- Then inhale, pause... exhale.
- When you pause, stay relaxed and passive.
- Let your hips and shoulders drop. Your spine remains relaxed and straight.
- Let your body continue to be expanded by the breath within you.
- Exhale slowly and naturally.
- Continue with this pattern for as long as you are comfortable and then return to normal breathing.

There are a number of classical rhythms that are used for retention. Before you try any of them find out how long you can *comfortably* pause. Gradually lengthen your pauses, always being sure that you are relaxed and quiet during and after your practice.

The rhythm that I have been taught is to inhale for a count of 5, hold 15, exhale 10; a ratio of 1:3:2. If you are comfortable pausing after your exhalation, you can inhale 5, hold 10, exhale 10, hold 5; the ratio is 1:2:2:1. One rhythm that is often used is inhale 4, hold 16, exhale 8 (1:4:2). Both of these ratios are much too long for most beginners to do with ease.

Take time to build up to these rhythms, gradually increasing the length of your retention. The retention should be easy and never forced, and you should feel calmer and quieter afterwards, not tense. Remember that the people who developed these patterns practised for hours daily over many years. *Never* strain in any of the breathing practices. All of the techniques should be adapted to your body and to the moment.

Alternate Nostril Breathing

Alternate Nostril Breathing alternates the breath between the left and right nostrils. It balances the left and right sides of our bodies, and the two channels of energy on the left and right sides of the spine (known in Sanskrit as the *ida* and *pingala* respectively). It is a calming and soothing technique which is recommended for insomnia.

It takes much less pressure and contact than you think to close your nostrils. A gentle touch with the *tip* of your finger at the end of the bony part of your nose (where the nostril starts to flare) is sufficient to close the nostril. Too much pressure will distort the flow of air.

When you begin, use the index fingers of each hand to close the respective nostrils, alternating hands. When you are comfortable with the breathing technique, you can close the nostrils with one hand. Touch the tips of your ring and pinkie fingers together to close one nostril and the tip of your thumb to close the other. The index and middle fingers remain relaxed.

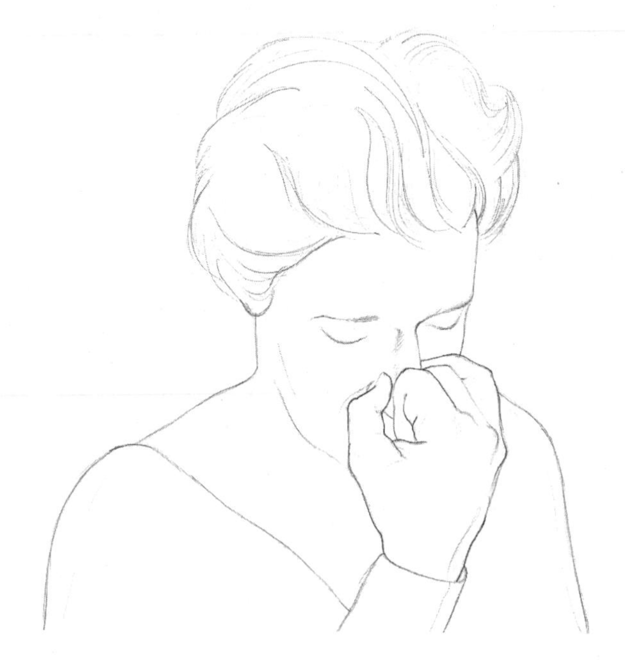

Bringing your arm up to control the breath through your nostrils should not distort your sitting posture. Your spine should remain straight and both shoulders relaxed and dropped. Your elbow should drop and your hand remain relaxed, so the touch on your nostrils is light and easy. You can put a cushion on your lap to support your arm.

If you are using one hand, you may find that your head turns toward that side. Open your eyes every once in a while and check to see that you are looking straight ahead. Classically, only the right hand was used for alternate nostril breathing, because of negative associations with the left side of the body. However, I have found it more comfortable and balancing to alternate the use of my hands.

Wait for your breathing to be steady and relaxed before beginning any of the alternate nostril practices. The techniques are given in increasing order of difficulty. Be sure that you are comfortable with each one before you go on to the next.

At first, most of your attention will be on your hands and organizing the changes. Wait until the basic technique is familiar, then focus on the flow of air in your nostrils. Let your pelvis drop as you exhale to stay grounded.

Alternate Nostril Exhalation (Anuloma Pranayama)

- Take a few normal breaths to establish an easy, steady rhythm.
- Inhale normally through both nostrils.
- Close the right nostril and exhale through the left.
- Inhale normally through both nostrils.
- Close the left nostril and exhale through the right.
- Continue with this pattern for as long as you are comfortable and then return to normal breathing.

Alternate Nostril Inhalation (Pratiloma Pranayama)

- Take a few normal breaths to establish an easy, steady rhythm.
- Exhale normally through both nostrils.
- Close the right nostril and inhale through the left.
- Exhale normally through both nostrils.
- Close the left nostril and inhale through the right.
- Continue with this pattern for as long as you are comfortable and then return to normal breathing.

Inhalation through the Right Nostril/ Sun Channel (Surya Bhedana Pranayama)

This practice is warming and energizing.

- Take a few normal breaths to establish an easy, steady rhythm.
- Exhale normally.
- Close your left nostril and inhale through the right.
- At the end of the inhalation, close your right nostril. Both nostrils will be closed momentarily.
- *Then* release your left nostril and exhale through the left.
- At the end of the exhalation, close your left nostril. Both nostrils will be closed momentarily.
- *Then* release your right nostril and inhale through the right.
- Continue with this pattern for as long as you are comfortable. Finish the practice with an exhalation. Return to normal breathing.

Inhalation through the Left Nostril/ Moon Channel (Chandra Bhedana Pranayama)

This practice is cooling and quieting.

- Take a few normal breaths to establish an easy, steady rhythm.
- Inhale normally.
- Close your left nostril and exhale through the right.
- At the end of the exhalation, close your right nostril. Both nostrils will be closed momentarily.
- *Then* release your left nostril and inhale through the left.
- At the end of the inhalation, close your left nostril. Both nostrils will be closed momentarily.
- *Then* release your right nostril and exhale through the right.
- Continue with this pattern for as long as you are comfortable. Finish the practice with an exhalation. Return to normal breathing.

Full Alternate Nostril Breathing (Nadi Sodhana Pranayama)

Full alternate nostril breathing combines the above techniques, changing nostrils at the end of the inhalation or the exhalation. Changing after the exhalation is grounding and cooling, and brings your awareness down to your pelvis. Conversely, changing after the inhalation brings your awareness to your upper body and is warming and more stimulating. Eventually you can combine Alternate Nostril Breathing with Inhalation and Exhalation Retention.

To Alternate after the Inhalation

- Take a few normal breaths to establish an easy, steady rhythm.
- Inhale normally.
- Close your right nostril and exhale and inhale through the left.
- At the end of the inhalation, close your left nostril, *then* release your right nostril and exhale through the right.
- With your left nostril still closed, inhale through the right.
- At the end of the inhalation, close your right nostril, *then* release your left nostril. This completes one breathing cycle.
- Continue with this pattern for as long as you are comfortable. Finish with an exhalation. Return to normal breathing.

To Alternate after the Exhalation

- Take a few normal breaths to establish an easy, steady rhythm.
- Exhale normally.
- Close your right nostril, inhale and then exhale through the left.
- At the end of the exhalation, close your left nostril, *then* release your right nostril and inhale through the right.
- With your left nostril still closed, exhale through the right.
- At the end of the exhalation, close your right nostril, *then* release your left nostril. This completes one breathing cycle.
- Continue with this pattern for as long as you are comfortable. Finish with an exhalation. Return to normal breathing.

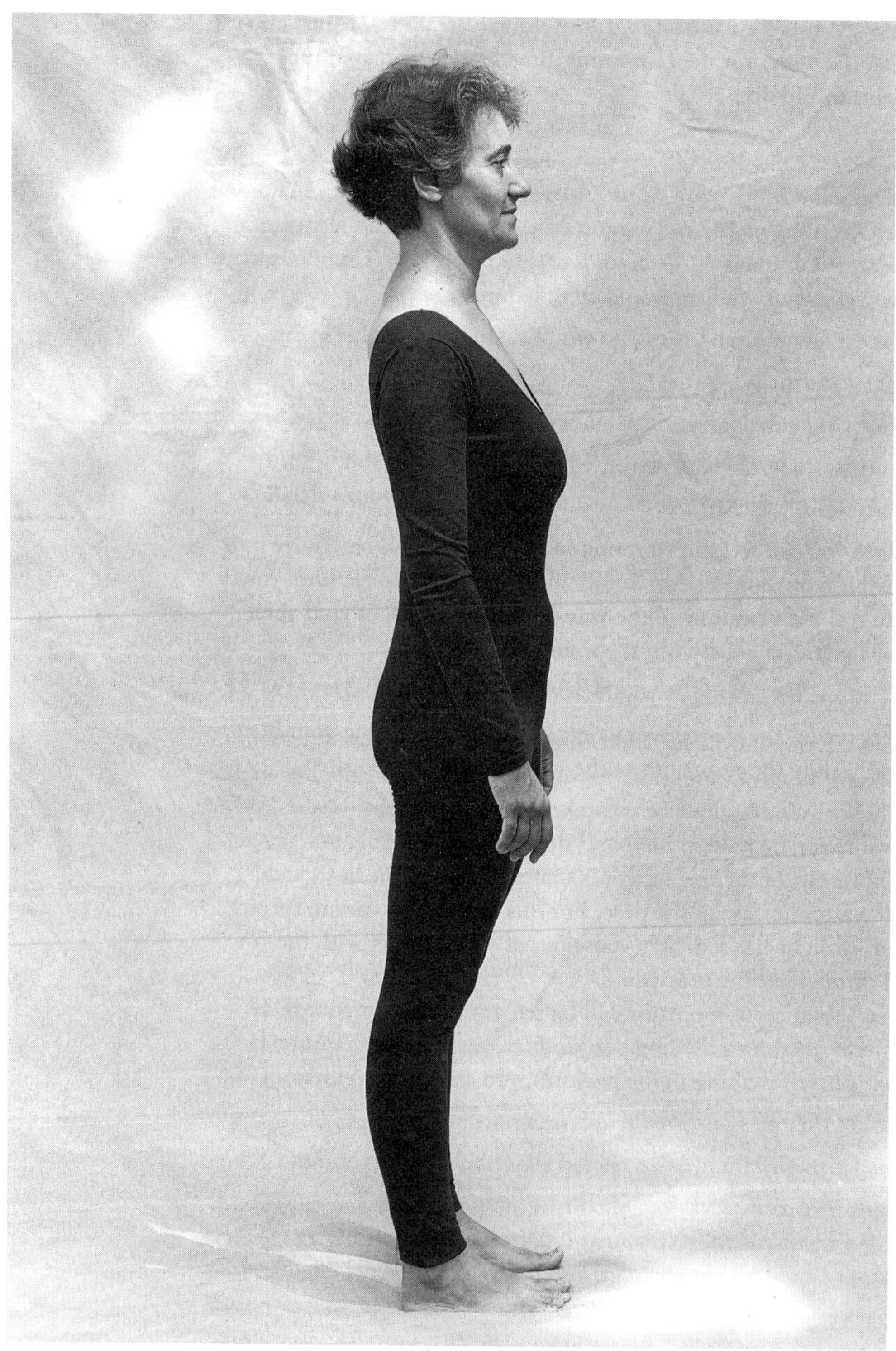

Standing Straight, Mountain Pose

CHAPTER 7

Learning to Stand

STANDING IS BASIC to our understanding of our relationship to the ground, to gravity and to the spine. The ability to stand upright is at the core of our evolution as human beings, rooted in the earth and growing upwards toward heaven.

Standing Straight, is the simplest standing pose, and the foundation for all of the other standing poses. It is a "pose" that we do every day.

When we stand, weight is transmitted down through our spines, into our pelvis, through our hip joints to our feet. Standing is a foundation for stability, mobility, and confidence. When the lower part of the body is grounded properly, the upper part of the body, including the mind, becomes light and agile. Energy is freed up. We learn to have our feet on the ground, to find connection to the earth and to grow upwards toward the sky.

It is well worth taking extended periods of time (at least 5–10 minutes) to practise Mountain Pose, as a standing meditation. Remember I told you about studying with Vanda, and how she told me to grow the roots, and then went away for twenty minutes? But I now feel that I have legs and that they are supporting me. There is no substitute for the time it takes to feel these connections and deepen them.

Finding Your Legs and Feet

Our feet are the foundation when we stand, and are designed to give us both stability and lightness. They bear the entire weight of the body and at the same time give spring and elasticity to our movement.

To support the weight appropriately and maintain their natural resilience, your feet need extension in the arches and flexibility in the muscles, tendons, ligaments and many small joints. Because of shoes and moving on hard, flat surfaces, our feet have lost their natural resilience and pliability. Move your feet, stretch your toes and roll your feet from side to side. Feel the weight shift as you move. Notice how the weight falls on your feet when you stand, and think about the way that you wear down the soles of your shoes. Wearing shoes has also shifted our sense of appropriate balance forward onto the balls of our feet. Therefore, we need to focus on the heels in standing poses. Leaning backwards to find your heels will make you feel as if you are falling. Imagine a strong magnetic force from the centre of the earth, pulling your heels into the floor.

Flat feet, bunions and other foot problems can be corrected through appropriate movement and exercise. If your arches tend to collapse, focus on weight dropping through the outer edges of your feet.

Ideally, our feet and knees face forward when we stand and walk. However, twist or tension in the sacrum, hips, knees, ankles or feet can cause your feet to turn out, or in. If you force your feet to be parallel too soon, without correcting the cause of the problem, you can cause further distortion and stress. It is more important to have your knees facing forward than your feet.

If your knees lock, bend them slightly to ease the tension at back of your knees. As you establish a connection through your heels, you will gradually be able to straighten your legs without stress.

Standing Straight, Mountain Pose (Tadasana)

- Start standing with your feet hip-width apart.
- Be aware of your weight being transmitted down your legs to your feet. Feel the contact of your heels with the floor.
- Focus on your breath. Start by following the natural rhythm of your breath. Notice if you are tense and if your breathing feels different than when you are sitting. You may find it more difficult to find the movement of your breath in your belly when you are standing than when you are sitting or lying down. Learn to feel the movement of your belly as you breathe.
- Let the back of your pelvis drop. There is no need to pull it down by tightening the buttocks. Feel that from the waist down you are being pulled into the ground, and from the waist up you are supported or growing upwards. The images that we used for sitting (p. 62) can also help you sense the lengthening of your spine when you are standing.
- Let your arms and shoulders relax.
- Feel as if the crown of your head is blossoming like a flower.

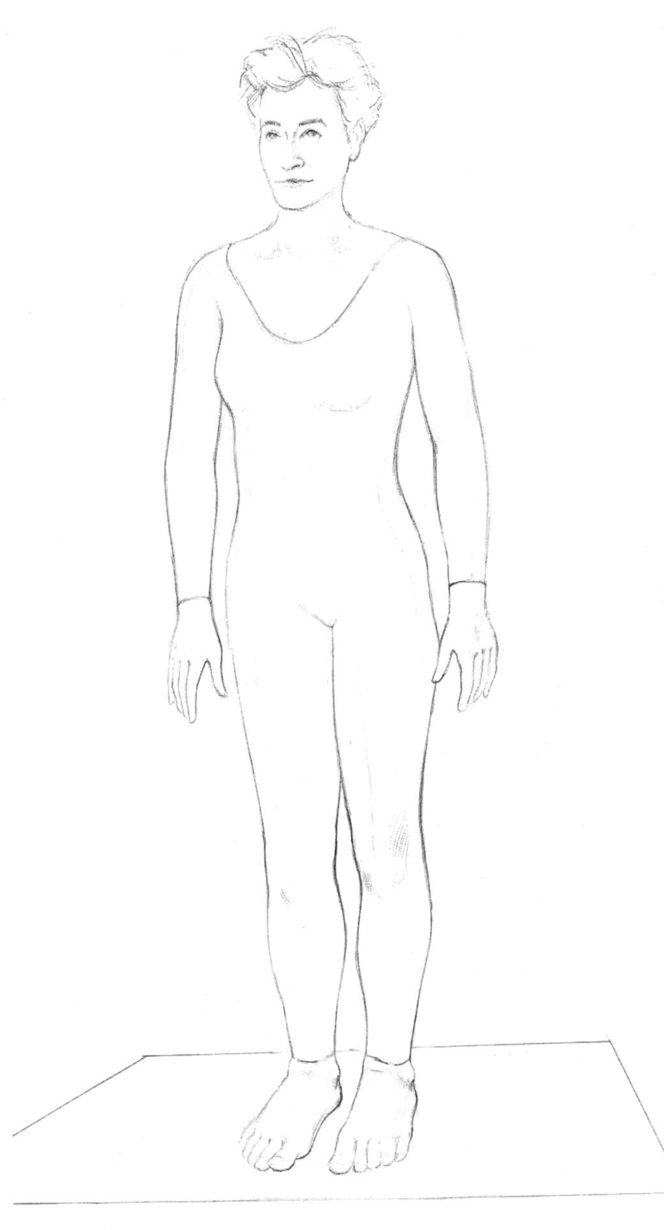

Releasing Your Pelvis and Lower Back

Alignment of your pelvis is essential when you are standing. Look in a mirror and adjust your position so that the line across your hip bones is horizontal. This usually means shifting weight to the non-dominant side (i.e. right-handed people shift to the left).

When we stand, the back of the waist is concave and usually tight and shortened. The curve of the spine should be long and shallow. So we need to practise dropping the back of the pelvis when we're standing just as we do sitting.

In some people the back of the waist is too straight. This is more difficult to correct, but the principle is the same. As you release your lower back and allow your pelvis to fall into place, the natural curve returns.

Fierce Pose is a very simple pose that strengthens your legs and hips as you learn to let your pelvis drop.

Fierce pose, Chair Pose (Utkatasana)

- Start by standing straight, with your legs a little more than hip-width apart.
- Bring your arms up over your head, keeping your arms and shoulders loose and relaxed.
- Bend your knees.
- With your knees bent, let the back of your pelvis drop.
- Stay in the pose, breathe and continue to relax.
- Return to standing straight by pressing down with your heels, as you exhale. Tuck your pelvis into a pelvic tilt as you come up.
- When you return to standing straight, release the pelvic tilt. See if you can feel new space in the back of your waist.

Lengthening Your Spine

The spine is the vertical axis and core of all poses. This is especially clear in the simplicity of Mountain Pose. Developing an awareness of the back of the body and a sense of the vertical axis takes time and practice.

To feel the line of your spine, stand against the edge of a doorway. Move your feet away from the corner until the back of your pelvis rests easily on the corner. The area between your shoulders should also touch the corner. The back of your head will also eventually touch, but do not arch your neck and force your head back. When you have a sense of the line of your spine, imagine it growing in both directions.

Freeing Your Upper Body, Neck and Head

The shoulders and upper back should be relaxed and passive when you stand. Rolling your shoulders, shoulder stretches and neck rolls help release the upper back. Move your shoulders as often as possible, for example, at a stop light while driving or during a break at work.

Unfortunately, most of the time we carry our heads in front of our body, creating tension as our back muscles tighten to counterbalance the weight of our heads. Beginners often look up to find the feeling of lift and lengthening, but this will only shorten the back of your neck. As your shoulders and upper back release, your head will balance more easily on your neck and shoulders. Practicing head and shoulder stands will help you free your upper body and feel the relationship of your head and neck to your torso.

The neck is the most delicate and mobile part of the spine and is very vulnerable. It is designed to support the weight of the head, and needs support and flexibility in the thoracic spine below. Let your head balance lightly on the top of your neck, and float freely in Mountain Pose, like a flower at the top of a stem.

Standing is a "pose" we do every day. Awareness of your feet, your spine and your breath as you stand or walk is a wonderful way to incorporate yoga into your daily life.

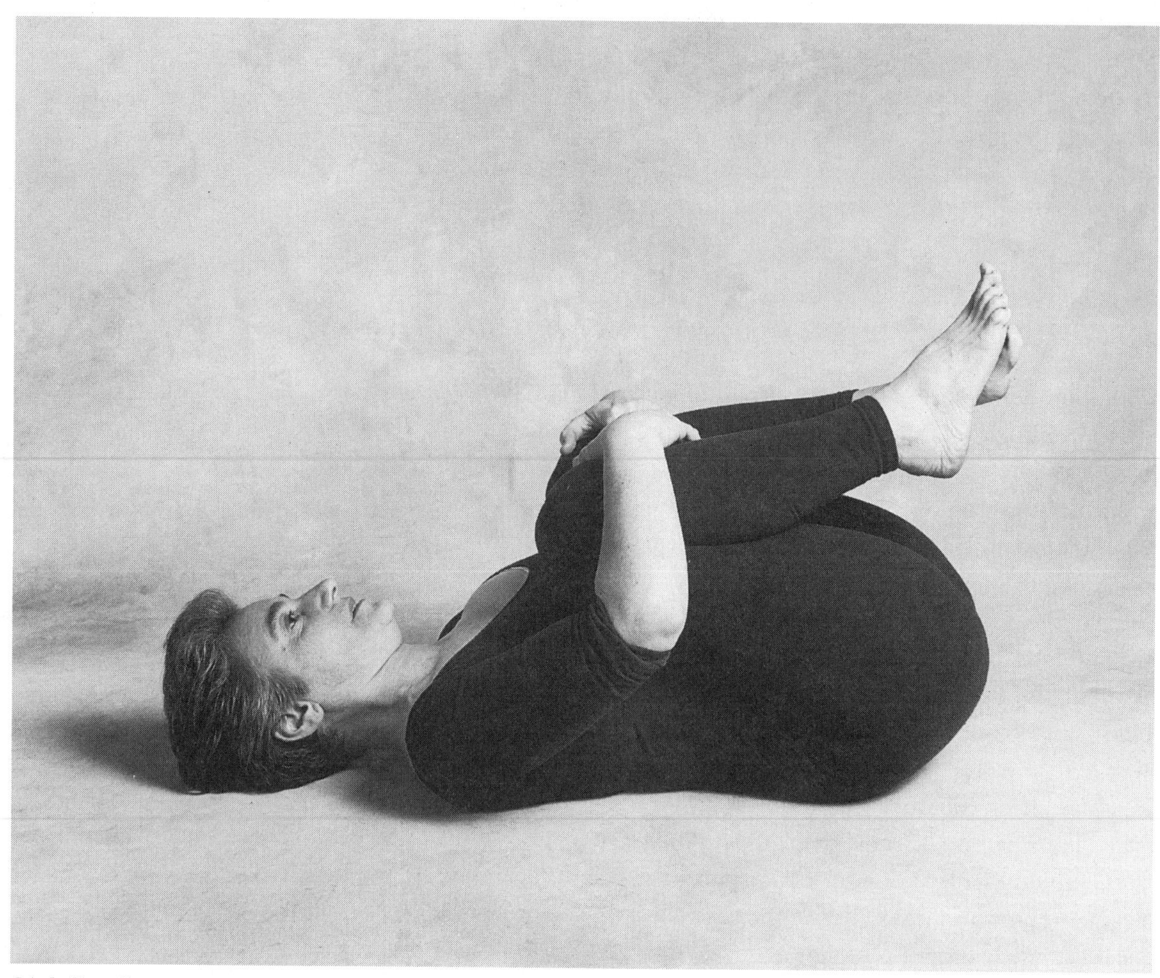

Little Boat Pose

CHAPTER 8

Simple Stretches

THESE SIMPLE POSES show you how to implement the basic principles of yoga in the postures. Bring the awareness of your breathing, the ground and the release of your spine into these basic poses.

Little Boat Pose (Pavana Muktasana)

(See photograph on opposite page.)

- Lie on your back with your knees to your chest.
- Wrap your arms around your legs.

This pose releases the back of your waist and lengthens your spine. Think of your arms as weights resting on your legs and helping them to drop. In order for your knees to drop toward your chest, you must soften and release your hips. See if you can feel the release of your lower back carry through your spine to your head. Then the back of your head will release away from your shoulders and your chin will drop.

Practice working with the rhythm of your breath.

- Remain passive as you inhale, letting your thighs lift a little away from your chest.
- Let your body rest back as you exhale.
- As you feel your back lengthen and the front of your thighs soften, draw your knees toward your chest. Use the minimum possible effort and leave your arms and shoulders relaxed.
- When you feel your body start to harden and resist, relax, wait, breathe and try again.
- One of the nice things about a simple pose like this is that there is no struggle to get into the pose, but simply the enjoyment as you move *with* the natural release of your body as you breathe.

Variations

- Cross your ankles (make sure you alternate the way they are crossed) or take your knees wider apart to alter the movement of your hip joint slightly.

  People who are overweight or have very stiff hips will probably prefer to take their knees wider. Pregnant women must keep their knees apart.

Little Boat Twist (Parsva Pavana Muktasana)

- Place your right arm on the floor at shoulder level.
- Holding your knees with your left arm, take your legs to the left for a gentle spinal twist.
- To stretch your neck, turn and look at your outstretched right arm. Drop your right shoulder toward the floor.

Remember that it does not take effort for the shoulder to drop; as your chest and arm muscles relax the shoulder will drop by itself. Continue to release into the back of your waist as you exhale. Notice the stretch on your outer right thigh and hip. When you repeat on the other side, be aware of any difference between the two sides. You can intensify the pose by keeping your knees close into your body.

CHILD'S POSE (PRANATASANA)

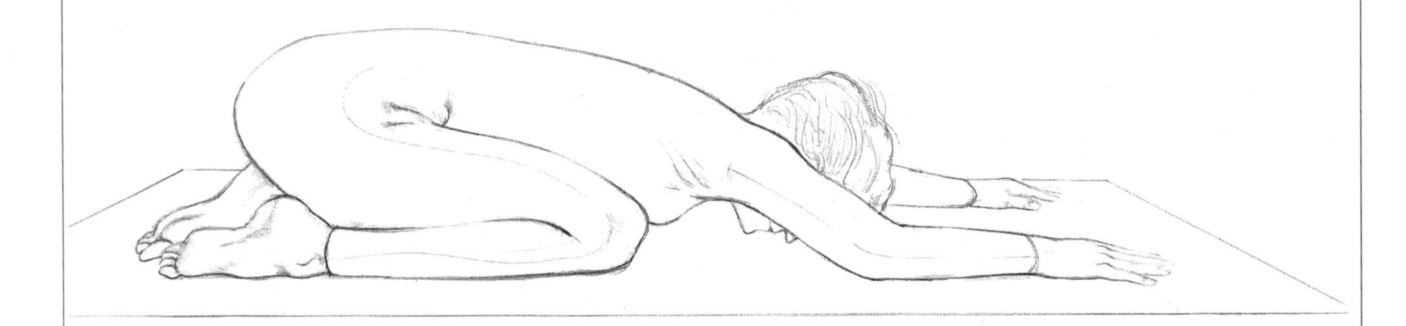

Child's Pose is Little Boat Pose turned over. Because your spine is now free, it is easier to feel it lengthen.

- Sit on your heels.
- Bend forward and rest your arms and head on the floor.

As you exhale, let your hips drop toward your heels. At the same time, let your head, arms and shoulders also drop. See if you can feel the ripple through your back as your spine releases. This is the beginning of "wave" described in the Introduction.

If you are very stiff or have knee problems, place a folded blanket between your hips and your heels or rest your upper body on a pillow.

Cat and Dog Poses

Cat and Dog poses are safe, simple poses. There are many ways to vary Dog and Cat Pose. You can stretch one leg or one arm at a time. You can lift one leg back. They are poses with a lot of freedom to stretch and explore, as cats and dogs do.

Cat Pose (Marjarasana)

Cat Pose explores the forward and back bending movements of the spine. The alternating movement will give you a sense of the wave.

There are many variations on the use of the breath in Cat Pose. The most common one is to exhale as you round your back and inhale as you let it relax. I prefer to do the movements on exhalations and relax on the inhalations since this is consistent with everything else I teach.

Cat Pose is recommended for pregnancy and menstrual problems.

- Start on your hands and knees, with your hands underneath your shoulders and your knees underneath your hips.
- Exhaling, curl your pelvis under and press down with the heels of your hands to round your back. Let your head drop.
- As you inhale, relax your spine and your arms, especially your elbows.
- When you relax your spine it will be concave, but do not let the back of your neck and your lower back compress. Your back will be gently and evenly curved.
- Alternate these movements for a dynamic and relaxing release of the spine.

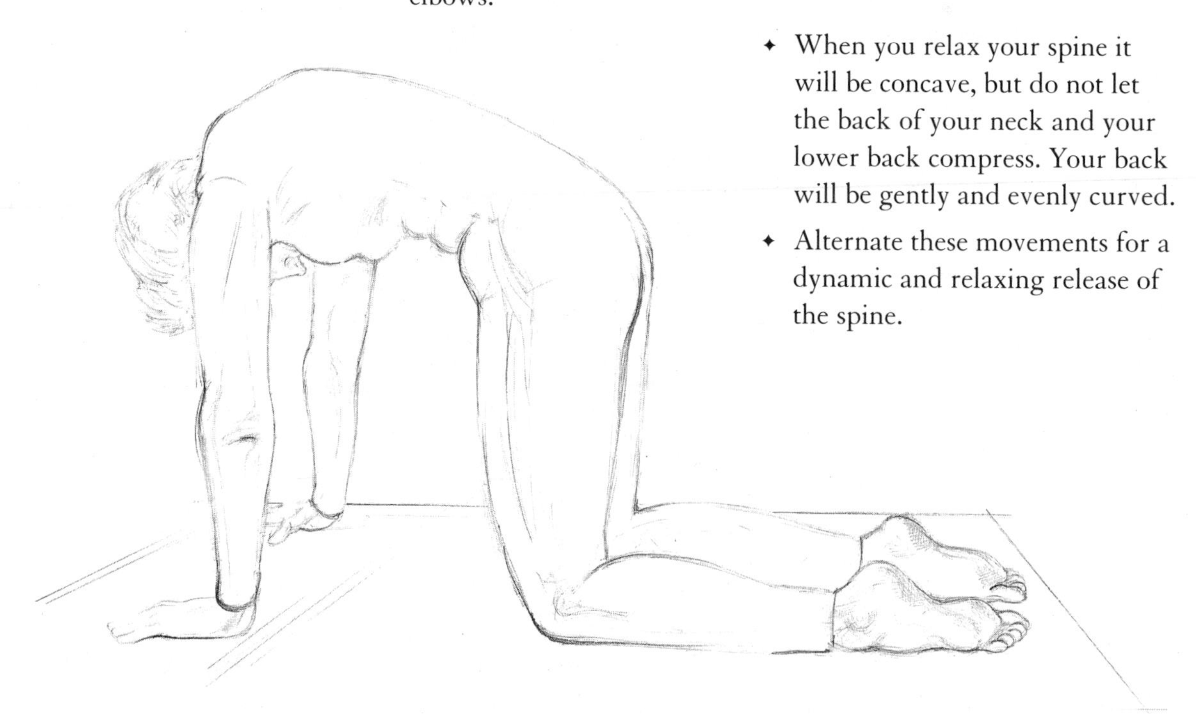

You can also do a more active backbend in Cat Pose which prepares you for Sun Salutation.

- Round your back as in Cat Pose.
- Then scoop your head down using an active movement to make your spine concave.
- Let the rest of your spine follow the movement.
- Be careful to keep the back of your neck and your lower back long as you bring your head up.
- To round your back again, pull your tailbone down and let the rest of your spine follow.
- Alternate these movements for a dynamic and relaxing release of your spine.

Variations

There are lots of ways to play in Cat as cats do. You can move sideways to stretch your side ribs, make circles with your spine, stretch your legs or your arms one at a time. See how many different ways you can find to vary this pose.

Dog Pose (Adho Mukha Svanasana)

Dog Pose is an intense stretch of the back of your legs, especially your calves. As your legs become more flexible, increase the distance between your hands and your feet.

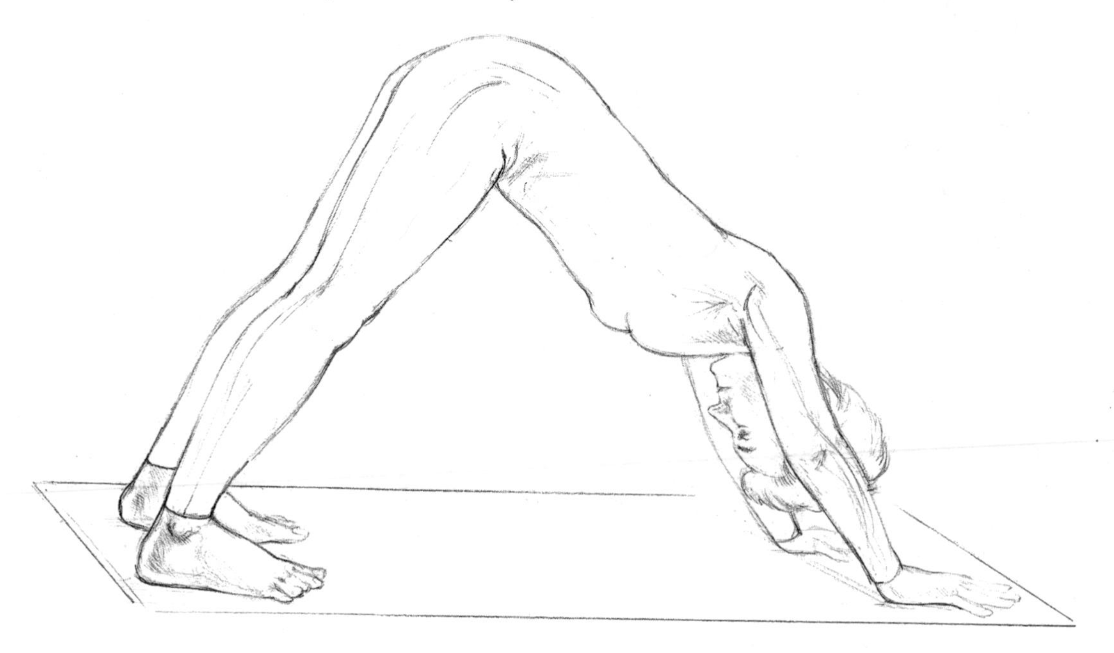

- Start in Cat Pose with your back rounded, or Child's Pose with your arms stretched out in front of you.
- Turn your toes under.
- As you exhale, straighten your legs.
- Continue the action that you learned in Cat Pose. Relax as you inhale. As you exhale, take your abdomen well back and press down with the heels of your hands, sending the weight back onto your legs.
- Take your heels down.
- To come down, bend your knees and return to Cat Pose or Child's Pose.

As your heels come down, they will tend to slide together. Keep them in line with each other (feet parallel). If you have weak arches, they will tend to collapse as you take your heels down. To strengthen your arches, take the outer edges of your feet down first and keep your arches lifting for as long as you can.

Garland Pose, Squatting (Malasana)

This pose is an intense stretch on the ankles and the back of the pelvis, and requires a deep release of the hips. It strengthens the inner thighs, and prepares you for Crow Pose. It is also a good preparation pose for labour and birthing.

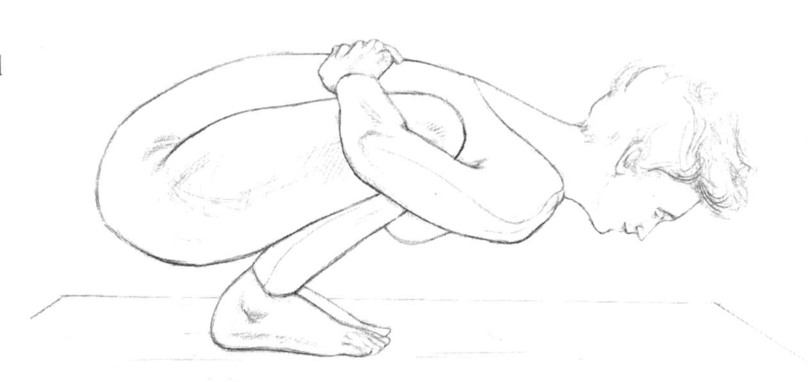

- Start standing straight, with your feet hip-width apart.
- As you exhale, drop forward (Standing Forward Bend, p. 111).
- Bend your knees and take them wide apart.
- Drop your upper body forward between your inner thighs. Your heels will probably come off the floor. If you have difficulty balancing, place a folded blanket under your heels.
- Stay forward, releasing and lengthening as you breathe. Let your elbows drop as much as possible.
- Then, leaving your upper body forward, slowly take your heels down, as far as you can. Focus on bringing the weight to the inner feet.
- When your arms have dropped below your knees, wrap them around your legs and catch your hands behind your back. If you can't grasp your hands, lay a belt across your back and hold it.
- Continue to lengthen your spine and take your heels down as you exhale. As your spine lengthens and your shoulders release, you will be able to reach around further.
- Draw your knees in toward each other, closing the gap between the inner thighs and the rib cage as you exhale.
- When you are ready to come up, release your hands and straighten your legs back into the Standing Forward Bend.

The pose is more difficult with the feet close together. If your hips are stiff, take your feet wider apart.

Lunge (Anjaneyasana)

Lunge Pose is part of the traditional Sun Salutation. This pose stretches the front thighs and opens the hips.

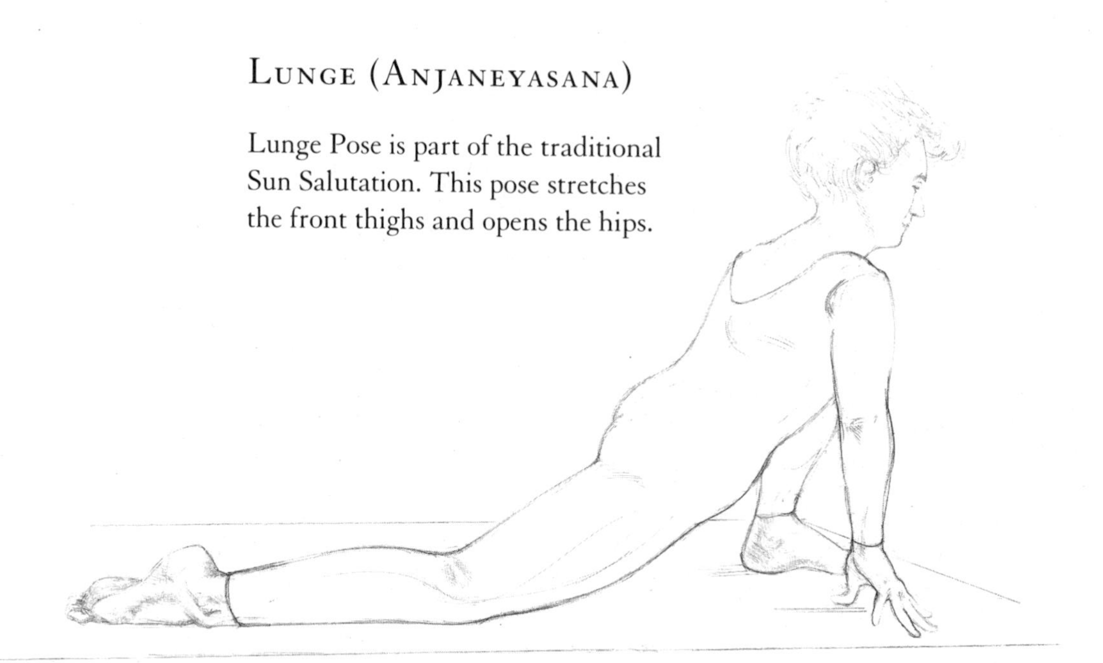

- Start on your hands and knees.
- Bring one leg forward so that your foot is between your hands. Your front knee can be directly over your heel or over your toes, as long as there is weight on your heel.
- Stretch the other leg back behind you. Your back leg can be straight or bent. It is easier to sustain the pose when your back leg is bent. When it is straight, the back thigh is strong and the leg is extended through the heel.
- Adjust the position of your torso to keep the line of your spine long and straight. As your hips become more flexible you can be more upright in the pose without shortening the back of your waist. Let the back of your pelvis drop as you exhale.
- Keep the back of your neck long and the back of your head in line with your upper back. If your pelvis is vertical, you will be looking straight ahead; otherwise you will probably be looking at the floor.
- The position of your arms is secondary. Do not round your back to keep your hands flat on the floor.
- To intensify the pose, press your front heel down and actively tilt your pelvis forward as you exhale.
- Repeat on the other side.

Pigeon Preparation Stretch (Eka Pada Raja Kapotasana)

Although this pose is a forward bend, it is a useful warm-up for prone backbends like Cobra because it wakes up the back of the pelvis and brings the sitting bones into clear focus. Once you are comfortable in it, it is an extremely restful pose that will also help your sitting postures.

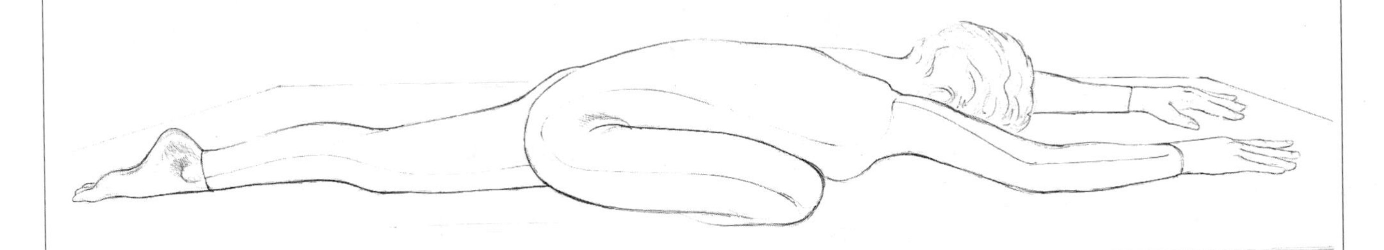

- Start in the Lunge Pose.
- Using your hands for support, bend your front leg sideways until the outside of your thigh is resting on the floor, as in Half Bound Angle Pose (see p. 191).
- Bend forward and rest your body over the bent leg.
- Adjust your position until the back of your pelvis is horizontal.
- Breathe and lengthen as your body releases to the floor. The stretch on the bent leg side of your pelvis will be intense.
- Stay in the pose for as long as you want, and then repeat on the other side.

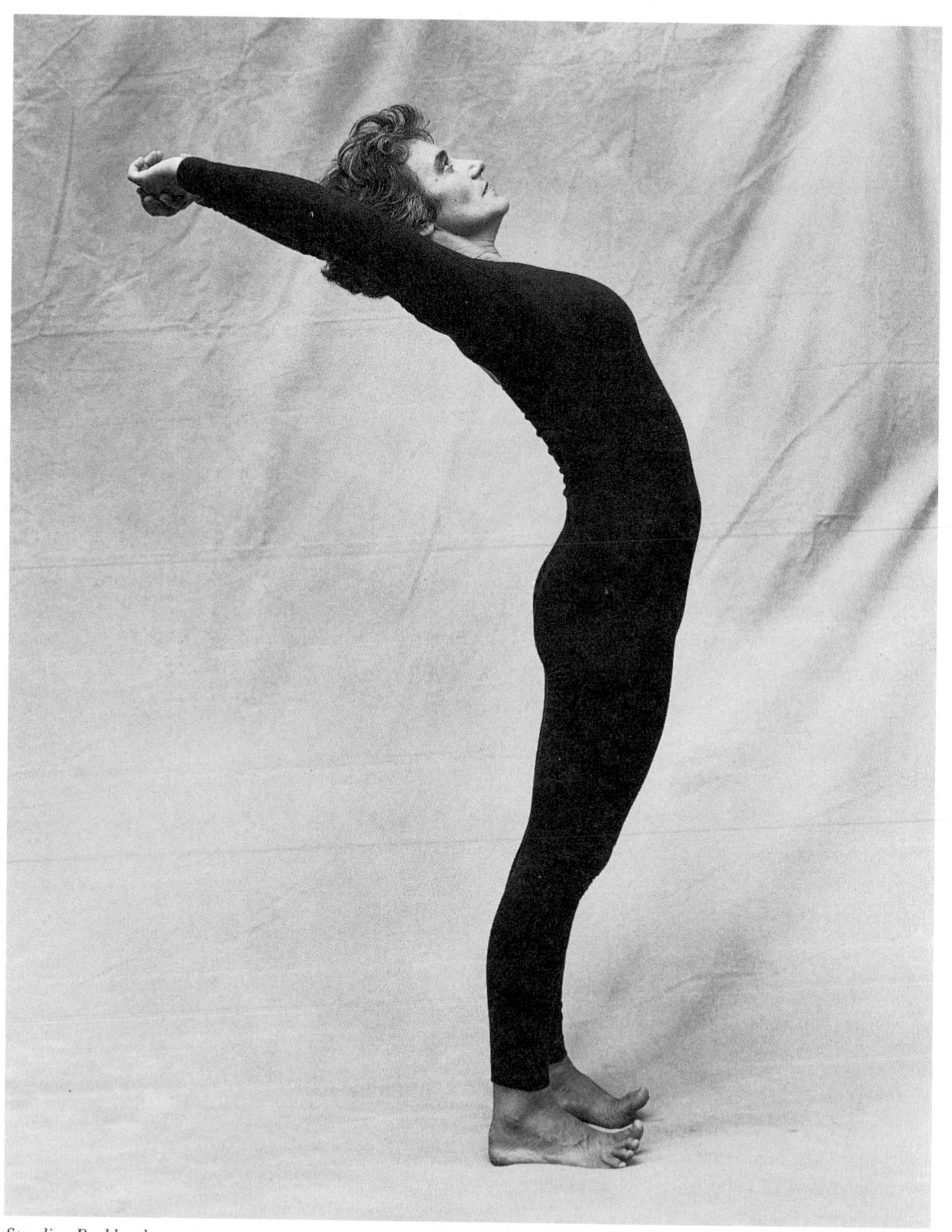

Standing Backbend

CHAPTER 9

Sun Salutation: The Wave

SUN SALUTATION, *Surya Namaskar*, is a warming and energizing series of poses which alternates forward bends and backbends in a flowing and fluid sequence. As the name implies, it was traditionally done in the morning. The undulating motion as you go from one pose to another is a wonderful example of the wave of the spine with the breath. To emphasize this wave, I have added a movement between the Plank Pose and the Dip which releases the spine and makes it easier to come up into the backbend.

All the poses in Sun Salutation are rooted from the waist down. Sustaining this awareness throughout protects your spine and gives a simple, consistent focus to your practice.

In Sun Salutation, we do poses on the inhalation as well as the exhalation. Remain relaxed and grounded during your inhalations as well as during your exhalations.

Ideally, the distance between the hands and feet is established on the first Lunge and remains unchanged. If you are a beginner, it will take some time before you are able to maintain this distance throughout the sequence.

You can use Sun Salutation as the core of your practice because of the variety of poses it contains. It is a good series to do when you have very little time to practise. Follow Sun Salutation with Shoulderstand and a twist, and your practice will contain the key movements of the spine.

Guidelines

- *Start Slowly*
  When you are learning the sequence or warming up, go through it slowly. Take time in each pose to breathe, lengthen your spine, and ground the pose.
- *Breathing*
  When you start to move on each breath, you will probably find it easier to move on the exhalations, and pause in the poses to inhale. When you are at ease with the flow of the poses, you can move on the inhalation as well. Your breathing should remain smooth and natural throughout. Co-ordinate the movements with the length and rhythm of your breath.
- *The Flow*
  Then, start to focus on the transitions between the postures. The movement of your spine should be smooth, round and flowing.
- *Your Breath and Your Spine*
  Finally, you can focus completely on the movement of your spine with your breath.

The Sequence

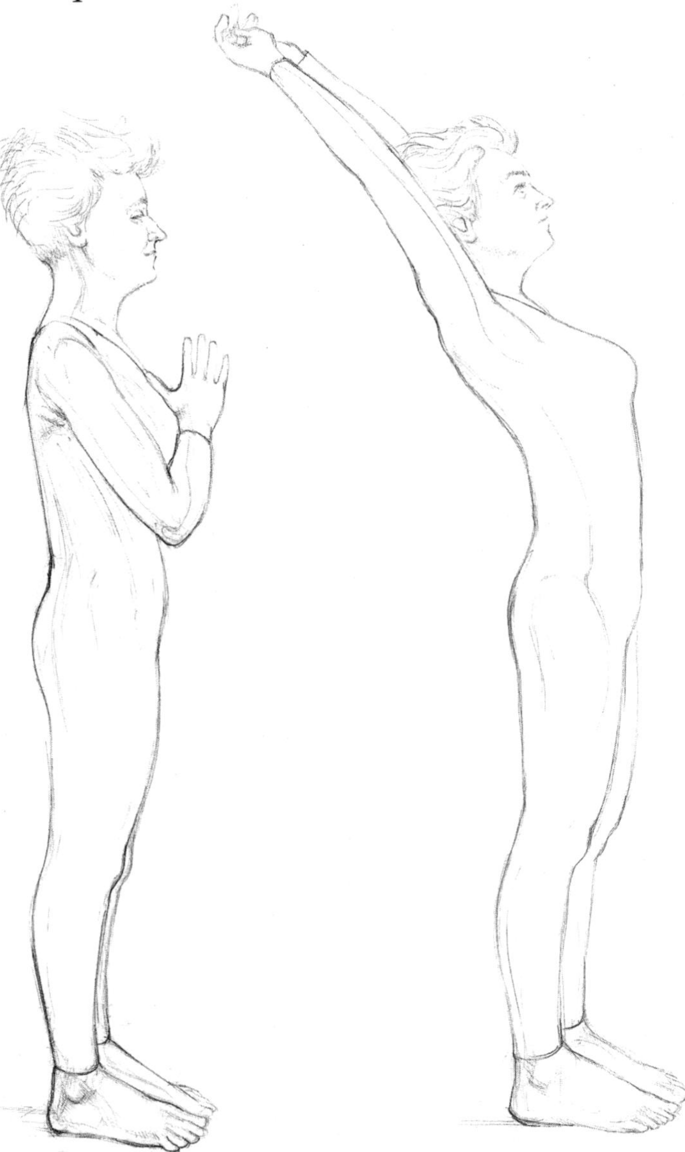

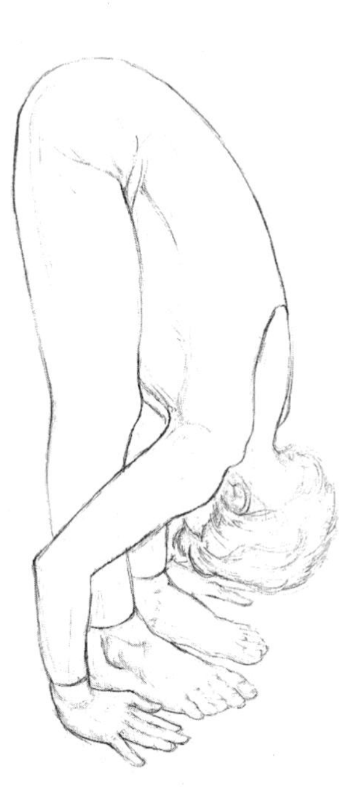

- Start Standing Straight with your hands in Prayer Position. Exhaling, drop your weight into your heels.

- Inhaling, drop your arms and bring them up over your head in a circular movement, making a long gentle arch with your back.

- Exhaling, drop into a Standing Forward Bend (p. 111).

- Inhaling, bend your knees, and step your right leg back into the Lunge position (p. 94).

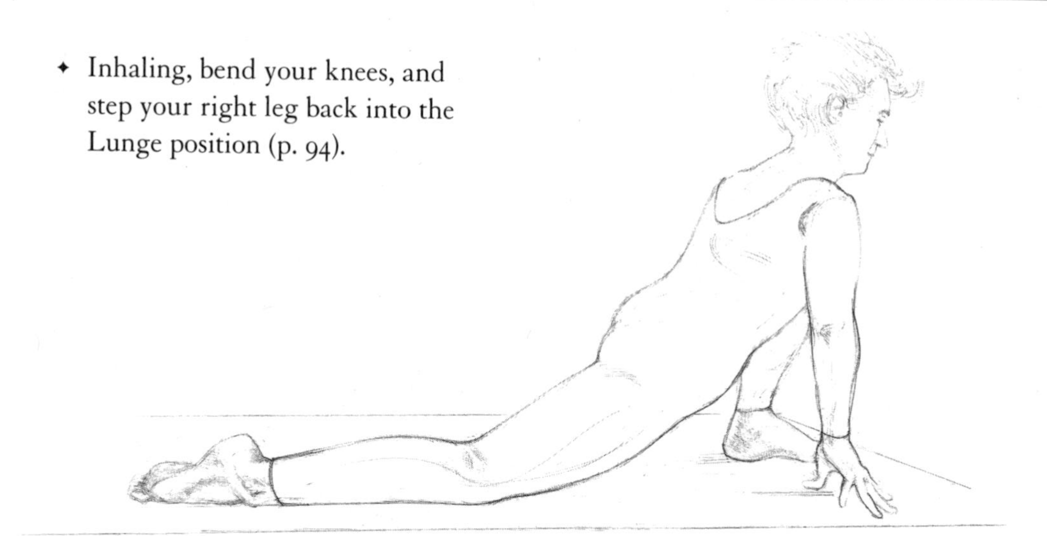

- Holding your breath, step your other leg back, into Plank Pose (p. 128).

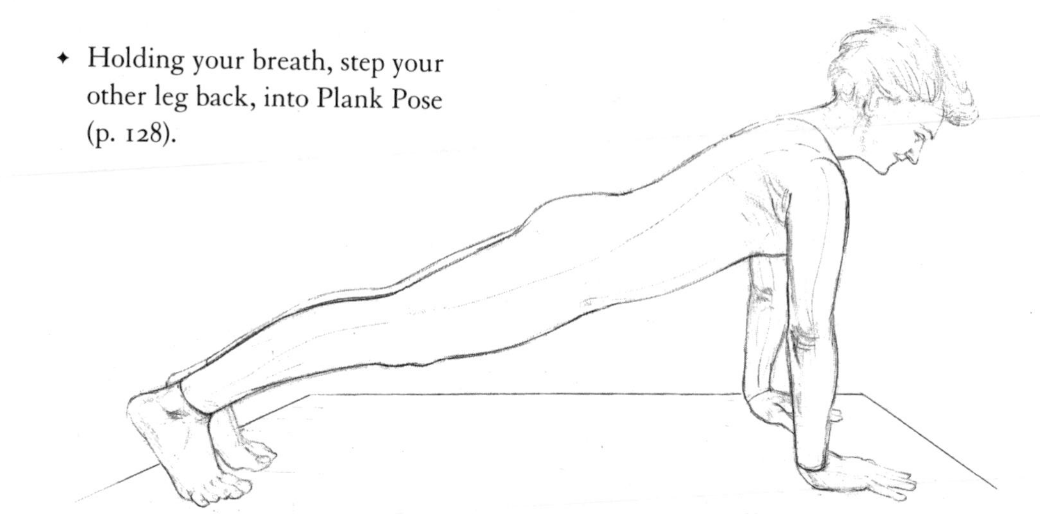

- Exhaling, bend your knees, and come down into Child's Pose (p. 89).

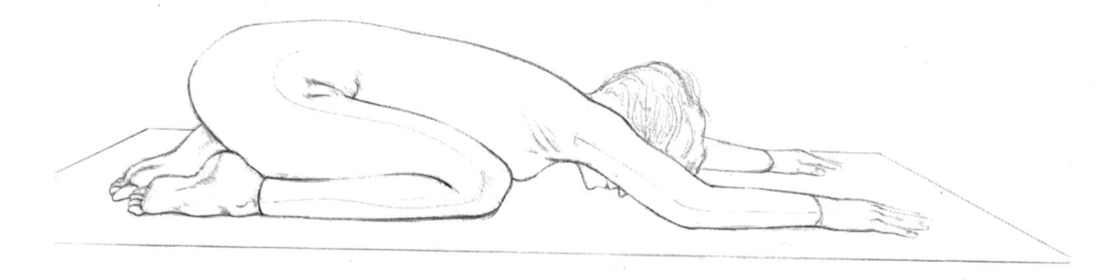

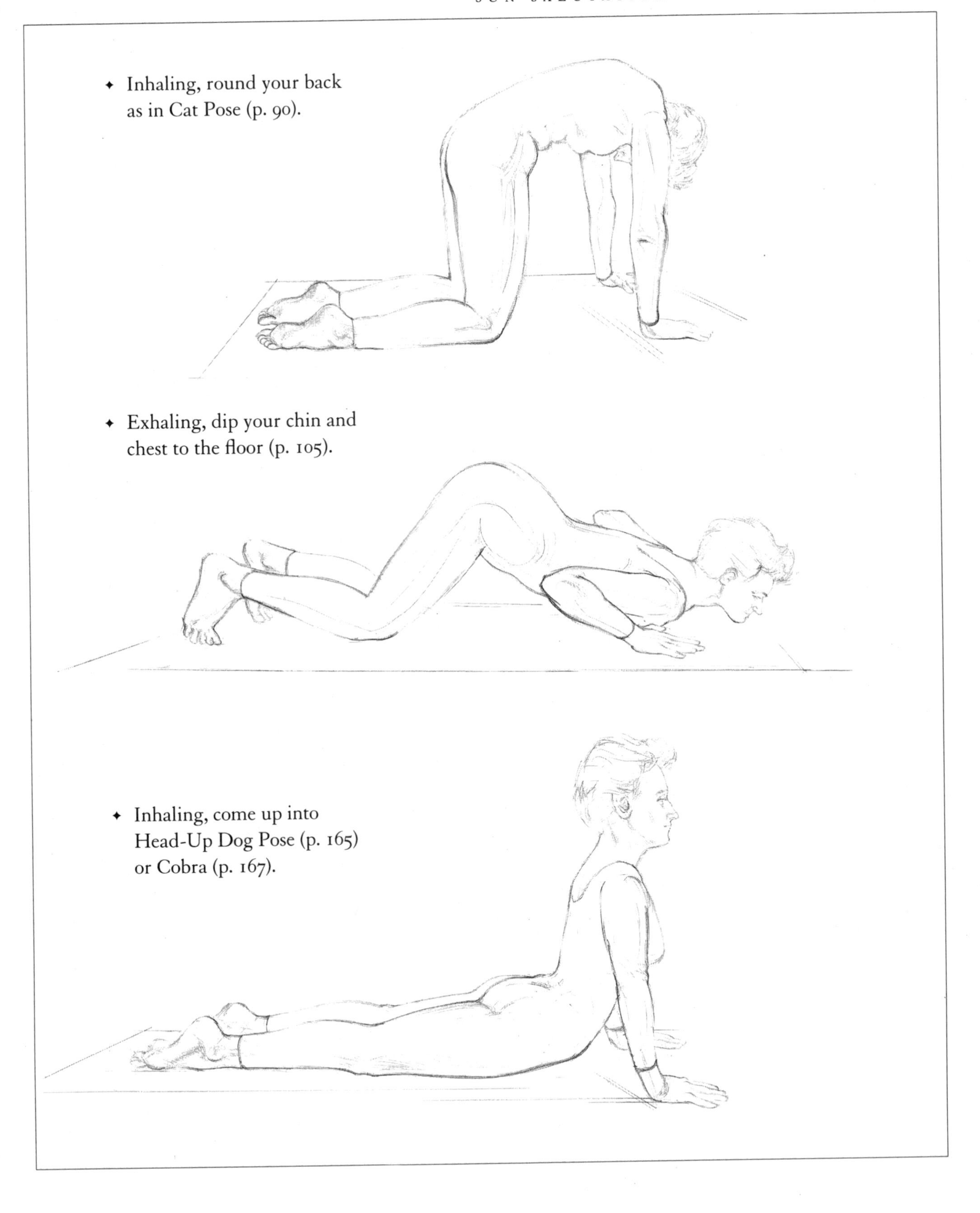

- Inhaling, round your back as in Cat Pose (p. 90).

- Exhaling, dip your chin and chest to the floor (p. 105).

- Inhaling, come up into Head-Up Dog Pose (p. 165) or Cobra (p. 167).

- Exhaling, press down with your wrists to move back into Head-Down Dog Pose (p. 92).

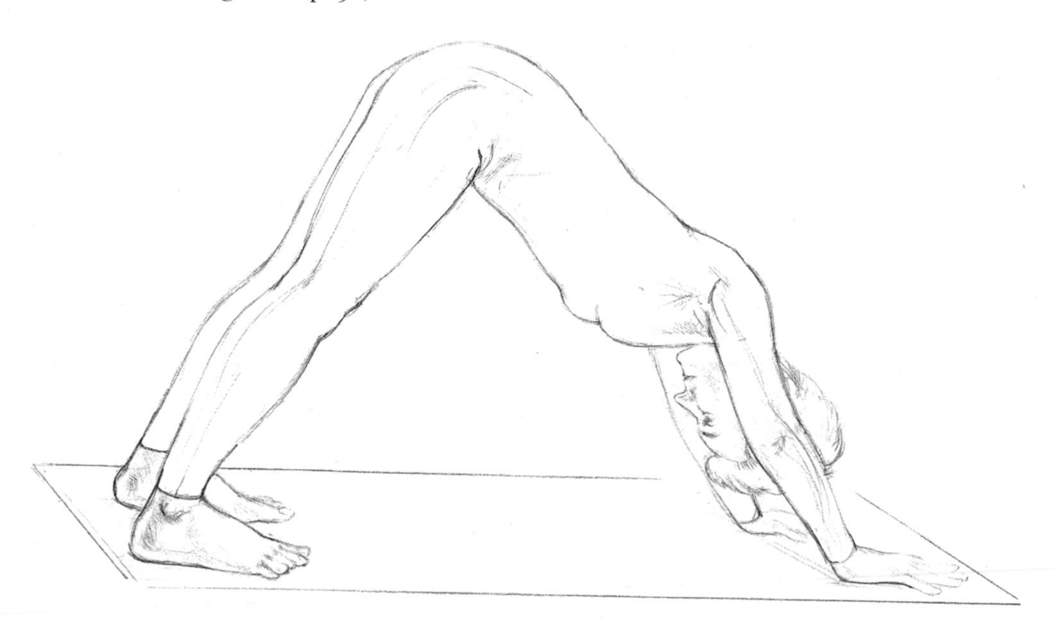

- Inhaling, step forward again into the Lunge position.

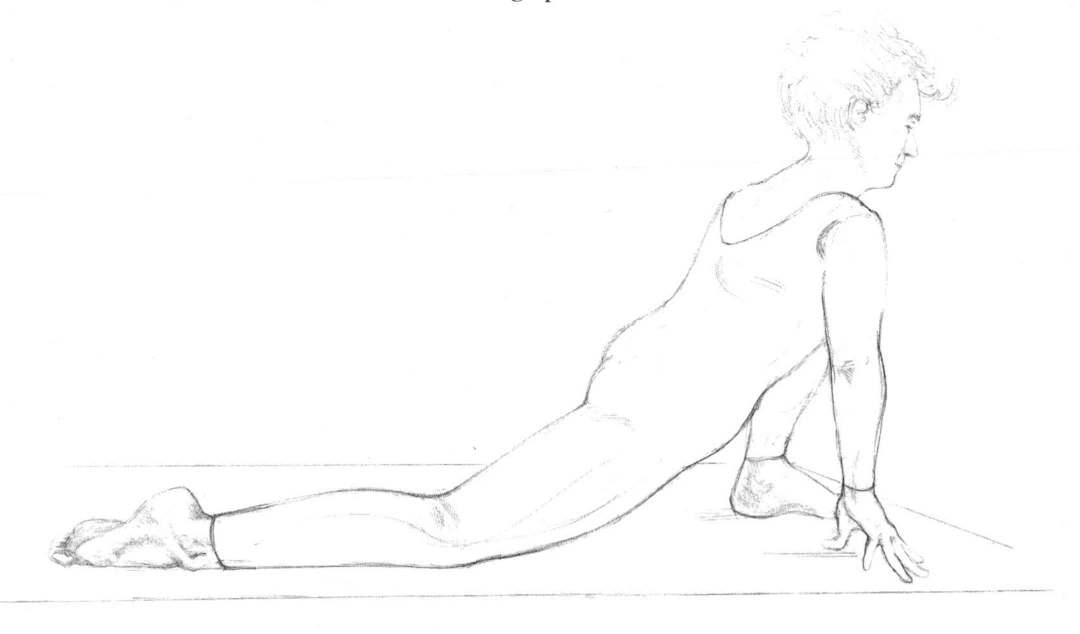

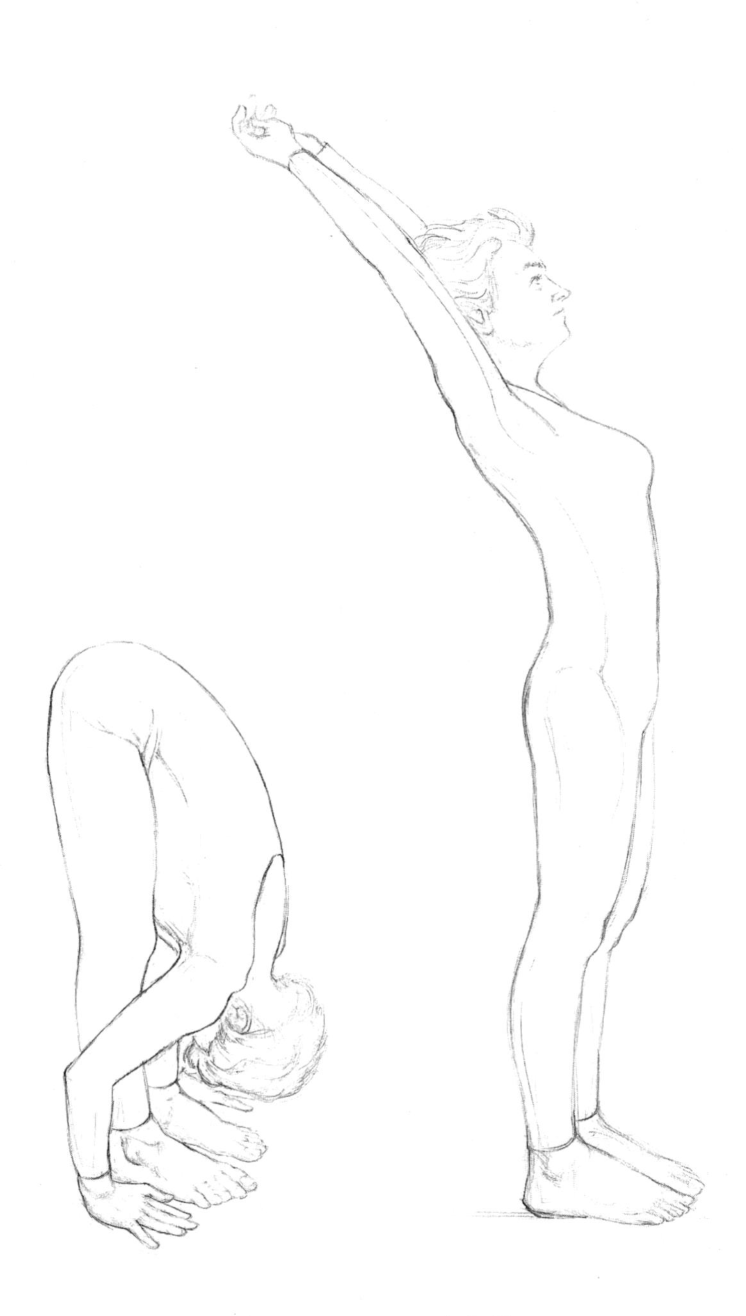

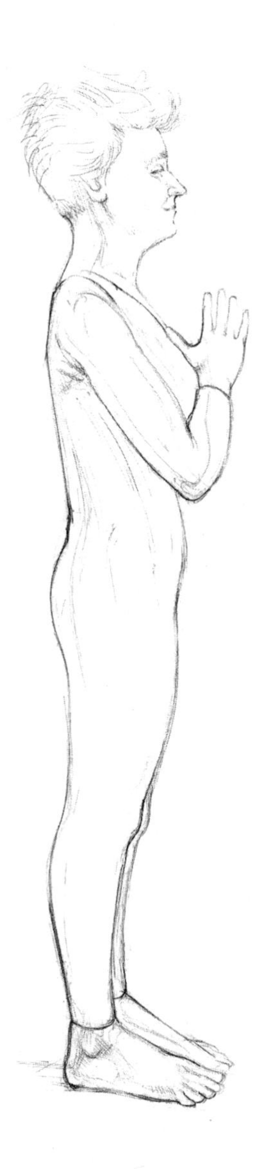

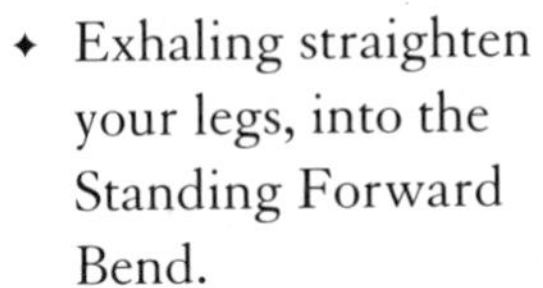

- Exhaling straighten your legs, into the Standing Forward Bend.

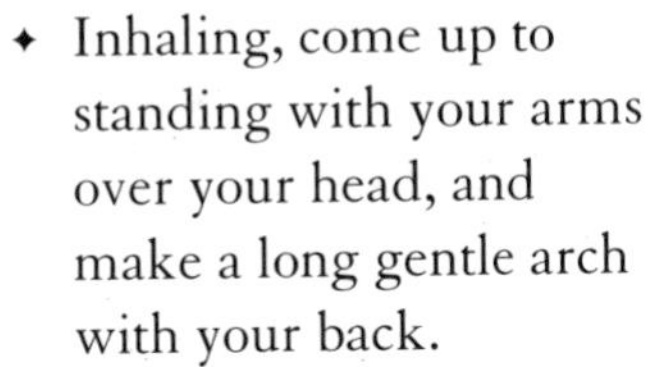

- Inhaling, come up to standing with your arms over your head, and make a long gentle arch with your back.

- Exhaling, come back to Standing Straight and bring your hands into Prayer Position.
- Repeat, starting with the left leg.

The Postures

Standing Straight, Prayer Position (Tadasana, Namaste)

When your hands are in Prayer Position, your shoulders, shoulder blades and elbows remain relaxed and dropped. The palms of your hands also stay soft.

Standing Backbend (Prstha Vakrasana)

Let the momentum carry your arms up. As your arms come up over your head, stretch your legs. With your back thighs strong, arch back slightly. Your arms are relaxed and loose as if suspended from the ceiling. Arching back from standing requires strong roots in your legs, length in the back of your waist and movement in your upper back.

Standing Forward Bend (Uttanasana)

If possible, place your hands on the floor beside your feet. This establishes the position of the hands for the entire sequence. If you are unable to reach the floor with your legs straight, place your hands beside your feet as you bend your knees to step back.

Lunge (Anjaneyasana)

The position of your front knee can vary. Do not sacrifice the weight on your heel to take your knee forward. The line of the spine remains straight. Your back leg can be straight or bent. I often keep it straight on the first Lunge as this leads directly into the Plank Pose, and bend it when I come forward at the end of the series.

Plank Pose (Chaturanga Dandasana)

There needs to be a clear distinction between this pose, which is straight, and Head-Up Dog Pose and Cobra, which are arched. The action in both poses is the same, but the positions themselves are different. If you are stiff you will tend to be straight in both poses. If your lower back is weak or overly flexible, you will likely collapse in the waist.

Child's Pose (Pranatasana)

When you bend your knees from Plank Pose, leave your hands where they are. It doesn't matter if your hips do not reach down to your heels. You can either leave your toes turned under or have the tops of your feet on the floor.

If you are doing Sun Salutation very slowly, Child's Pose is a wonderful place to stop and breathe.

Cat Pose (Marjarasana)

Rounding your back into Cat Pose opens the upper back so the dive down into the Dip is easier.

Dip, Eight Parts Pose (Astanga Namaskar)

In this pose the goal is to have eight parts of your body touch the floor: feet, knees, hands, chin and chest. To do this you need a great deal of flexibility in your upper back and shoulders which takes time to develop. Practice Cat Pose to make this part of the sequence easier.

Head-Up Dog Pose or Cobra (Urdhva Mukha Svanasana or Bhujangasana)

Head-Up Dog Pose is an easier and safer backbend than Cobra, where there is a strong tendency to constrict the lower back.

Head-Down Dog Pose (Adho Mukha Svanasana)

This pose counterbalances the backbend immediately, and lengthens the lower back if there has been any compression.

Lunge (Anjaneyasana)

Many people find stepping forward into the Lunge from Dog Pose the most difficult movement in the series. Try taking your abdomen well back, as if you were doing Cat Pose, to lift your pelvis and release your hips. You may find it helpful to think of your knee and chest coming forward, rather than your foot. Leave as much weight as possible on your back leg, so the leg coming forward is lighter. And remember to breathe!

With time you will be able to return to the original position, with your foot between your hands. The knee should come forward in a straight line. If you have stiff hips, you will find your legs making a circular motion.

Standing Forward Bend (Uttanasana)

To keep the back of your neck long as you come from the Lunge, drop your head before you straighten your legs.

Standing Backbend (Prstha Vakrasana)

To come up, bend your knees, round your back, as in Cat Pose, and press down with your heels. As you come up, straighten your legs, keeping your pelvis under. Then your waist will be long when you come back to standing. Leave your arms loose, so they follow the movement of your spine.

Standing Straight, Prayer Position (Tadasana, Namaste)

Bring your hands back into Prayer Position in a relaxed, circular motion.

Adaptations

Beginners

In learning to do Sun Salutation, take care not to compress the back of your waist in the backbends. It will take time for you to develop the length in your lower back, the strength in your back thighs, and the flexibility in your upper back that you need to do these poses well and safely. In the meantime, there are several adaptations that you can make.

- Instead of the Standing Backbend, stand straight with your arms over your head.
- If your lower back is weak, do not stay in the Standing Forward Bend for long.
- Replace the Plank Pose with Head-Down Dog Pose. Exhale to go into the pose, and inhale while you are in it, instead of holding your breath.
- Do shallower dips. Don't worry about getting your chest to the floor.
- Head-Up Dog Pose or Cobra can be replaced by Cat Pose. Or, you can keep your knees on the floor and your back straight.

More Experienced Students

There is a multitude of variations on Sun Salutation. You can vary the rhythm and energy of your breathing or stay longer in some of the poses. Classically, Sun Salutation is done twelve times on each side every day. Continuous repetitions will give you cardiovascular exercise which is not found elsewhere in yoga. "Strong" systems of yoga, like Iyengar yoga or Astanga yoga, jump from one position to the next. This makes for a more vigorous workout, and a more muscular action, but sacrifices the wave.

You can improvise and incorporate more poses into the series. Virtually any pose can be added into the sequence. Feel free to adapt Sun Salutation to your own level and to meet the needs of your body, your mood and your energy.

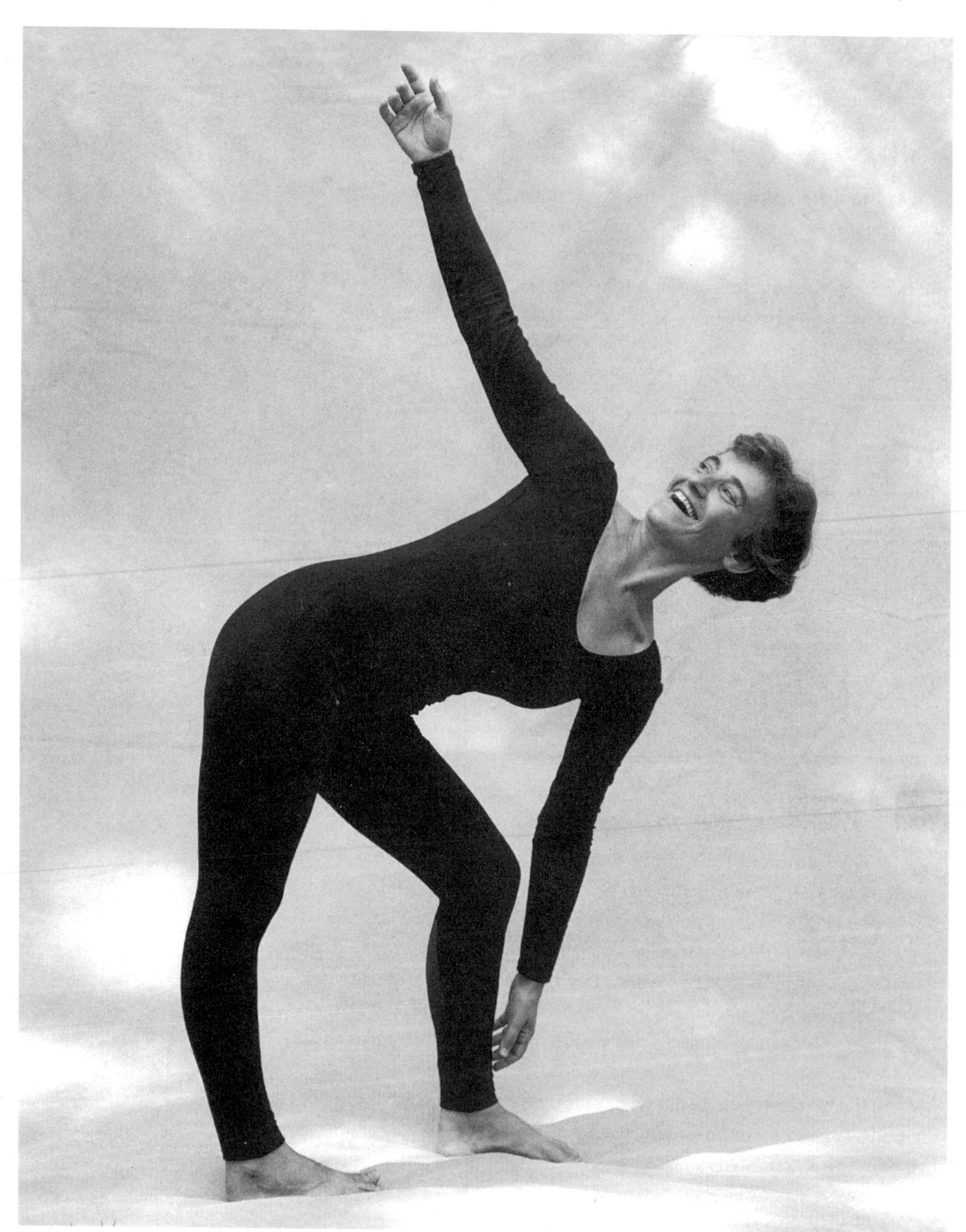

Side Angle Pose

CHAPTER 10

Standing Poses

VANDA MADE A DRAMATIC CHANGE in the standing poses, shortening the distance between the feet considerably. This change has been central for me. It gave me permission to experiment and explore in all of the poses. It has confirmed the fundamental principle that the postures are not set in stone. They can and are being constantly adapted and changed.

In order to understand these standing poses I have approached them from a variety of positions. I have gone into the poses from standing straight, as I describe in the instructions. I have also used the Triangle Forward Bend with my hands on the floor as a base. From there I have turned away from the front leg into Triangle Pose and towards the front leg into the Triangle Twist. (I have used a similar approach to the Side Angle Pose and Twist.) I have found that this approach reduces confusion about turning the hips and highlights the need to rotate the upper back.

I want to encourage you to experiment for yourself, to follow your own body and its needs. The purpose of the standing poses is to find stability in standing, and to explore a variety of leg and hip positions. Feel free to adapt the positions to your own body proportions and capabilities. The question is not "Am I doing the correct position?", but "What is the pose doing for me?"

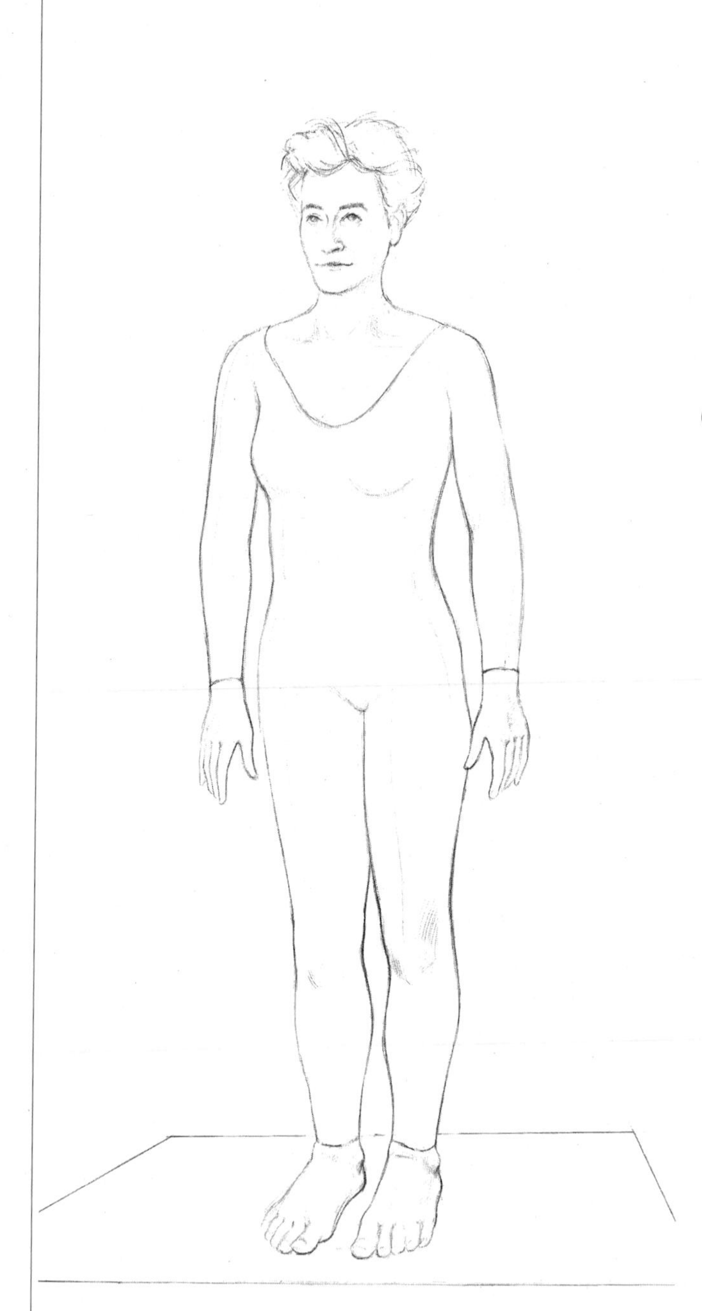

Ask yourself:

- *Am I more grounded? More stable on my legs? More secure?*
- *Are my legs freer and more aligned?*
- *Is my spine freer?*
- *Can I breathe easier?*
- *Are my shoulders looser?*

Guidelines

- *Focus your attention on your breathing.* Any tension in the pose will be reflected in the rhythm of your breath. Adjust the pose until you are relaxed and steady. If your feet wobble, take time to steady yourself and become quiet in the pose before going on.
- *Once you are established in a pose, you can be more active, working with the rhythm of your breath to make the poses more dynamic.* Focus on the heel of your back leg (or the standing leg in the balancing poses). Relax as you inhale, letting the back of your leg soften, especially if you tend to lock your knees. As you come to the end of your exhalation, press down with your heel and stretch your leg. This action sends a wave of extension through your spine. If your spine is free, you will feel the movement carry through to the back of your head, lengthening your spine and releasing your shoulders.
- *Stay in the pose as long as you can continue to breathe and lengthen, and then change sides.*

Standing Forward Bends

Basic Standing Forward Bend (Uttanasana)

Although this pose is an intense stretch of the back of the legs, it is a resting pose for your heart, since your head is dropped below your heart. Use it to relax your upper body and clear your head. Be careful if you have a weak lower back.

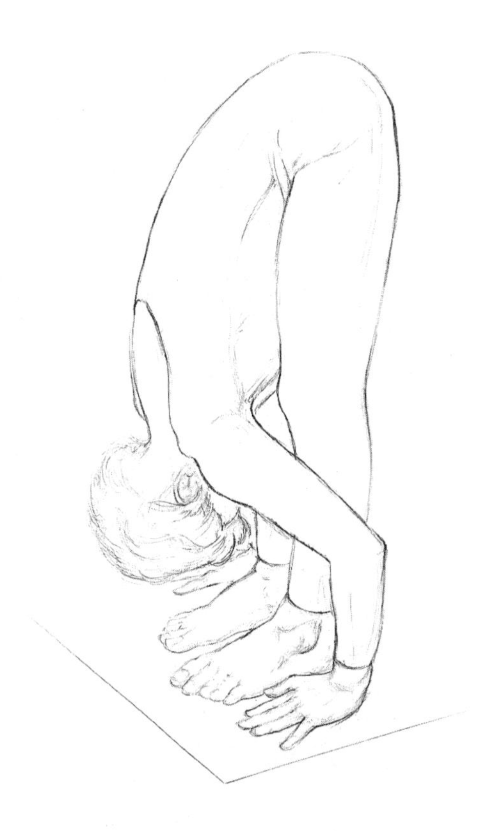

- Start standing straight.
- Exhaling, drop your upper body forward. Let your head and neck relax, and your arms hang loosely from your shoulders.
- Focus your attention on the movement of your belly as you breathe.
- As you exhale, stretch the back of your legs from your heels to drop further forward.
- Come up, exhaling, with the feeling that the back of your pelvis is being pulled down. Let your spine remain loose and relaxed, and follow the movement of your hips.

Variations

There are many variations of the Basic Standing Forward Bend. Here are a few suggestions. Feel free to improvise.

Balance (Urdhva Prasarita Ekapadasana)

- For an intense stretch, lift one leg behind you.
- Keep your toes pointing toward the floor.

Half Lotus (Ardha Baddha Padmottasana)

- Put one foot in Half Lotus (p. 189) and then drop forward.

Legs Wide (Prasarita Padottanasana)

- Spread your legs wide and bend forward.

Triangle Forward Bend (Parsvottanasana)

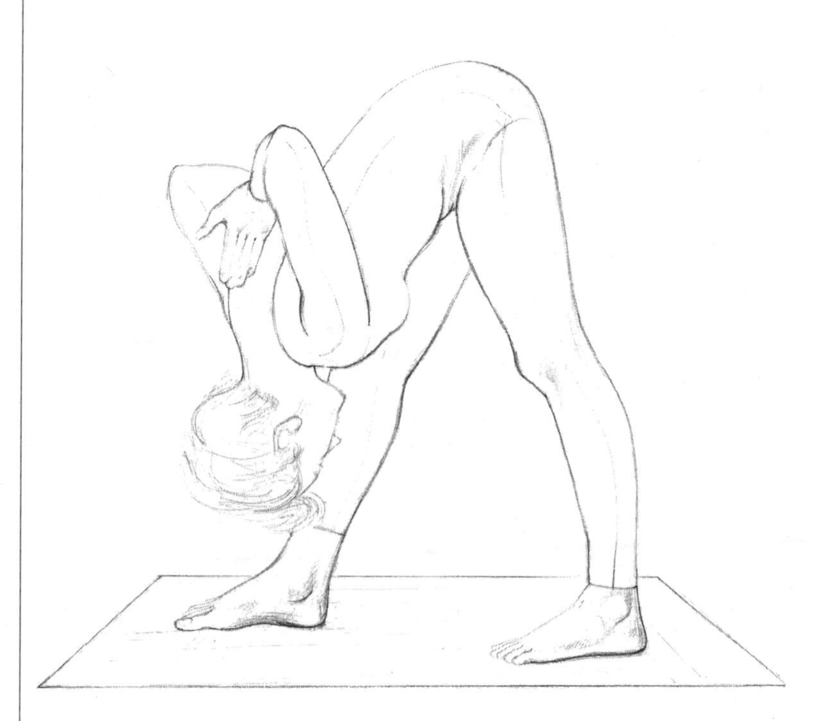

- Start standing straight.
- Step one leg forward.
- Leaving your back leg anchored, exhale and bend forward. As you go down, you will feel increasing stretch and weight on your front leg. However, the "roots" of the pose remain in the back heel.
- As you exhale, extend your back leg to intensify the pose and drop further. Relax as you inhale.
- Come up, exhaling, with the feeling that the back of your pelvis is being pulled down. Let your spine remain loose and relaxed, and follow the movement of your hips.
- Step back to standing.
- Repeat on the other side.

Variation

This pose can also be done with your hands in Prayer Position behind your back.

- Take your hands behind your back, palms together and fingers pointing down. Turn your hands so that your fingers point toward your back. Continue turning until the outer edges of your hands are touching your upper back.

  If you are unable to bring your hands into this position, clasp your elbows behind your back. When you change legs, put the other arm on top.

Warrior Poses

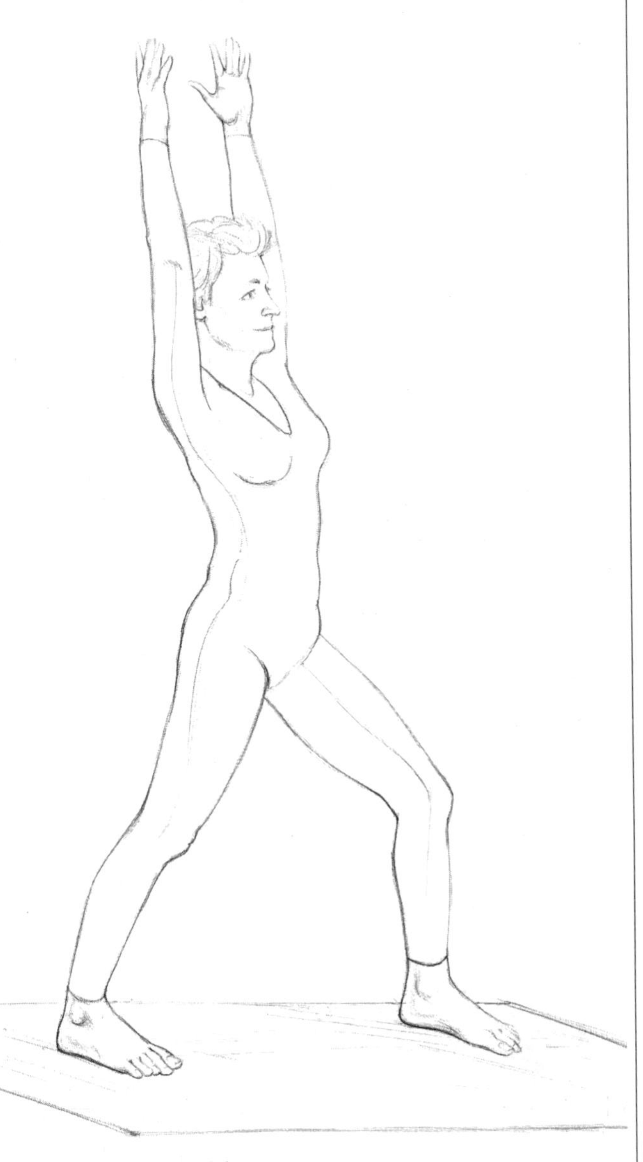

As the name implies, the Warrior Poses are based on fighting stances, and are similar to the stances in Tai Chi and the martial arts. The strength and power of these poses is in the legs and pelvis. The upper body remains light and free. When done well, these poses are strong and stable, with very little strain or effort.

Warrior I (Virabhadrasana I)

- Start standing straight.
- Exhaling, bring your arms up over your head, keeping them loose and relaxed. Drop your shoulders as you bring your arms up.
- Step one leg forward. Keep the weight or roots in the back leg.
- Exhale and bend your front knee, but do not lunge forward.
- Keep the line of your spine vertical and the back of your pelvis dropped. You may feel the stretch on the front thigh and calf of your back leg.
- To come up, exhale, straighten your front leg, and step back to standing straight.
- Repeat on the other side.

Adjust the position of your feet so that your stance is natural and stable. At the beginning, your back foot will probably be slightly turned out. As the pose becomes more familiar and your pelvis releases, turn your back foot in until your feet are parallel.

This Warrior Pose prepares you for standing backbends. To be more active in the pose, extend your back leg with your breath, then tuck your pelvis under as the extension reaches the top of your leg. Let the wave of extension carry through your spine, releasing your neck and shoulders as your spine lengthens.

Warrior Balance (Virabhadrasana III)

This pose is a strong standing balance. It is easier for stiff people.

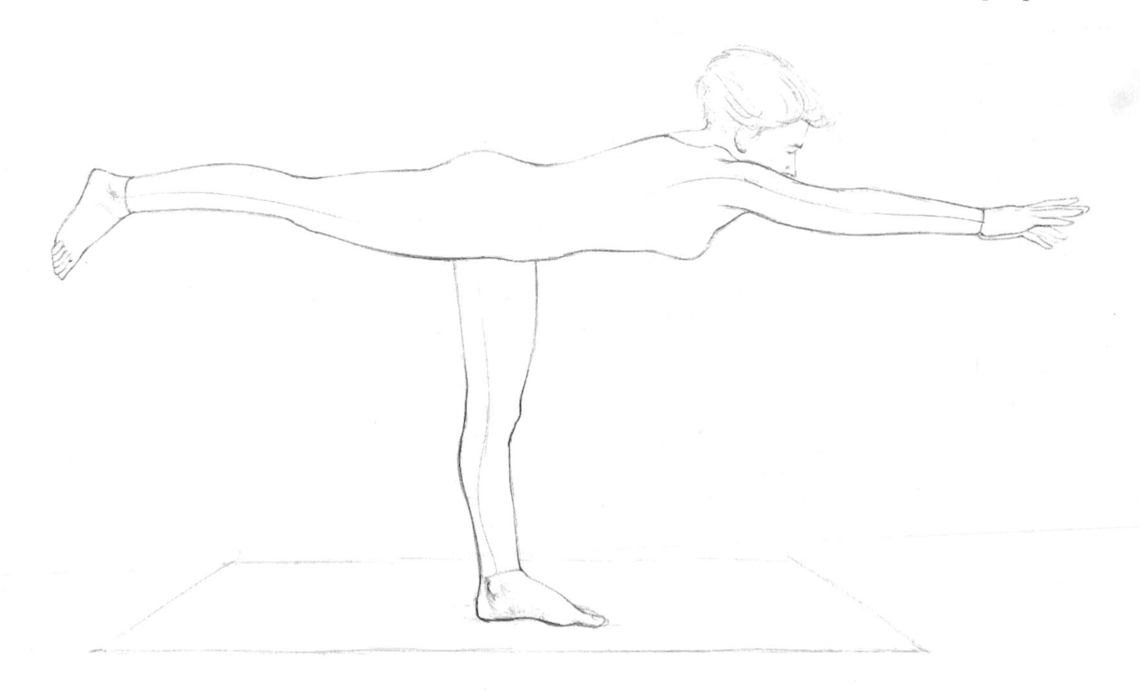

- From Warrior Pose I, exhale and shift your weight forward onto your front leg.
- Then straighten the front leg and bring your back leg up off the floor.
- Support your spine with a deep strong breath as you lengthen and extend. The dynamic thrust and energy move from the belly to the back heel.
- Keep your shoulders relaxed and lengthen your arms away from your shoulders.
- Exhaling, come back into Warrior I, then step back to standing.
- Repeat on the other side.

Keep your pelvis horizontal and your toes pointing toward the floor. Only go as far as you can, while remaining steady and elongated. If necessary, place your hands on a table or the back of a chair. Lengthening your back leg as you exhale makes it easier to balance.

Warrior Pose II (Virabhadrasana II)

This pose is a preparation for the Side Angle Pose. In this pose, the pelvis remains vertical; in the Side Angle Pose, the pelvis moves sideways.

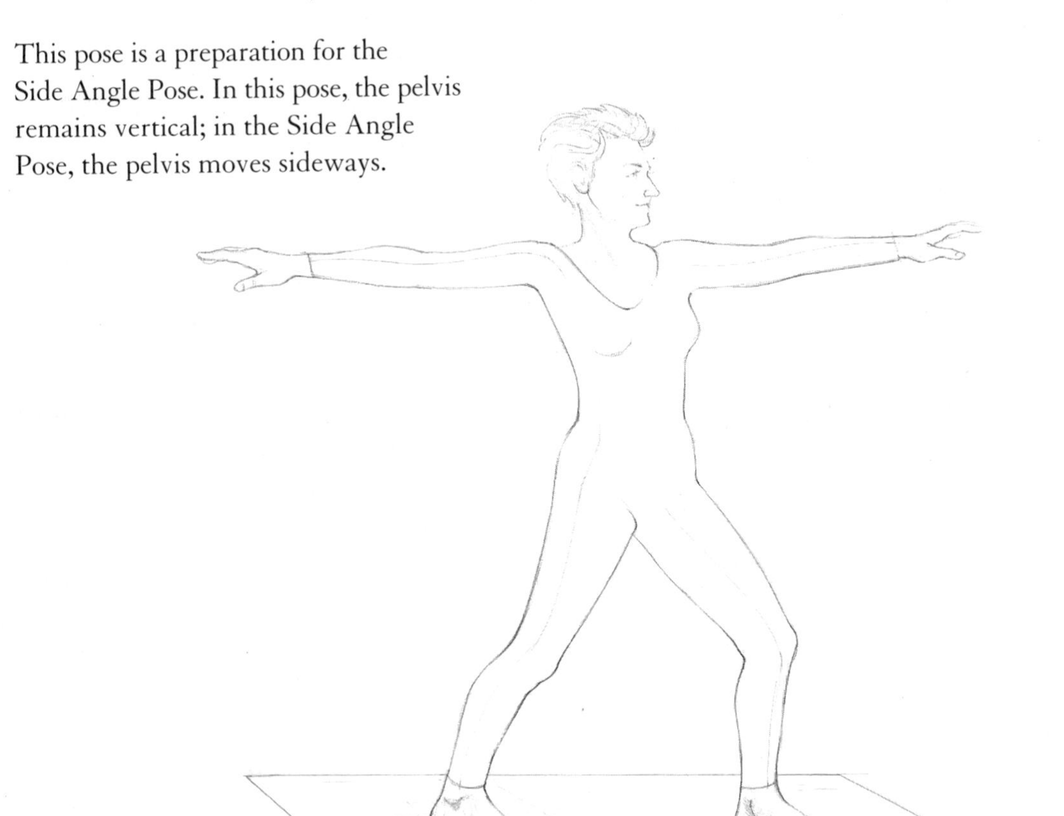

- Start standing straight.
- Step your left leg forward. Keep your weight on the back leg.
- Bring your arms up sideways, just below shoulder level and turn your upper body to the right.
- Bend your front knee, so it faces forward over your toes.
- As you exhale, stretch your back leg and bring your pelvis under.
- To come up, exhale, straighten your front leg and step back to standing straight.
- Repeat on the other side.

Leave your arms loose and relaxed, with the weight dropping away from your shoulders. Focus on the release of your back arm away from your spine to bring the weight onto your back heel.

Side Angle Poses

The Side Angle Pose and the Triangle Pose are very similar in action and function. These poses are sideways extensions of the spine, which stretch the sides of the pelvis and the sides of the legs.

Side angle Pose (Parsvakonasana)

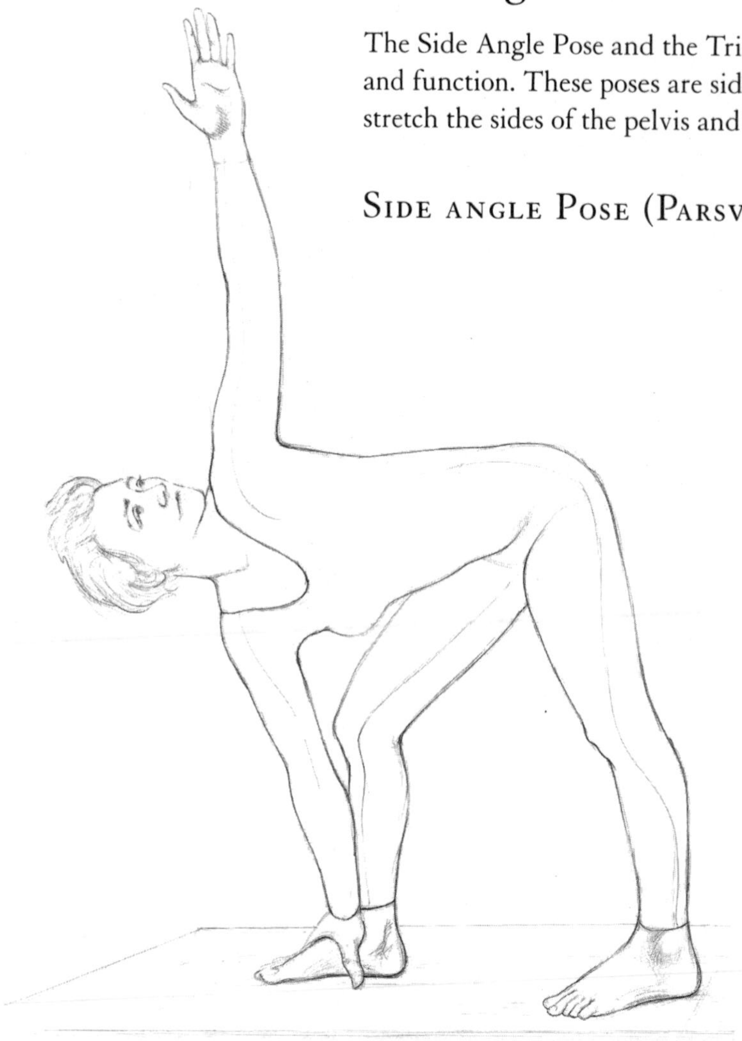

- Start in Warrior II Pose, with your right leg forward.
- Exhaling, release your left hip and stretch sideways to bring your right hand down beside your right leg.
- Keep your spine straight, with your head in line with the back of your pelvis and your neck relaxed.
- Your arms and shoulders remain relaxed in the pose. The lower arm drops from the shoulder, and your upper arm will lift out of your shoulder joint as your spine releases.
- As you exhale, stretch your back leg from your heel to release and lengthen your spine.
- Exhale and come up.
- Repeat on the other side.

When you are in the pose all your weight is over your front leg. However, the back leg should remain stable and weighted.

Even if you have a clear sense of the line of your spine when you are upright, you may lose it when you bend sideways. Use a mirror to see if your spine is straight.

Most people lean forward in this pose. Let yourself rest back into the support of your spine, as you do when you are standing. You will not fall backward. You can do the pose with your back near a wall to establish the feeling of support and to find the correct alignment.

In addition to the downward pull on the back leg and the extension of the spine, the lightness and lift of the poses carries through the upper arm. As your upper back, neck and shoulders release, let your upper arm float out of your shoulder joint.

If you have neck problems or very stiff shoulders, you may not be able to find a comfortable position for your upper arm. If necessary, rest your upper arm on your side. If your neck is long and relaxed, turn your head and look up.

Triangle Pose (Trikonasana)

Triangle Pose is similar to the Side Angle Pose, except that the front leg is straight.

If you have lower back problems, be careful. Going down too far can strain the sacroiliac joint.

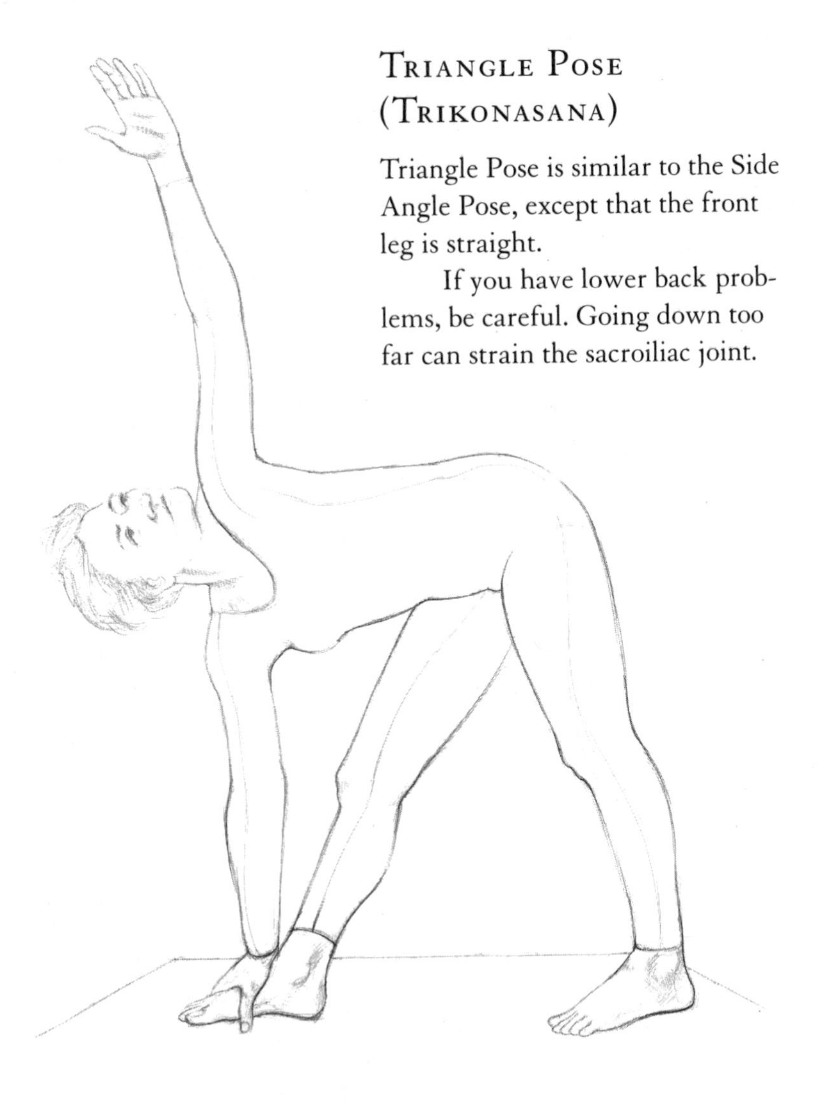

Standing Balances

The standing balances teach us about our legs. They help you learn to feel your feet and become aware of the contact of your feet with the floor. These poses also help to give you a feeling of weight and support on each leg independently. When you come back to Standing Straight, you will feel that you have two legs supporting you. Weakness or misalignment in the legs that you may not be aware of normally is highlighted by the increased weight, so you have an opportunity to build strength and better alignment in your legs.

If you are agitated or stressed, it will show in these poses. Breathe. Steadinesss and grounding, alignment and extension are more important than balance. Use a wall or chair for support until you are steady and quiet, then work on balance.

Some people find it helpful to focus on a point to steady their balance. Keep your forehead relaxed and your gaze easy and passive.

Practise Standing Straight, taking time to grow roots. Then see what happens when you lift one leg off the floor. Experiment with different positions for the bent leg. Bend your knee to your chest, take it out to the side, or catch your foot behind you (Simple Dancer Pose).

Ask yourself:

- *What happens to the contact of your foot with the ground?*
- *What happens to your shoulders and your breathing?*
- *Which poses feel easy and steady?*
- *Which ones wobble?*
- *Are you steadier standing on your right leg or your left?*
- *When you come back to standing on both legs between the standing balances, what new awareness do you have about your legs?*
- *How do these poses change your understanding of being rooted and stable, yet relaxed?*

Tree Pose (Vrksasana)

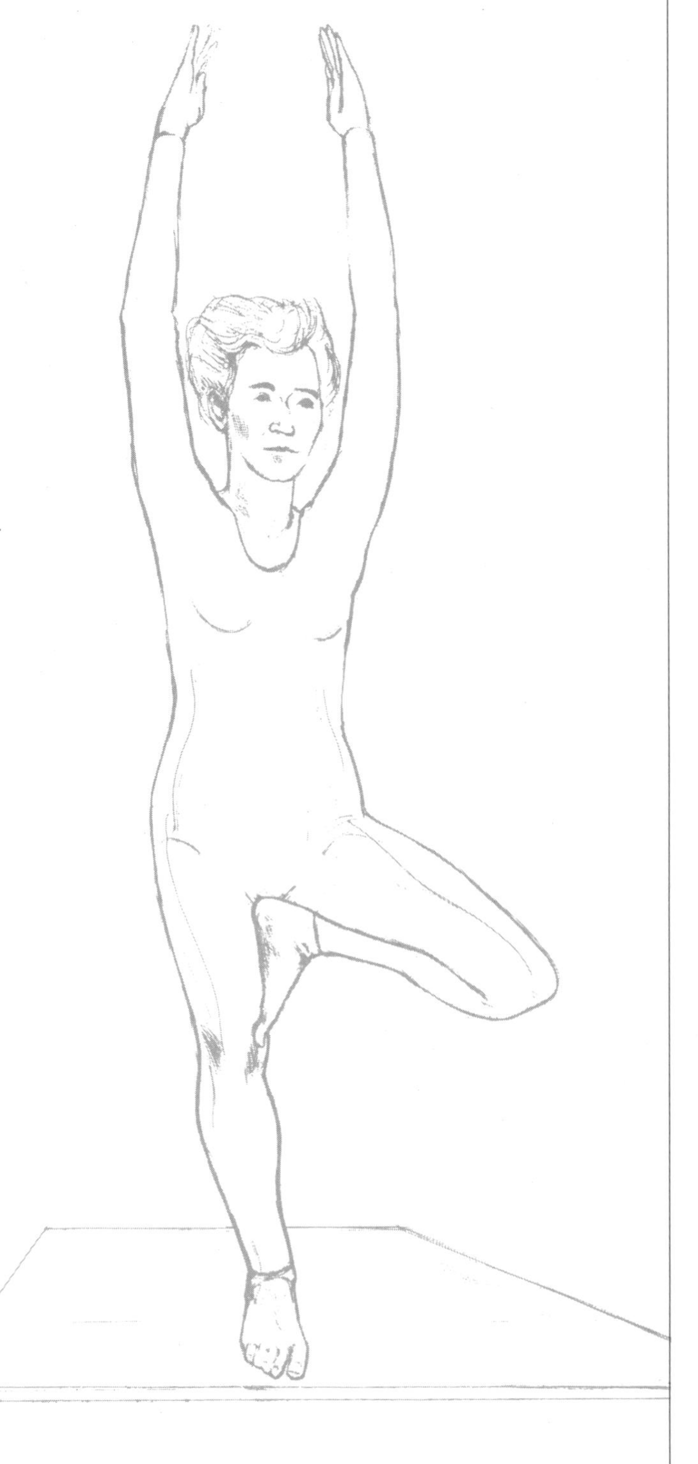

- Start by standing straight.
- Bend one leg and place the heel as high as you can on the inner thigh of your straight leg. If you can, bring your heel right to the top of your thigh, there is a notch where it "fits." If necessary, hold your foot with one hand to prevent it from slipping. Or put your foot lower on your leg.
- As you exhale, press down firmly on the outer heel of your standing leg to strengthen and stabilize your pelvis.
- Dropping your bent knee away from your hip helps to lengthen your waist.
- When you are balanced, bring your arms over your head or into Prayer Position.
- Stay in the pose, with your breathing steady and your gaze relaxed and passive.
- When you are ready, return to standing straight.
- Repeat on the other side.

Variation

- Bend one leg in Half Lotus, and place it on the front thigh of your standing leg.

  This variation is much easier to align and stabilize than the basic pose if you have flexibility in your hips to do Half Lotus.

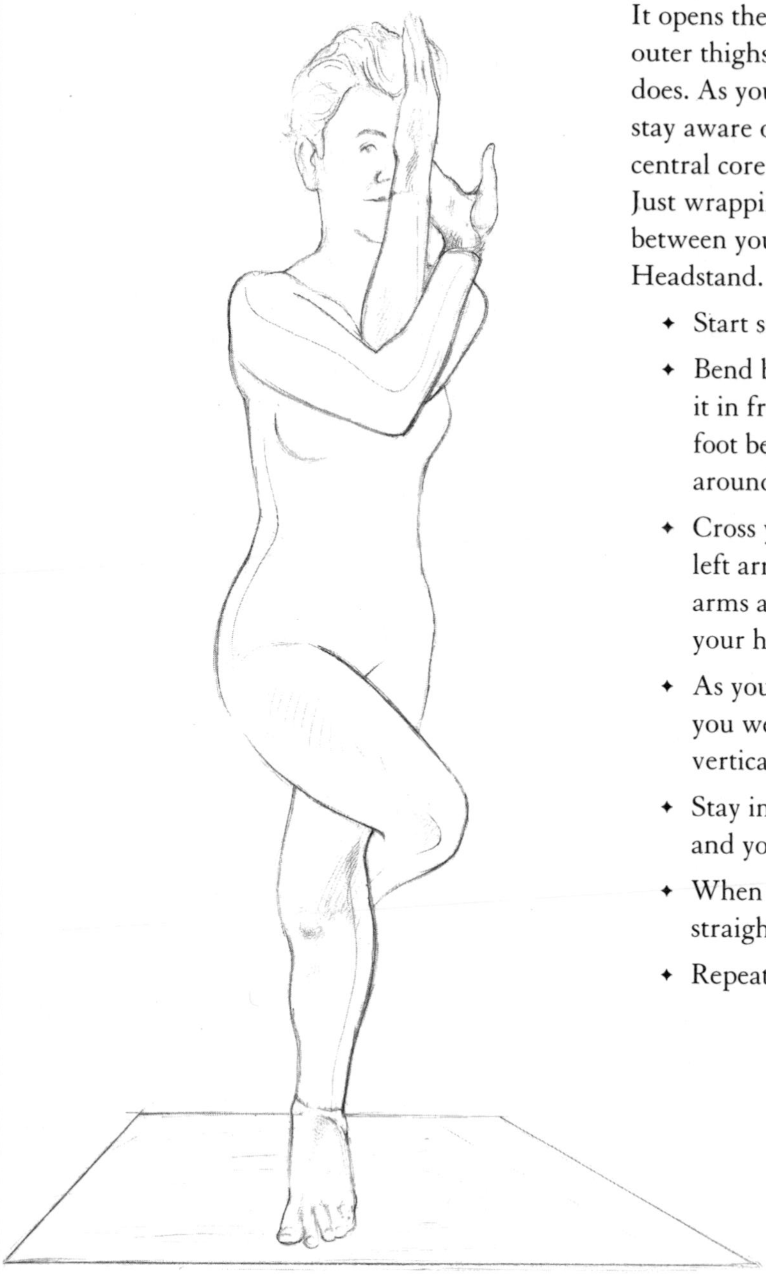

Eagle Pose (Garudasana)

This pose is easiest for people with long limbs. It opens the back of the pelvis and stretches the outer thighs, as Cow's Head Pose (see p. 186) does. As you wrap your limbs around each other, stay aware of the line of your spine, which is the central core of the pose that you wrap around. Just wrapping your arms is a good way to stretch between your shoulder blades and prepare for Headstand.

- Start standing straight.
- Bend both legs. Lift your right leg and place it in front of your left. Then wrap your right foot behind your left calf, hooking your foot around the calf muscle.
- Cross your arms in front of you, with your left arm over your right. Wrap your forearms around each other so that the palms of your hands face each other.
- As you stay in the pose, drop lower as if you were sitting down, keeping your spine vertical.
- Stay in the pose with your breathing steady and your gaze relaxed and passive.
- When you are ready, return to standing straight.
- Repeat on the other side.

Half Moon Pose (Ardha Chandrasana)

This is a wonderfully free and spacious pose. It opens in all directions. If you have trouble balancing, try it with your back against a wall so that you can feel the freedom it gives.

- ✦ Start in the Standing Forward Bend.
- ✦ Lift your right leg up so you are standing on your left leg. Keep your right leg long and extended. 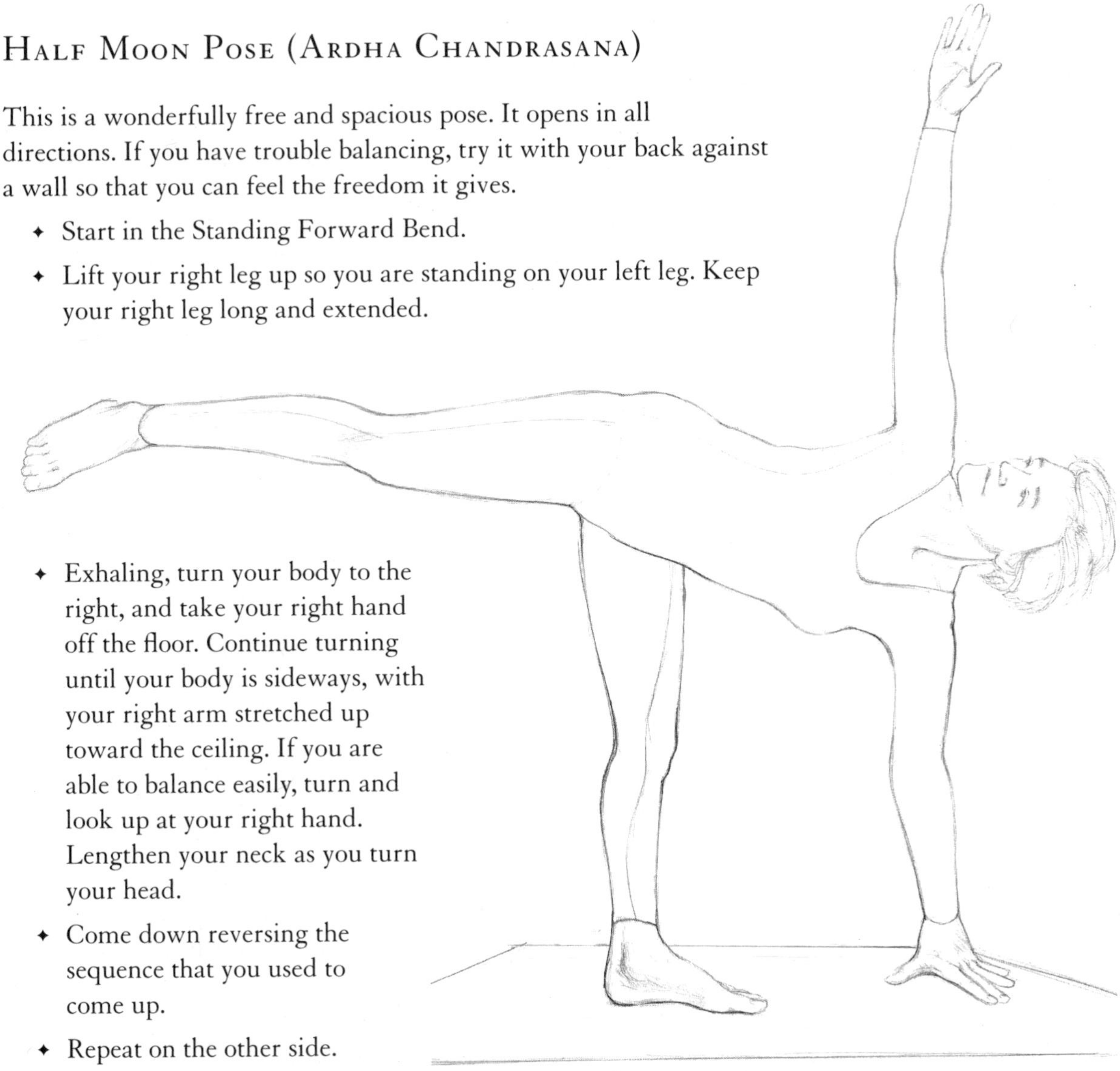
- ✦ Exhaling, turn your body to the right, and take your right hand off the floor. Continue turning until your body is sideways, with your right arm stretched up toward the ceiling. If you are able to balance easily, turn and look up at your right hand. Lengthen your neck as you turn your head.
- ✦ Come down reversing the sequence that you used to come up.
- ✦ Repeat on the other side.

Variation

Half Moon Twist (Parivrtta Ardha Chandrasana)
This pose is similar to Half Moon Pose, however, balance is more difficult, and the stretch on the outer hip of the standing leg is intense.

- ✦ From the Standing Forward Bend turn toward the standing leg instead of away from it.

You can also come into these poses from the Side Angle Pose and Side Angle Twist (see p. 123). Shift your weight forward onto your front leg, and then straighten it to come up.

Standing Twists

When you have established a secure foundation in the basic standing poses, and the principles are clear, you are ready to go on to the standing twists. These more challenging poses require strong anchoring in the back leg and a clear sense of the axis of the spine.

The Standing Twists can be done during pregnancy because the abdomen is open and free.

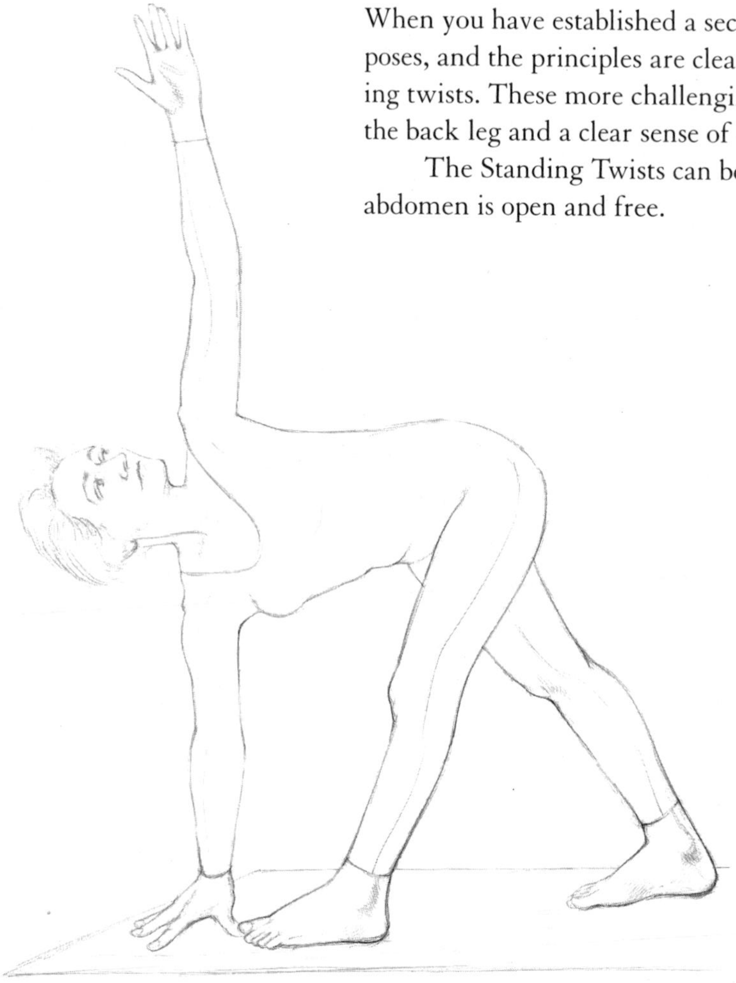

Triangle Twist (Parivrtta Trikonasana)

The triangle twist is easier than the Side Angle Twist so try it first.

- Start standing straight.
- Step your one leg forward.
- Exhaling, bring your arms up, then turn and face your front leg.
- Exhaling, extend your back leg and press your back heel to turn your hips further.
- Keep your back heel anchored. The vertical line of your spine remains undisturbed as the rotation takes place around it. If you start to feel strain in your back knee, you have turned too far.
- When you have turned as far as you can, go down.
- Keep your back leg as vertical and anchored as possible, with weight on the outer edge of the back foot. As you go down, you will feel increasing stretch and weight on your front leg. However, the "roots" of the pose remain in the back heel.
- Come up on an exhalation.
- Repeat on the other side.

Side Angle Twist (Parivrtta Parsvakonasana)

This pose is the same as the Triangle Twist, except that the front leg is bent. There is a tendency to straighten the front leg while concentrating on the back one. You will probably find this pose more difficult than the Triangle Twist. You can also come up into the twists from the Triangle Forward Bend. Try both and see which you prefer.

It took me a long time to understand these new positions. In these poses the pelvis is almost horizontal which broadens the back of the sacrum. Focusing on the back leg releases the psoas muscle (see p. 63) creating tremendous inner freedom and space.

It takes many years to develop the flexibility in your hips and upper back that these standing twists require, so you will find that movement into the posture is minimal at first. They are also somewhat confusing, since it is not easy to bend at the hip, and retain the line of the spine while turning. Do not go further down into the pose than you can do correctly; it is best to come back up a bit in order to be in correct alignment. Avoid the temptation to round your back and curve into the pose, rather than lengthen.

Your arms and shoulders remain relaxed in the pose. The lower arm drops from the shoulder. Your upper arm will lift out of your shoulder joint, as your spine releases. If you have neck problems or very stiff shoulders, you may not be able to find a comfortable position for your upper arm. If necessary, rest your upper arm on your side. Look up at your hand, if you can do so without causing strain in your neck or shoulder.

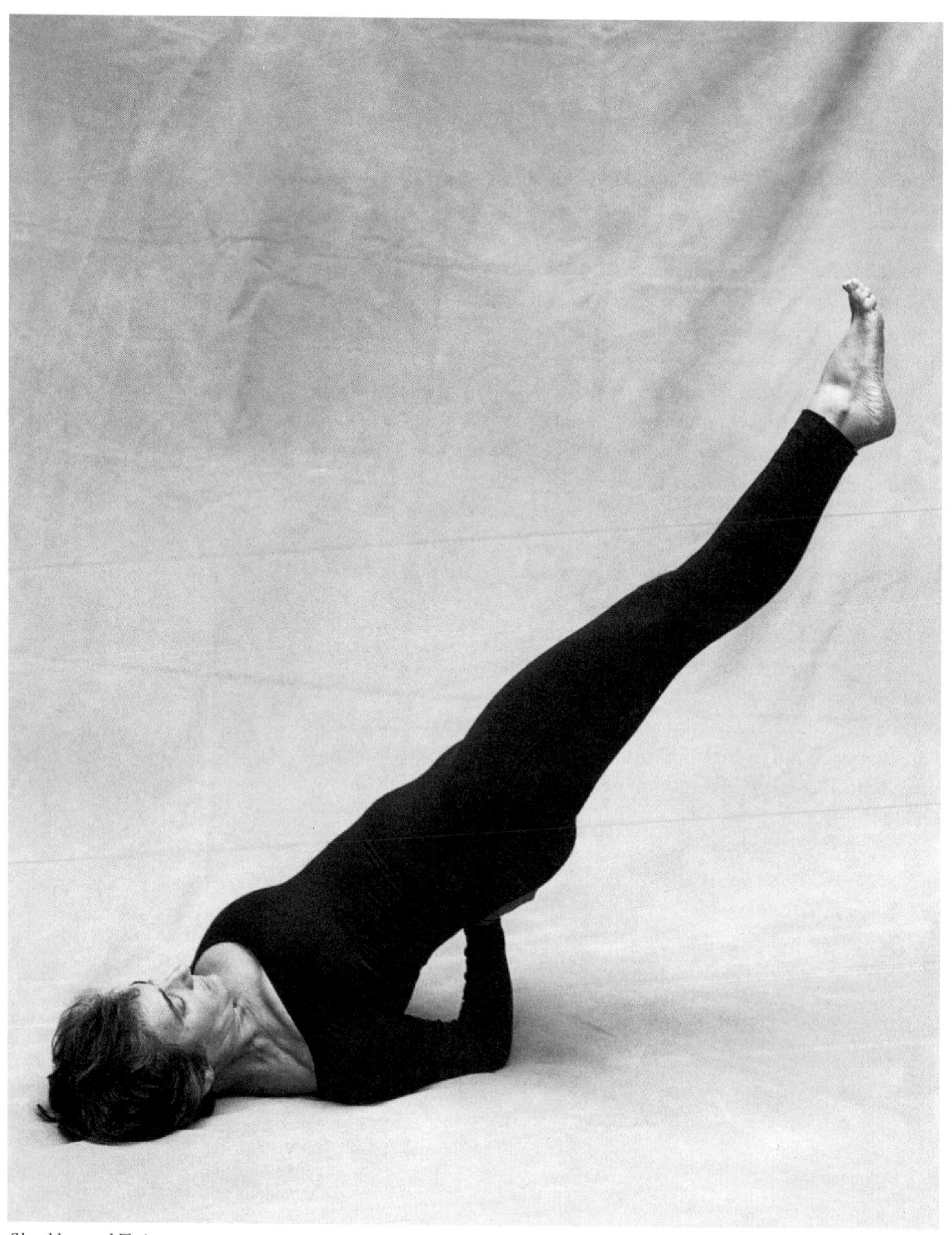

Shoulderstand Twist

CHAPTER II

Inverted Poses and Arm Balances

Caution: Inverted poses should be avoided by people with high blood pressure, eye or ear problems, and women who are menstruating. Stop or modify the pose if you feel compression in your neck or pressure in your face, throat or eyes.

INVERSIONS ARE A CENTRAL PART of yoga practice. Being upside down is unfamiliar, so inversions challenge us in new and interesting ways. These are strong, stable poses which are generally easier for men than for women. It takes time to learn to find your centre when you are upside down. Headstand, especially, is confusing at first, and highlights any weaknesses or imbalances in our bodies. As you learn to function in a reversed relationship to the gravitational field, you deepen your understanding of the vertical line of the spine. With practice, you will be able to develop a clear sense of this line. As your inverted poses become more centred and balanced, you will be able to find ease, poise and equilibrium in them.

Each time you start a new pose, come back to the basic principles: take time to breathe and to feel the base of the posture on the ground. Relax as you drop weight into the base, and feel yourself being pulled into the earth. Practise this way until you can feel your arms securely underneath you without tension. Notice any tension that arises when you start to think about your arms supporting you, and let it go.

Guidelines

Caution: If there is any indication of stress in an inverted pose, come down. Signs of stress are redness in your face, bulging of the veins in your neck or forehead, unnatural brightness or strain in your eyes, overheating, difficulty breathing or a choking feeling in your throat.

You can look in a mirror for signs of stress in Headstand. Ask someone to look at you in Shoulderstand, since you may not feel the pressure.

Head and Shoulderstand are the basic inverted poses. They are centring, grounding and balancing poses and have a wide range of physical and psychological benefits. Using the arms and shoulder girdle as a foundation, they release and strengthen the upper body. They clear the mind, and are beneficial for the heart, circulation and digestion. They can be used to correct misalignment and the compensations associated with injuries in the legs and hips, since the legs and pelvis are not weight-bearing. However, they must be done with caution to protect the neck.

If you are just starting yoga, learn Shoulderstand first. It is easier to approach, since your head is not inverted, you can see your body and you have the support of your arms.

Once you are able to do both poses, do Headstand first. Shoulderstand is a more intense stretch on the neck than Headstand. It will relieve any compression that may have been caused by the Headstand. Headstand is traditionally considered to be strong, masculine and heating; it is counterbalanced by Shoulderstand, which is surrendering, feminine and cooling.

While inverted poses are strong, they are not rigid. As always, the strength of the pose is in the roots, the action of your breath and the extension of your spine. The elongation and release with the breath continues. Once you are secure and stable, you can become more dynamic in the positions, just as you did in the Standing Poses. Think of your wrists in Handstand, and your elbows in the other inversions as heels. Then your arms and shoulders become like legs and hips. With practice, you will be able to relax your body, including your arms, as you inhale, without collapsing. As you exhale, press down with your "roots," and take your abdomen well back to support and lengthen your spine. The action of your breath and belly needs to be deeper upside down than standing, but the effect is the same. The pose becomes longer and lighter. There is less pressure on your arms. As in any other pose, the goal is to be light and free, with minimum effort to sustain the position.

There are a lot of variations of Head and Shoulderstand. I will describe a few in detail and suggest some others. You can start the variations when you are at ease and stable in the basic pose. The precautions in the variations are the same as for the basic postures.

You can start variations in Shoulderstand and Plough quite early on. Single Leg Stretch in Shoulderstand and Plough with Knees Bent are the most basic and easiest. The Headstand variations are generally strenuous and demanding. They require increased stability, strength and elongation.

When you start to practise the variations, begin with the poses that keep your body in a straight line. Be sure that you are balanced and lengthening in those before you do any that involve twisting. The twists are unusual because the neck remains straight and the twist starts in the thoracic spine, between the shoulder blades.

Some poses are surprisingly easier upside down than right side up. For example, in the straight leg variations it is easier to extend the lifted leg when you are inverted than to make a similar movement when you are lying on the floor. The Bound Angle Pose and even Lotus Pose are much easier upside down than sitting, because the weight of the body is not resting on the hip joints.

If you have hand, wrist, elbow, arm or shoulder injuries, you will not be able to do the inverted poses. However, you can practise Cat Pose and let the weight drop into your hands without putting pressure on them. If you have wrist injuries, practise Cat and Dog with your elbows bent as in Elbow Balance.

If you are already practising inverted poses you can continue to do them safely during pregnancy; however, pregnancy is not the time for learning them. If you feel any pressure or experience breathing problems, come down immediately. You may be able to continue Headstand when you can no longer do Shoulderstand. You can be substitute Supported Shoulderstand for as long as it is comfortable.

Finding Your Arms — Plank Poses

In Plank Pose and Sideways Plank, you will start to support the weight of your body on your arms. In these poses, your body should be in a straight line, from the back of your head, through the back of your pelvis, to your heels. Use a mirror to check your alignment.

These are strong, straight poses, but they are not rigid. The rhythm of the breath and the wave of release of your spine continue in these poses as well. Relax and learn to trust your arms to support you.

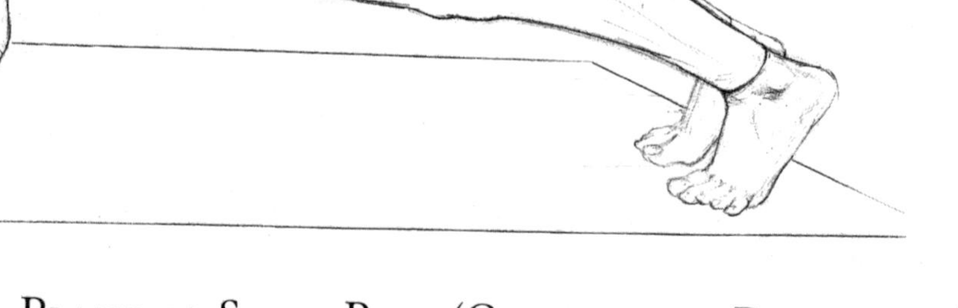

Plank or Stick Pose (Chaturanga Dandasana)

- Start lying face down on the floor, with your toes turned under.
- Place your hands, palms down, on the floor beside your ribs.
- Exhale, and push up.
- Relax as you inhale. As you exhale, take your abdomen well back, press down with the heels of your hands and extend your heels away from you. As the back of your waist lengthens with your breath, tuck your pelvis under. The greater the extension in your spine the lighter the pose will be on your arms.
- Come down, exhaling.

You can bend your knees and come down into Child's Pose, or hold your body straight and bend your arms. If you have trouble pushing up from the floor, go into Dog Pose and then bring your weight forward until your shoulders are over your wrists.

Sideways Plank Pose (Vasisthasana)

- From Plank pose, exhale and roll to your left, so your weight is on your left hand and the side of your left foot is on the floor. Your right foot and leg will be resting on your left.
- Take your right hand off the floor, and stretch your right arm up toward the ceiling. It should remain loose and relaxed.
- Turn and look at your right hand.

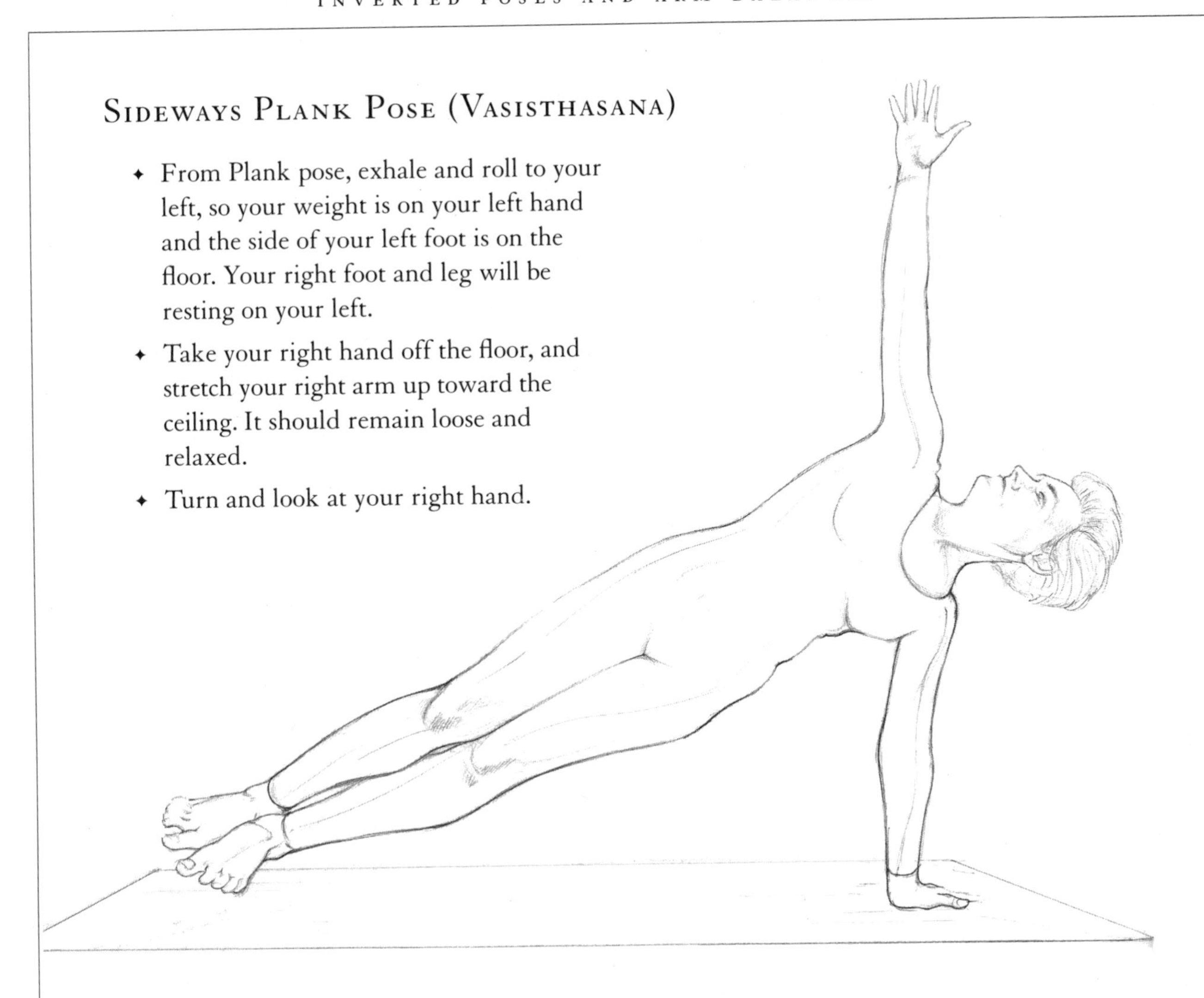

- Relax as you inhale. As you exhale, take your abdomen well back, press down with the heel of your hand and extend your legs away from you. As the back of your waist lengthens with your breath, tuck your pelvis under. The greater the extension in your spine the lighter the pose will be on your arm.
- To come out of the pose, turn back toward the floor. Place your right hand on the floor so you are in Plank Pose, bend your knees and come down.
- Repeat on the other side.

Handstand and Elbow Balances

Handstand and Elbow Balance are dynamic and energizing poses. They open the shoulders and free the upper back. They enable you to find the strength in your arms that comes from the core of your body as you find a connection to the ground through your arms.

The head drops freely in these poses and there is no danger of compression in the neck. If you are unable to do Head and Shoulderstands because of neck problems, you can still do these.

Handstands are very safe poses, but they are usually intimidating because so few people have confidence in their arms. Women find them particularly daunting. This fear is almost always without foundation and has very little to do with actual strength. There are very few people whose arms won't hold them once they are able to get into the pose. Once you can do Handstand, you can try Elbow Balance, which is a more intense stretch of the shoulder girdle.

If you lack confidence in your arms, the very idea of Handstand will be frightening. This fear will block the dynamic thrust you need to kick up. Most people are pleasantly surprised once they are up — the pose is easier and more fun than they thought it would be.

To get the feeling of your arms supporting you, try standing a couple of feet away from a wall, with your back to the wall. Bend forward and place your hands on the floor, shoulder-width apart. Walk your feet up the wall. Stay in this pose for as long as you can and then walk down.

To prepare to kick up, do Dog Pose with one leg up and back. Practise bending and straightening the standing leg. Wait until this movement is smooth and easy, before you try to kick up. Keep the lifted leg straight as you come up. It is carried upwards by the thrust of the kicking leg. A strong Rapid Abdominal breath or "Ha" will help give you energy as you kick.

Handstand, Head Down Tree Pose (Adho Mukha Vrksasana)

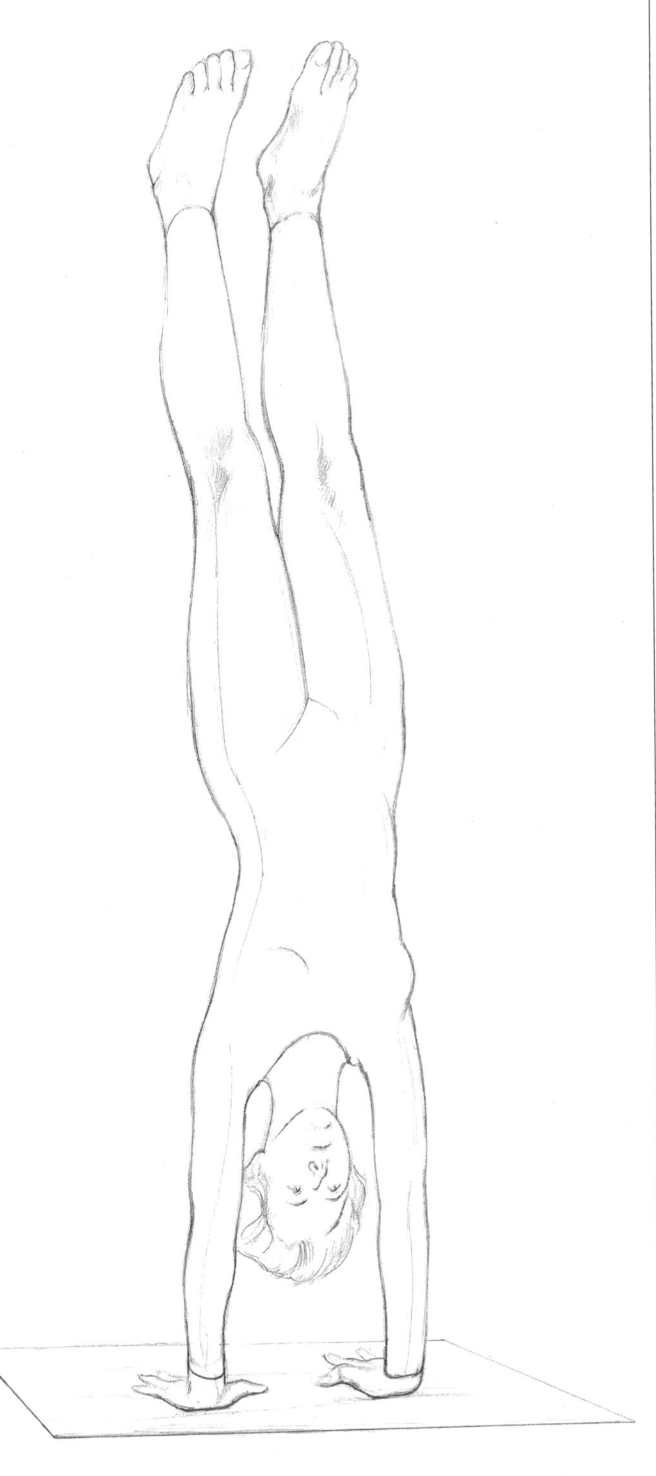

- Start standing straight, facing a wall.
- Bend forward and place your hands on the floor, shoulder-width apart, palms down.
- Take time breathing and dropping weight into your arms and wrists.
- Step one leg back. Bend your front leg, then straighten it quickly, using it as a spring to come up.
- When you are in the pose, let weight drop down into your wrists.
- Let your head drop, so the back of your neck remains long and loose.
- Keep the line of your spine long and straight. Do not arch your back.
- Let your elbows relax as you inhale. As you exhale, press down with the heels of your hands to rebound upwards. Use a strong breathing action in your abdominal muscles to support the back of your waist. The back of your legs and your inner knees should also lengthen and lift as you exhale. This extension may take you off the wall into a freestanding balance.
- To come down, bring one leg down and the rest of the pose will follow.

At first your feet will rest against the wall. Keep your lower back long and lift your legs and pelvis away from the back of your waist as you exhale. To balance without arching you need to be very grounded and centred.

Elbow Balance, Peacock Tail-Feather Pose (Pincha Mayurasana)

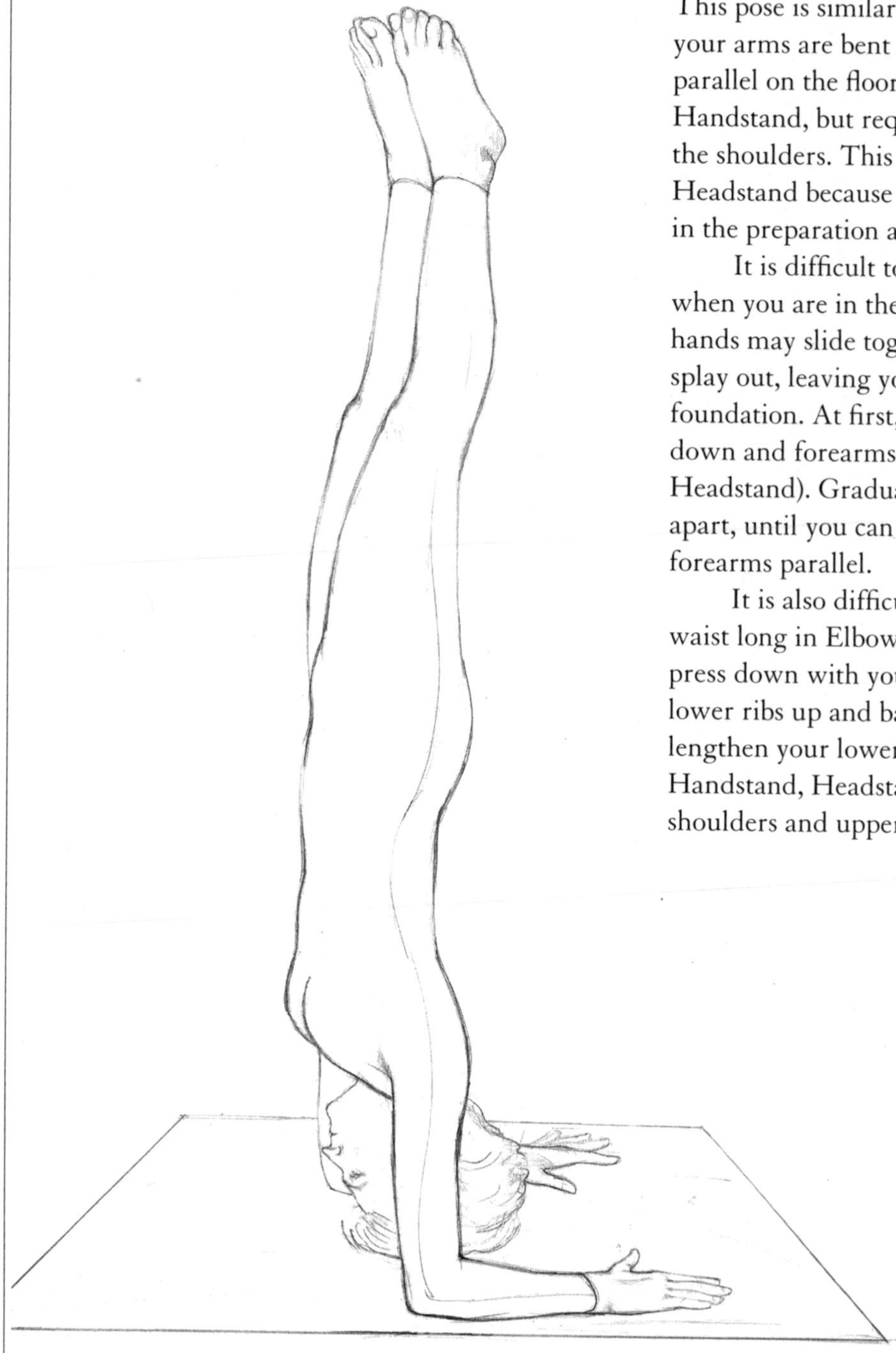

This pose is similar to Handstand, except that your arms are bent so that your forearms are parallel on the floor. It is an easier kick than Handstand, but requires more opening in the shoulders. This pose is different than Headstand because your head is off the floor, in the preparation and the full pose.

It is difficult to keep your arms parallel when you are in the pose. As you come up your hands may slide together and your elbows splay out, leaving you without a secure foundation. At first, practise with your palms down and forearms in a triangle (like Headstand). Gradually take your hands further apart, until you can do the pose with your forearms parallel.

It is also difficult to keep the back of your waist long in Elbow Balance. As you exhale, press down with your elbows to move your lower ribs up and back. If you are unable to lengthen your lower back in the pose, practise Handstand, Headstand and Wheel until your shoulders and upper back are freer.

Headstand (Sirsasana)

Headstand is a classic yoga posture. When you tell people you do yoga you often may be asked, "Do you do Headstand?" For most people Headstand is very intimidating. It takes a long time to learn to orient your body with your head upside down. You will probably need to spend at least six months in the preparation stages before going up into the full pose.

Before starting Headstand or Headstand Preparation, do some shoulder stretches, Dog Pose and Standing Forward Bend to release your shoulders and lengthen your neck. Repeat the Standing Forward Bend immediately after Headstand to undo compression. Then do Shoulderstand to further release and stretch your neck.

Headstand will highlight any structural weakness or imbalance in your body. Weakness in the lower back is intensified and any twist or scoliosis is magnified. At the same time, by changing the relationship of the body to gravity, Headstand provides an excellent opportunity for correction. If you are practising alone use a mirror, or have someone look at you from time to time.

For all the difficulties and risks with Headstand, its benefits are well worth the time and effort required. It is considered a masculine pose, the father of all poses, and brings with it inner strength, clarity, steadiness, courage and balance. In this sense it is counterbalanced by Shoulderstand, the mother of all poses, which is softer, more soothing and more surrendering.

Preparation

The foundation in Headstand is a triangle formed by the forearms. The elbows are the anchoring points, and the forearms lengthen toward the wrists, which are also weighted.

- Start in Child's Pose.
- Place your elbows on the floor shoulder-width apart or narrower.
- Clasp your hands and interlock your fingers so that your forearms form a triangle. Your hands should be relaxed and your fingers passive.
- Take a long time in this position, breathing, lengthening your spine and letting your arms and shoulders drop.
- From this position shift your weight forward, until your shoulders are above your elbows and you are on your hands and knees. Let your head drop away from your shoulders. It does not matter at this stage if your head is on the floor.

As you stay in Child's Pose, be aware of the ease and relaxation in your neck, arms and shoulders. Continue to let your arms release out of your shoulder joints, and let your forearms drop to the floor. Imagine what it might be like to have that kind of ease in the full Headstand. As you go through the various stages to come up into the pose, notice when you start to tighten and hold. See if you can release and let go again.

It is essential that your elbows and your wrists are in contact with the floor; the position of your hands and wrists can vary, depending on what is most comfortable for you. I have used a number of different positions for my hands: the outside of my wrists on the floor, my palms flat on the floor and the wrapping of my hands around my head. This last position is very common, but it gives the least support and is the weakest of the three. There is a strong tendency to hold the head. No matter which position you use, any tension in your hands and fingers is an indication of an insecure foundation in the forearms.

Cat Pose Headstand Preparation

Practise the Cat Pose with your arms in Headstand position to learn the action of the arms and upper back. It is a wonderful way to learn the movement in a position that is safe and easy.

- From the preparation position, come up onto your hands and knees.
- As you exhale, press down with your elbows and wrists and round your back, as in Cat Pose. Let your head drop. Feel the space and movement between your shoulder blades.
- As you exhale, strongly draw your abdominal muscles back toward the back of your waist, and feel the pull down on your pelvis. You will need this strong action in the next stages of practice.
- Relax as you inhale, letting your spine become concave.

Dog Pose Headstand

This pose is more tiring than Headstand, but it is safer and more stable.

- When your shoulders are wide and the base of your pose is stable, straighten your legs as in Dog Pose.
- Exhaling, take your abdomen well back, just as you did in Cat Pose, to lift your hips away from your shoulders, and take your heels down.
- Gradually walk your feet in closer to your head, continuing to lengthen from your elbows to your heels.

It takes time to find the direction of movement along your spine with your head down. If you are unable to lengthen your spine in this pose, then you will tighten your shoulders to support the weight.

The closer your feet are to your head, the more you will need to lengthen your spine. Otherwise, your upper back will round and collapse. To protect your neck, practise this pose in a doorway with the back of your head against the edge of the door frame. You can then tell when your upper back is rounded. When you find you are unable to lengthen further, walk your feet away again or come down.

Going Up

Your first Headstand is a significant landmark in your practice. When you are ready to do a pose, it comes easily — even Headstand. Any fear is an indication that you are not ready, and need to take more time establishing your base and lengthening your spine.

Start with a wall behind you. At first you can kick up. Later, you will be able to simply lift your legs as your spine lengthens with your breath. When you are comfortable coming up with your knees bent, you can try it with your legs straight.

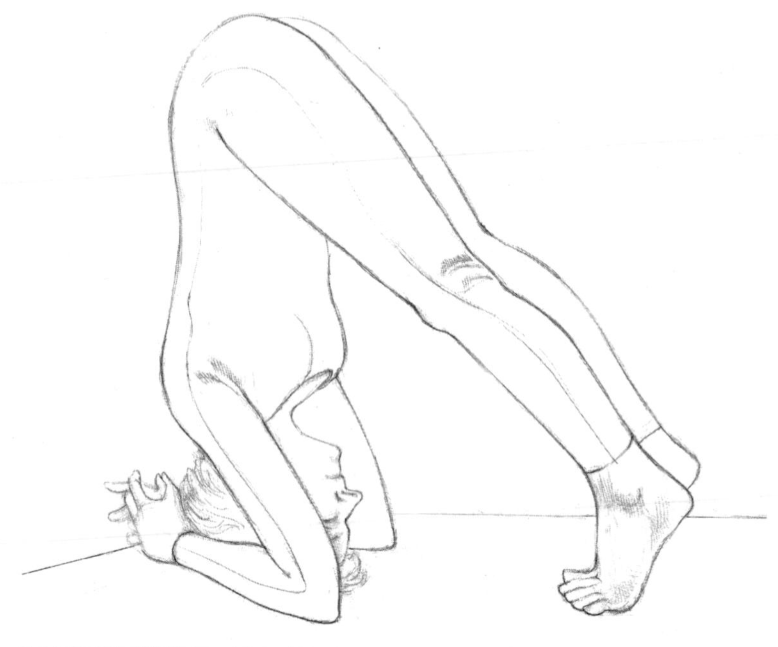

- From the Dog Pose Headstand, place your head on the floor between your inner wrists.
- Be sure your chin is in line with the notch between your collar-bones so that your head is straight.
- Let the weight drop into your elbows, so the back of your neck lengthens and the back of your shoulders broadens.
- As your spine lengthens, your sitting bones are lifted higher and higher, away from your elbows.
- Shift your hips back slightly and tuck your knees to your chest. (You may need a little hop at first.)
- Continue to breathe as you slowly straighten your legs up toward the ceiling. If there is any feeling of strain or pressure, come down immediately.

Be particularly attentive as you are going up into the pose. Even if you are very experienced, the foundation and orientation that you have taken so long to build can easily disappear in the few seconds it takes to go up. Stay conscious of your breath and the base of the pose as you come up.

If you have long arms, you may find that your head does not touch the floor when your elbows are anchored and your shoulders open. Place a small folded towel between your arms to provide a contact point for your head.

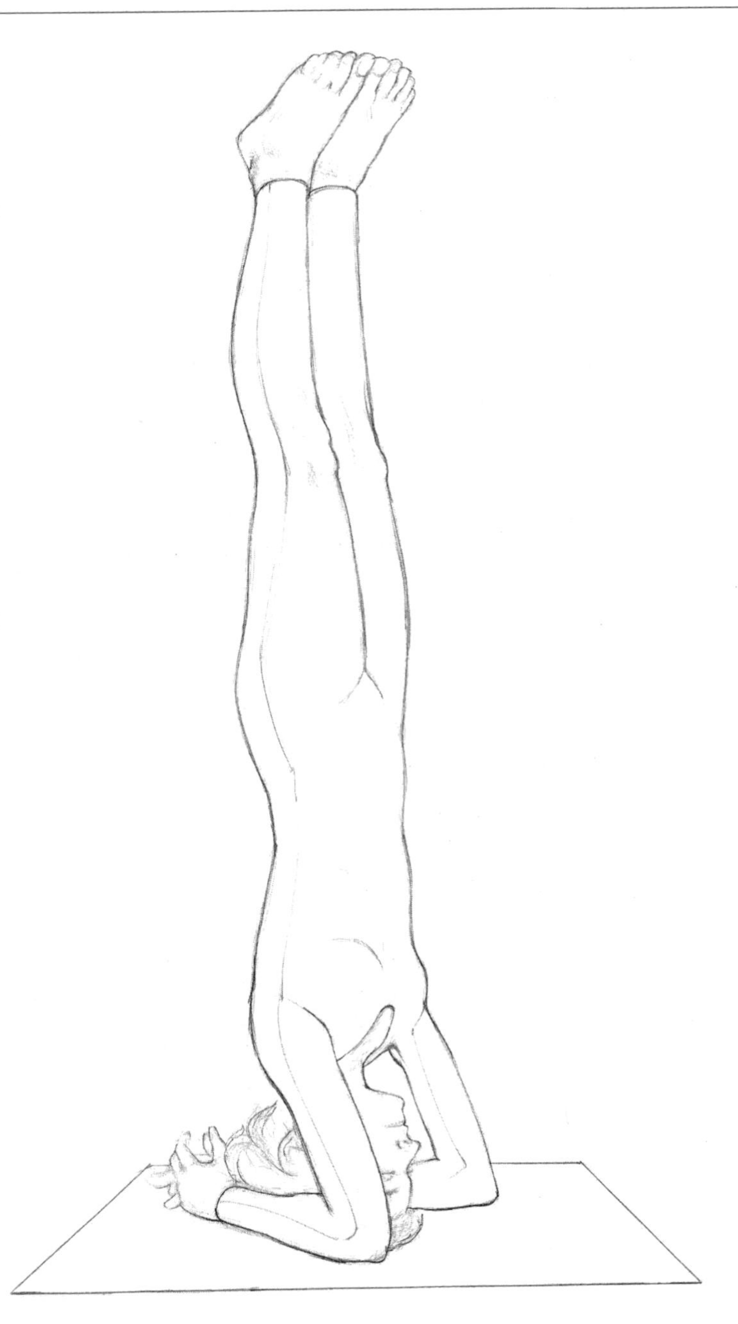

In the Pose

At first, being up in Headstand is surprisingly disorienting. However, the simplicity of the method is very helpful in finding your way around. Use the awareness of your breath and your forearms on the ground to orient yourself. When you are grounded, long and centred, you will gradually be able to balance. There is very little value in being balanced in a tense and crooked pose.

- Be aware of your breathing and the contact of your elbows with the floor. Release the back of your skull toward the floor to lengthen your neck.
- As you exhale, press down with your elbows.
- When you are quiet and centred, start to focus on lengthening your spine. Exhale deeply, drawing your abdominal muscles well back.
- Lengthen the back of your legs and your inner legs as you exhale.
- Carry this extension through to the soles of your feet. Your calves and feet should remain relaxed.
- When you are ready, come down slowly. Continue to breathe and lengthen your spine as you come down.

Headstand highlights any weakness, distortion or imbalance in the body. You can seriously damage your neck by doing crooked Headstands over a long period of time. When you are able to balance freely in Headstand, use the mirror to see if your pose is straight. Before you go up, spread your legs slightly and check to see that your head, shoulders and hips are straight before you go up. Check again when you are in the pose.

Ask someone to look at the back of your neck when you are up. The curve of your neck should be long and smooth.

There is a lot of confusion about weight and pressure on the head in Headstand. The line of gravity goes through the crown of your head in the pose. There is contact of the head with the floor and weight, but not pressure or tension. Just as standing does not create pressure in the feet, there should be no feeling of pressure on your head in Headstand.

If you have a stiff upper back and strong arms, you will probably do Headstand easily. But Headstand is not about strong arms and shoulders; it is about having a stable base and a long, light and free spine. Even if you are experienced and comfortable in Headstand, you are probably holding your neck and shoulders to support it.

As you learn to lengthen your spine, you will find lightness and freedom in the pose. As in all of the positions, the anchoring of the pose on the ground, the stability of the structure and the elongation of the spine all combine to free and balance the posture. Then you will find that your arms, neck and shoulders are also relaxed and at ease.

Headstand Variations

There are many ways you can play in Headstand once you are relaxed and stable. You can spread your legs wide like you do in the Wide Angle sitting pose, then bend your knees and bring you feet together in Bound Angle Pose, wrap your legs around each other as in Eagle Pose or bend your knees so your feet drop behind you like Hero's Pose.

The variations described here are some of the more difficult ones that need special care and instruction.

Single Leg Stretch (Eka Pada Sirsasana)

- Start in Headstand.
- Focus your attention on one leg. Take time to lengthen upwards through that leg.
- Then, exhaling take the other leg down toward the floor. Begin by taking your leg down a little, so you do not lose balance.
- As you exhale, lengthen the lower leg away from you. It is more important to stretch your leg straight than to reach the floor.
- Stay in the pose as long as you can continue to lengthen the lifted leg. Then, exhaling, come back up into Headstand. Repeat on the other side.

The lifted leg is more important than the one that drops. There will be a tendency for this leg to lean backwards and turn out. As you lengthen, bring it forward and turn it in.

When you are comfortable working each leg independently, you can integrate the movements in one breath. Remain passive as you inhale. As you exhale, drop the weight into your elbows, and take your breath well back toward the back of your waist to lengthen your spine and release the upright leg upwards. As your lower leg drops, lengthen it. All this will happen by itself, if your breath is deep enough and you are relaxed in the pose.

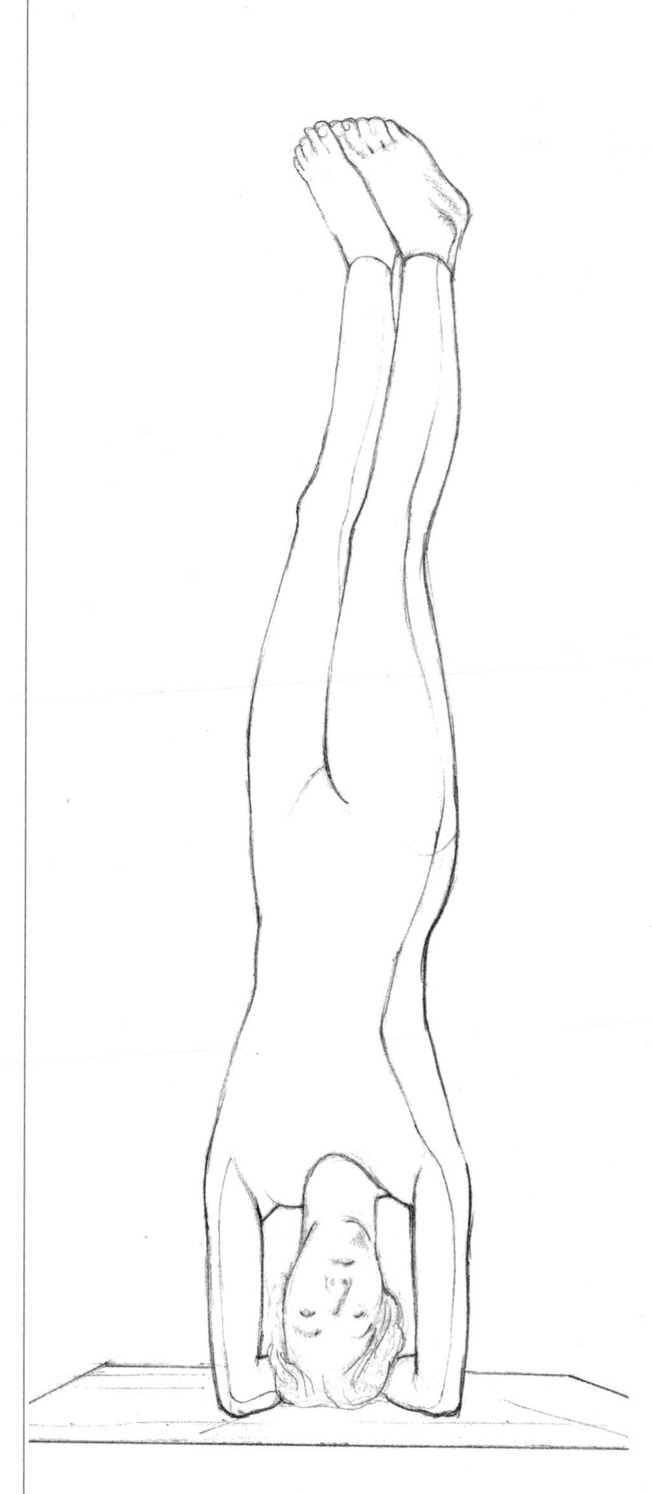

Headstand Twist (Parsva Sirsasana)

In this pose, the body rotates around the central axis of the spine. The shoulders remain horizontal, and the root of the twist is in the upper back.

- Start in Headstand.
- As you exhale and your spine lengthens, turn your whole body to the left.
- Stay in the pose, breathing and lengthening.
- Exhaling, lengthen your spine as you come back to centre.
- Repeat on the other side.

Just turn a little at first so that your spine stays straight and balanced. It is more important to keep your spine straight than to turn to the maximum. As you turn, anchor your left elbow strongly, so that your right shoulder does not collapse. Lengthen your right side, to keep the back of your waist long and balanced.

Once you have mastered this pose, you can combine it with Lotus in Headstand and Hero's Pose in Headstand.

Variation

Scissors Twist (Parivrttaikapada Sirsasana)

- Take your left leg back and your right leg forward, an equal distance from the centre line of your body. Begin with only a small distance between your legs. Your front leg will want to go down more, because it is easier.
- Turn your body to the left, so your right leg crosses in front of you.

  This pose is even harder to keep straight than the Headstand Twist, so be very careful.

Lotus in Headstand (Urdhva Padmasana Sirsasana)

In order to do this pose, you must be able to get into Lotus easily, since you cannot use your hands to help you. To warm up:

- Lie on your back with your legs in Lotus or Half Lotus.
- Place a folded blanket under your knees so the back of your waist rests on the floor. Rest in this position, following your breath and letting your legs drop away as the front of thighs and hips stretch.

If you are very secure in Headstand Preparation, you can bring one leg into Half Lotus before you go up.

- While you are in the preparation pose, bend your right leg; use your left hand to pull your right foot into Half Lotus. Bring it high up on your left thigh.
- Then hop up into Headstand. Your right foot will be closer to the left hip, which makes it easier to cross the left leg over. If you cannot come into full Lotus, bend your left knee and let your left foot drop behind your right thigh.

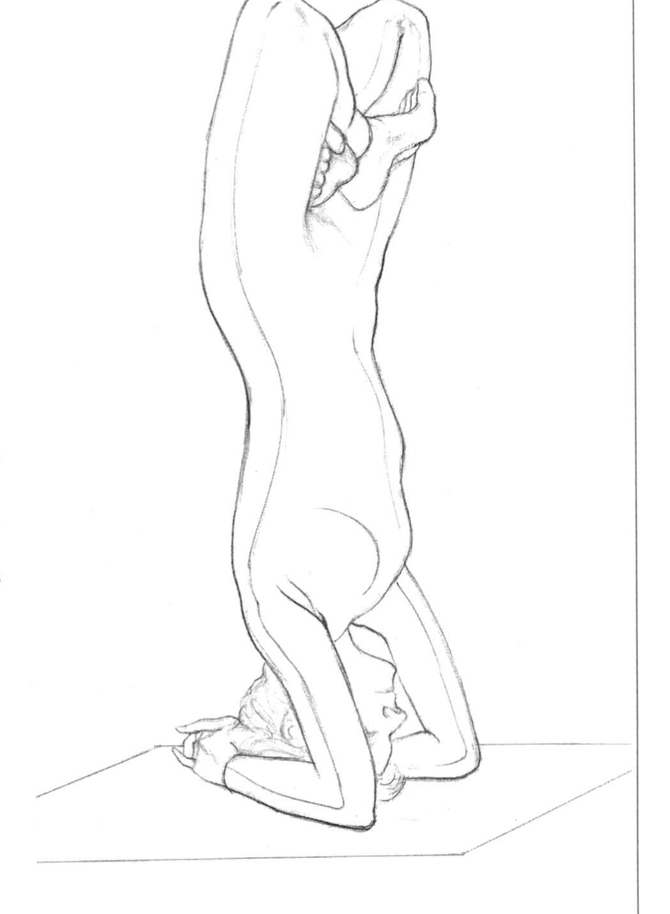

Full Pose

- If your hips are very flexible, you can go into Lotus in Headstand.
- In Headstand spread your legs wide apart, then bend your right leg and, exhaling, place it on your left thigh, as close to your left hip as possible.
- Exhaling, take your right knee back as far as possible, and bring your left foot in front of your right knee. Wriggle your foot toward your right hip.
- Breathe and lengthen as you do in Headstand.
- Straighten your legs, back into Headstand. Repeat with your legs crossed the other way.

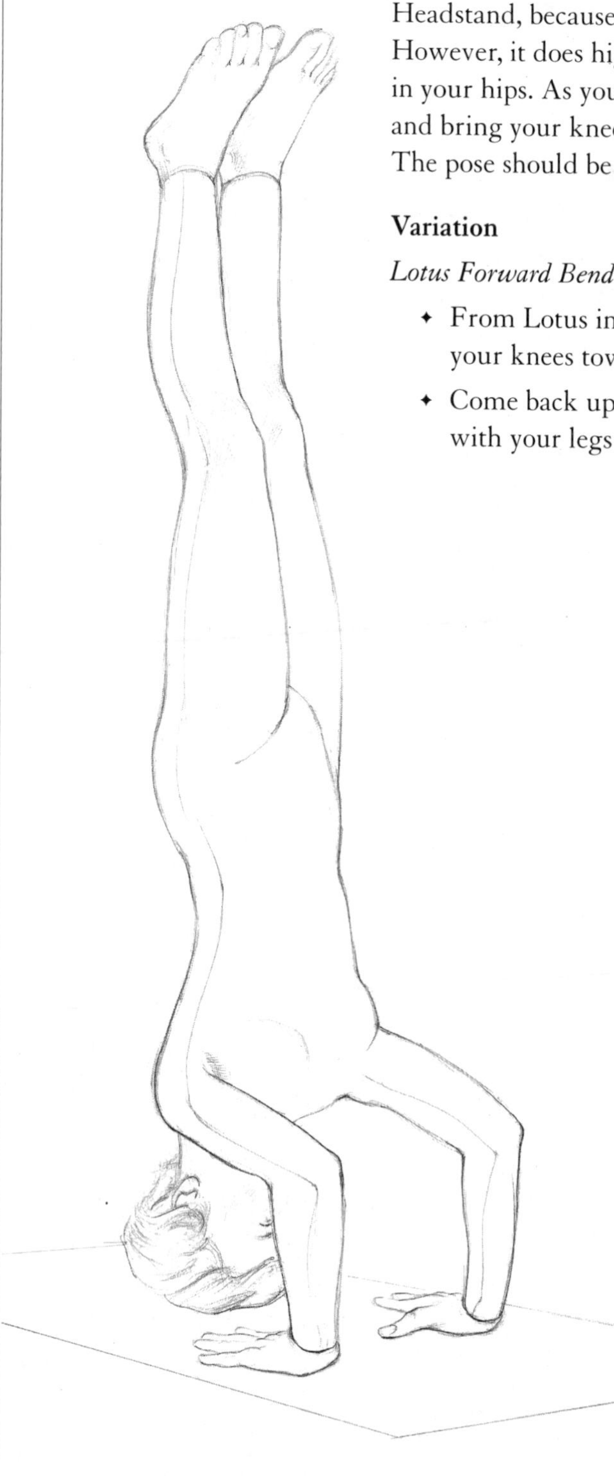

You may find Lotus in Headstand easier than the basic Headstand, because it is more compact and the hips are stronger. However, it does highlight any sway in your lower back and tightness in your hips. As you exhale, take your abdominal muscles well back and bring your knees toward each other and up toward to the ceiling. The pose should be as straight as possible.

Variation

Lotus Forward Bend in Headstand (Pindasana in Sirsasana)

- From Lotus in Headstand, exhale, lengthen your spine and bend your knees toward your chest.
- Come back up into Headstand and straighten your legs. Repeat with your legs crossed the other way.

Tripod Headstand (Sirsasana II)

Some people find this position easier than the basic Headstand.

- Kneeling, place your hands on the floor shoulder-width apart.
- Place your head on the floor in front of you, so that your head and your hands form a triangle. Drop your weight into your wrists.
- As you exhale, draw your elbows in toward each other and toward the floor.
- Exhaling, straighten your legs and come up as you do in the basic Headstand. You can rest your shins on your upper arms until you are ready to go up further.
- When you are in the pose, your arms should be relaxed and stable and your spine lengthening.
- Come down slowly, exhaling.

If your hands and head are too close together, it will be difficult to balance; if they are too far apart you will not be able to put your wrists securely on the floor.

Shoulderstand (Sarvangasana)

Beginners' Preparation Poses

Inverted poses are unique to yoga practice, and take some time to get used to. The idea of inversion is frightening for many people and, unlike the standing or sitting, is not part of their daily lives. Start gradually, until you are used to the idea and the feeling, and have a sense of what is happening to your body in the pose. Remember, never force yourself into a pose. If you feel strain, pressure or fear in any of these poses, come down or modify the pose until you are comfortable and can breathe easily.

When you are ready to come up into any of the inverted poses (Supported Bridge, Half Shoulderstand, Shoulderstand or Plough), use a blanket to create a soft base for the pose. The blanket should be neatly folded and should be large enough to provide a sufficient foundation for the pose. Lie with your head and shoulders toward the folded side. If you find the stretch on your neck too intense, lie with your shoulders on the edge of the blanket and your head on the floor. Do not use more than two blankets. If the pile of blankets is too high, you will not be able to anchor your elbows.

Legs Resting on the Wall

You can start to prepare your body for inverted poses by lying with your legs resting up against a wall. This pose benefits circulation in the legs, and stretches the hamstrings while supporting the spine. It is soothing and restful for most people; however, if even this small inversion causes stress, come down.

You can spread your legs wide, do the Bound Angle Pose or bend your knees and put your feet on the wall while you are in this pose.

- Sit on the floor beside the wall.
- Swing around to bring your legs up. You may need to wriggle closer to the wall. It is more important to have your pelvis on the floor and your spine supported, than to be right up against the wall.
- Stay in the pose, focusing on your breathing for as long as you are comfortable.
- To come down, bend your knees and roll to one side.

Supported Inverted Practice (Viparita Karani)

The next stage is a supported inversion. This pose opens your chest and starts to bring weight onto your arms and shoulders. It is very restful. You can practise this pose when you are exhausted or ill. It is beneficial for colds or coughs because it opens and clears your chest.

It is also a good pose for pregnant women who are no longer able to do Shoulderstand. It is restful and creates space in the diaphragm, allowing them to breathe more easily. Gentle inversion improves circulation in the legs, and takes pressure off the bladder and pelvic floor. This pose is also used to try to turn a baby from breech position. It should be avoided in the last six weeks of pregnancy.

- Start by lying with your legs up against the wall.
- Lift your hips and place a firm cushion or folded blanket under your hips.
- If you are comfortable, you can stay in this position for quite a while.
- When you are ready to come down, lift your hips and remove the support.
- Then, bend your knees and roll to one side.

Supported Bridge Pose (Setu Bandhasana)

This pose brings you up onto your shoulders. When you go up, check again for pressure or tension in your head and neck.

If your lower back is in pain, and you have trouble rolling up into Shoulderstand from the floor, you can go up from this position.

- Start by lying with your legs up against the wall.
- Check to make sure that your head is straight (your chin is in line with the notch between your collarbones) and the back of your neck is long and relaxed.
- Bend your knees and put your feet on the wall.
- Do a pelvic tilt and come up into Supported Bridge Pose.
- Place your hands on the back of your pelvis to support your hips.
- To come down, let your elbows slide apart and then gradually roll down.

Half Shoulderstand

- Start by lying on the floor with your knees bent over your chest, and your arms straight on the floor, palms down. Take time to let your arms lengthen away from your shoulders as you breathe.
- On an exhalation, press down with your hands to come up, as if you were going to do a backwards somersault.
- Place your hands on your back for support.
- Rest the weight of your hips in your hands, like a cup and saucer. Your body will be slanted away from your shoulders and your neck is free.
- If you are relaxed and comfortable, straighten your legs.
- To come down, let your elbows slide apart and then gradually roll down.

This is a very safe position for the neck. It places the weight of the pose appropriately on your elbows. As you start to come up into the full Shoulderstand, leave this feeling of weight in your upper arms.

You can also come up into Half Shoulderstand from Supported Bridge Pose by taking your feet off the wall one at a time. To come down, put your feet back on the wall, and roll down from there.

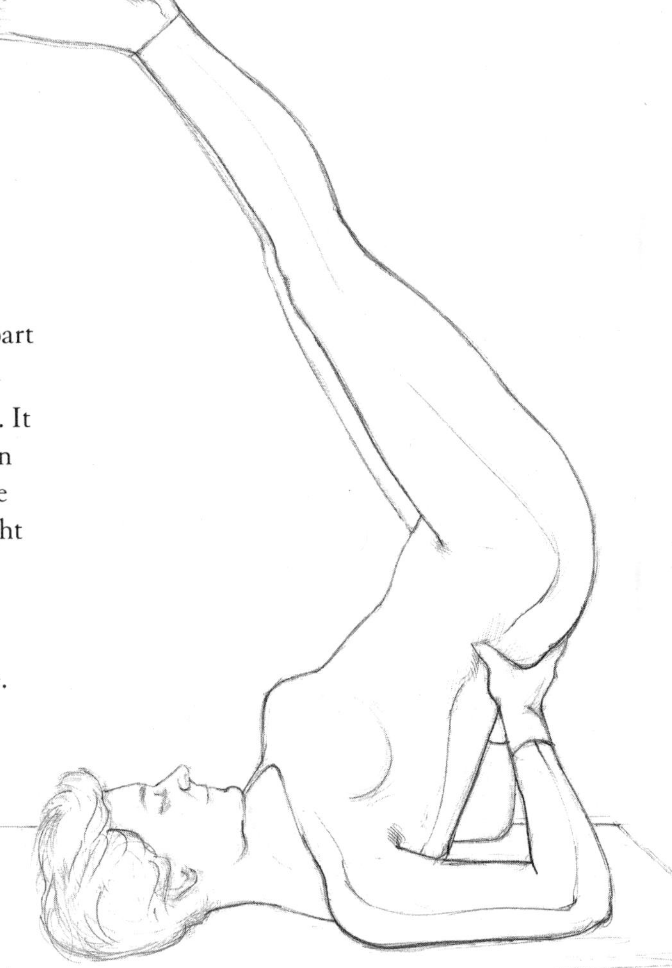

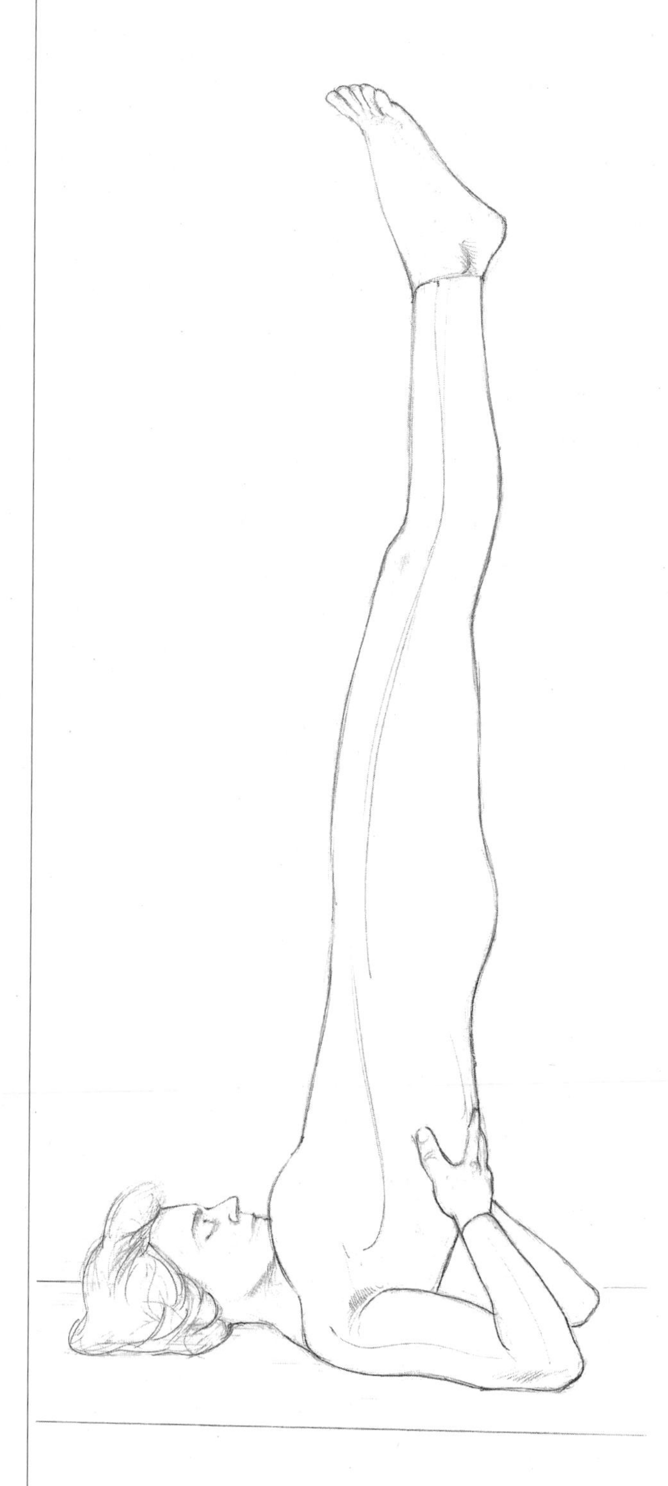

Shoulderstand (Sarvangasana)

With practice, Shoulderstand can be sustained for long periods of time. It is a very soothing, healing and restful pose.

- Start in Half Shoulderstand.
- As your shoulders and upper back release, gradually move your hands down toward your shoulder blades.
- Use the action of your exhalation to support your lower back and lift your pelvis and legs away from your shoulders.
- Carry the extension upwards through the back of your legs and along your inner leg to your inner ankles. Your calves, ankles and feet should remain relaxed, and be carried upward by the support from below. It is a common mistake to try to lift the pose up from the calves and feet.
- Stay in the pose for as long as you want, letting your neck continue to release and your back lengthen.
- To come down, let your elbows slide apart and roll down slowly, vertebra by vertebra, lengthening your spine as you roll down to the floor.

If your elbows splay out in Shoulderstand, you will lose the foundation and the pose will collapse. You can use a belt to support your arms. Tie the belt so that it is wider than your shoulders, and place it on the floor beside you where you can reach it easily. Go into Half Shoulderstand or Plough, and slip the belt onto your arms above your elbows. Then place your hands on your back. Take the belt off before you come down.

I find Shoulderstand an extremely variable pose. Some days I go up quite easily, and others I feel like I am right back at the beginning. Be present to your body in the moment; adjust the pose to how you are that day.

Moving your hands down toward your shoulder blades makes the pose straighter and more vertical. Do not force yourself to be straight too soon, as you can easily strain your neck.

One of the purposes of Shoulderstand is to develop the strength and awareness in your spine to support you upright. As always this comes from the action of your breath, and cannot be achieved through tension in your arms or legs.

If you feel strain in your lower back when you come down, bend your knees to your chest and rest for a while. Keep your Shoulderstands short until you have the strength in your lower back to give you adequate support. You can do Half Shoulderstand or Plough Pose as alternatives, until your back is stronger.

Shoulderstand Variations

Single Leg Stretch in Shoulderstand (Eka Pada Sarvangasana)

- From Shoulderstand, exhaling, extend one leg upwards.
- Take the other leg down toward the floor. As you exhale, lengthen the back of your leg, so it stays straight.
- Stay in the pose as long as you can continue to elongate the lifted leg, then on an exhalation come back up into Shoulderstand.
- Repeat on the other side.

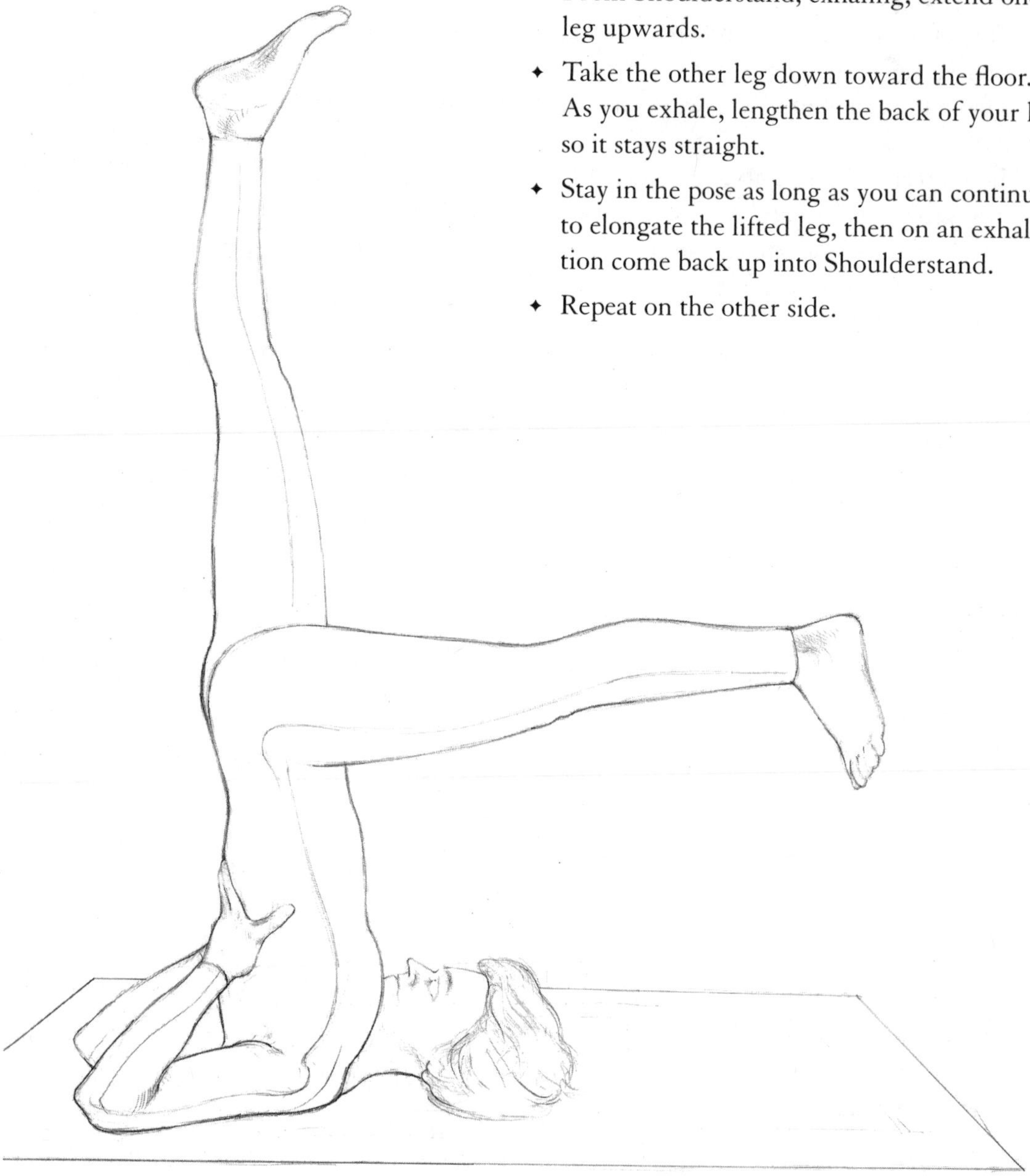

The lifted leg will tend to lean backwards and turn out to counterbalance the weight of the dropping leg. As you lengthen your leg, bring it toward you and turn it in. Continue to focus on the upright leg; extend it upwards on the exhalation as your spine lengthens. The extension of your spine is far more important than reaching the floor with your foot.

When you are able to lengthen your spine with your breath, you will find that all of the movements are integrated into one wavelike action. The rhythm is: remain passive as you inhale. As you exhale, drop your elbows, lengthen your spine and extend the lifted leg. *Then*, drop and lengthen the lower leg.

Shoulderstand Twist (Parsva Sarvangasana)

This pose is an open twist in Shoulderstand (see photograph on p. 124). It is much more strenuous than the corresponding Lotus variation, even though the latter looks much more exotic.

- Start in Shoulderstand. Bend your knees to your chest.
- Round your back, and then turn to place one hand underneath your sacrum (the triangular bone in the middle of the back of your pelvis). When your hand is correctly positioned, your middle finger will be touching your tailbone.
- Exhaling, press your elbow down to open your chest.
- Gradually straighten your legs away from you.
- The action of your breath must be strong and dynamic to keep your lower back strong. Stretch your inner legs away from your hips. If you lose control, bend your knees and drop your feet to the floor.
- When you are ready, bend your knees back to your chest, and come back into Shoulderstand.
- Repeat on the other side.

The weight of your body rests on your hand so your elbow will be weighted. This may cause pressure on your wrists at first; the more you can open your chest, the lighter the feeling on your hand will be. Your other hand can rest on your back, or on the floor.

Plough and Variations

Plough is a more intense stretch on the neck and lower back than Shoulderstand and a more passive and relaxing pose. If you are a beginner or your neck is stiff, approach it gradually.

Plough and variations are all inverted forward bends and resting poses, especially the ones with the knees bent. They must be done with caution because of the intense stretch on the neck, upper and lower back. Since they are forward bends, they can be used to counterbalance backbends.

This sequence can be done before or after Shoulderstand or both. You will have more lift in Shoulderstand after doing these poses. If you do them twice, you find that they come much better the second time.

Plough (Halasana)

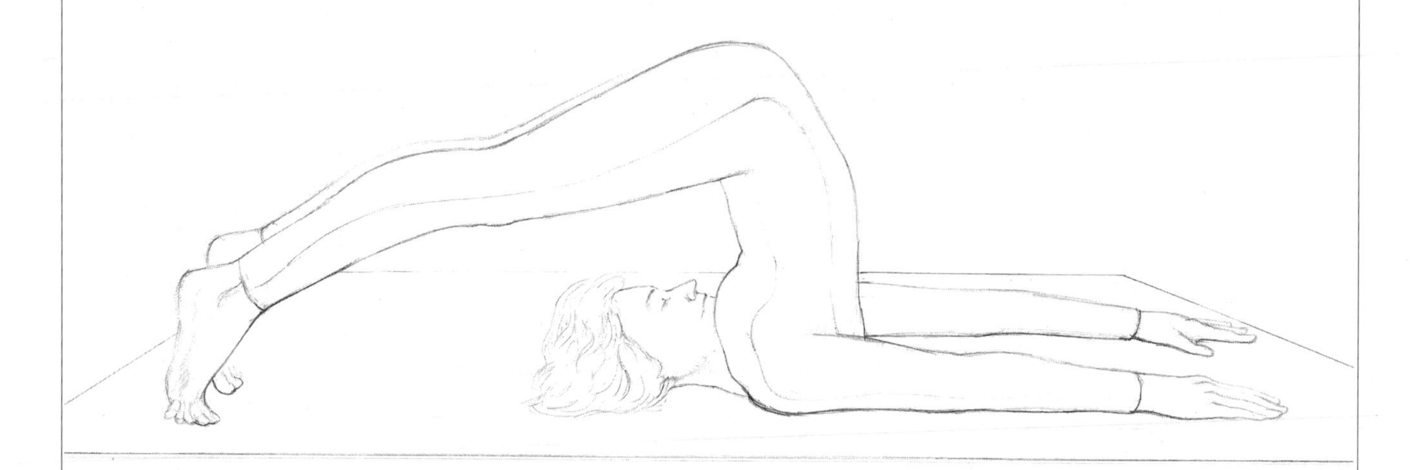

- From Shoulderstand, bring your legs down toward the floor behind your head.
- As you come down, use the action of your breathing to keep the back of your waist long and lifting.
- Your hands can remain on your back, as in Shoulderstand, or rest flat on the floor, palms down.
- As your neck, shoulders and spine release, lengthen your arms away from your shoulders, and walk your feet away from your head.

Plough with Bent Knees (Karna Pidasana)

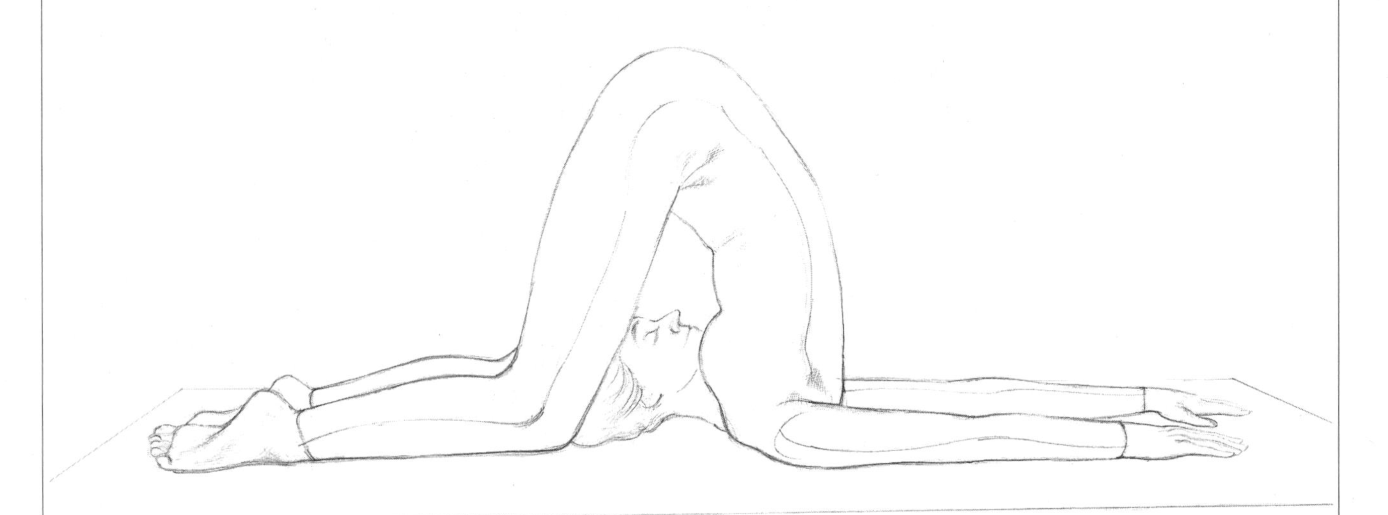

- From Plough, walk your feet as far away from your head as you can.
- Bend your knees and place them on either side of your head beside your ears.
- Stay in the pose as long as you are comfortable.
- When you are ready, straighten your legs, and come back into Plough Pose.

This pose is very introverted and restful, calming and quieting. It also stretches the lower back and is a good counterbalance to any compression in the lumbar that might take place during Shoulderstand. If your lower back is weak, be careful not to overstretch.

For a more intense stretch, keep your knees together, so they slide over the top of your head. For an even more restful pose, wrap your arms around your legs, close your eyes and rest.

Variations

Legs Wide in Plough (Supta Konasana)
This pose is an inverted form of the Wide Angle sitting pose. It is much easier to spread your legs apart when you are upside down, so it is a good pose to practise if you have trouble with the sitting poses. It is also beneficial for prolapsed uterus.

- From Plough Pose, spread your legs wide apart.
- Centre the weight on your feet, so that both the base of your big toe and the base of your baby toe are on the floor. Make sure that your elbows remain weighted on the floor.
- Legthen your spine and stretch your legs as you exhale.
- Bring your legs together into Plough or walk around to one side into Plough Twist.

Plough Twist (Parsva Halasana)

- From Legs Wide in Plough, walk your feet around to one side. Your feet should be in line with each other with the weight equal on both feet and distributed evenly across the balls of the feet; then your sitting bones will be level with each other.
- Leave the opposite elbow down and weighted.
- Repeat on other side.

Plough with Bent Knees Twist (Parsva Karna Pidasana)
The twist and stretch in this pose is in the upper back, between your shoulder blades.

- From Plough Twist, bend your knees beside your ear and rest there. Surprisingly, it is the knee nearer your head that is more difficult to drop.
- Straighten your legs back into Plough Twist.
- Repeat on other side.

Lotus Variations in Shoulderstand

It is easier to do Lotus upside down than sitting, because there is less weight on your hips. You may find that you can work on Lotus upside down when you are unable to do it sitting. All of these poses can be done with one leg in Half Lotus and the other leg bent behind it.

Lotus also makes the Shoulderstand more compact, and focuses the outer hips so they are easier to lift. When you come back into Shoulderstand after doing the Lotus variations, you will be much straighter and lighter in the pose.

Do as much of the sequence as you can, and then change your legs and repeat it.

Lotus in Shoulderstand (Urdhva Padmasana Sarvangasana)

- Start in Shoulderstand.
- Bring your legs into Lotus Pose.
- Exhale, lengthen the back of your waist and, as your hips release, extend your knees away from your hips and draw them toward each other. You are aiming to be vertical in the pose with your knees pointing to the ceiling and the back of your waist long.
- Continue on into Lotus in Plough, or straighten your legs and come back into Shoulderstand.

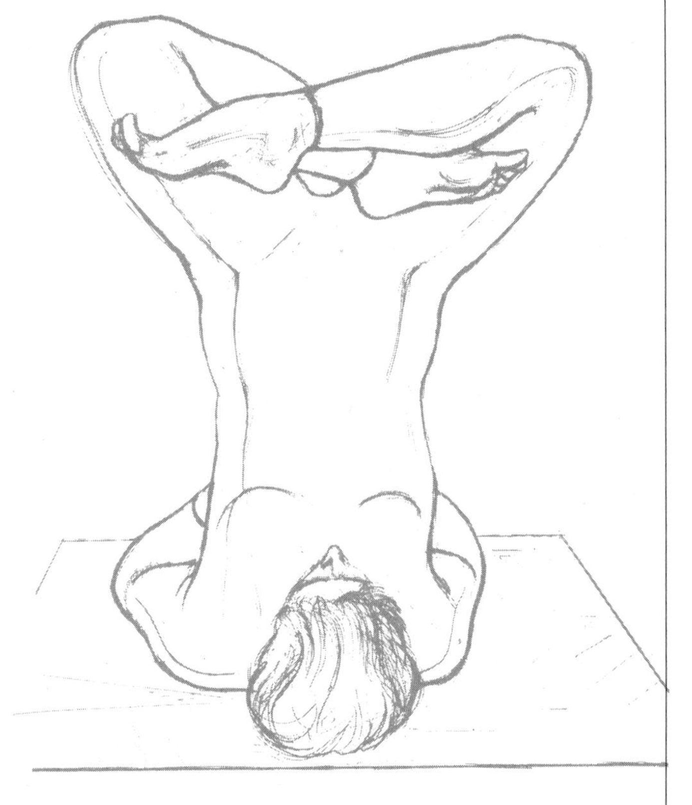

If you are secure in Shoulderstand, you can use your hands to cross your legs. Use your left hand to bring your right leg into Half Lotus, then put your hand on your back and use your right hand to pull your left leg into position. Be careful not to force your knees.

If you cannot get into Lotus when you are up in Shoulderstand, do it sitting and then somersault up into the Shoulderstand with your legs crossed.

Variation

Lotus in Shoulderstand Twist (Parsva Urdhva Padmasana Sarvangasana)
This pose is similar to the Shoulderstand Twist, but is much easier and more restful. It relieves any compression in your throat or upper chest after Shoulderstand.

Lotus in Plough (Pindasana in Sarvangasana)

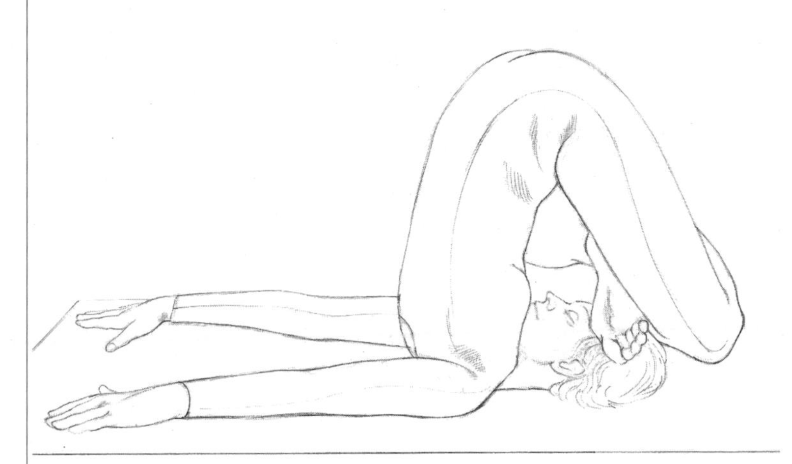

This pose is an intense stretch of both the upper and lower back, but it is also a resting pose.

- From Lotus in Shoulderstand, bend your hips and lower your knees toward the floor.
- Continue to breathe and lengthen your spine as you bring your legs down.
- Your arms must be weighted to counterbalance the weight of your legs dropping over your head.
- Rest in the pose for as long as you want, then come back up into Lotus in Shoulderstand.

Variation

Lotus in Plough Twist (Parsva Pindasana in Sarvangasana)
This pose is an intense twist and stretch of the upper back.

- From Lotus in Plough, turn your body to one side, and bring your knees down beside your head. The knee nearer your head is harder to drop.
- The opposite elbow must remain very heavy on the floor to keep the pose stable. As in Lotus in Plough, you may somersault if you lose control.
- Remain resting in the pose for as long as you want, and then on an exhalation come back up into Lotus in Shoulderstand.

Arm Balances

Caution: Because of the strong action on the abdominal and pelvic organs, these poses should be avoided by women who are menstruating, pregnant or post-partum. Do not attempt them if you have pelvic or abdominal problems such as cystitis or colitis, or are recovering from abdominal surgery.

Crow Pose is similar to Plough with Knees Bent, but is much stronger and more dynamic. Energy is gathered into the centre of the body, in contrast to backbends which are extroverted. The strong action of the abdominal muscles is a powerful massage of the internal organs.

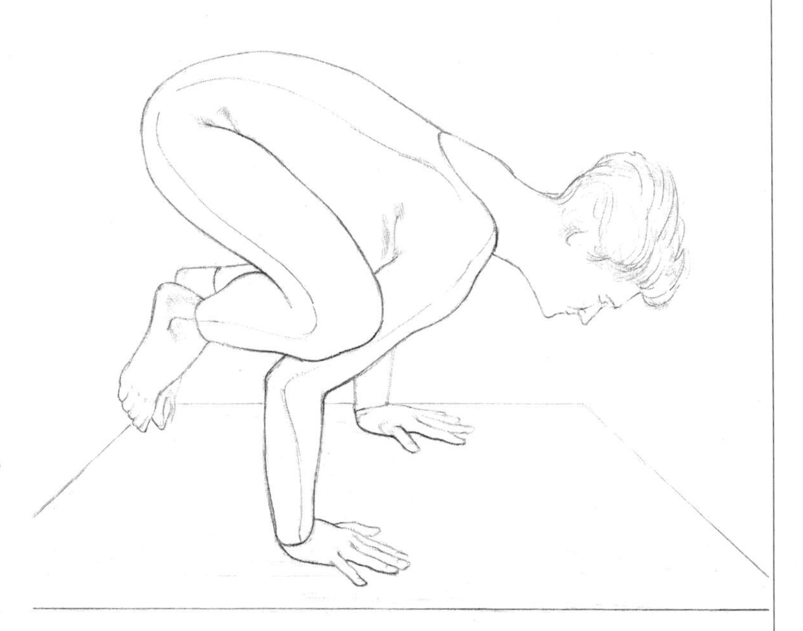

Like Handstand, these poses are rooted in the wrists, and confidence in the arms is essential. Therefore, they are usually easier for men who have strong arms and shoulders. Ultimately, however, the ability to do them comes from correct action and balance. Think of the weight of your body resting on your arms, and let your arms relax to take the weight.

The back rounds in these poses, which makes them a strong counterbalance to backbends. Finish with a backbend or do backbends in between the Crow Poses as counterposes.

These poses are lessons in humility. You may find yourself sprawled on the floor until you learn to draw your whole body into the centre — elbows, thighs and abdomen. You will need a positive attitude and a sense of humour to persist with them. There is a wonderful sense of accomplishment when they start to come together.

Crow Pose (Bakasana)

(see illustration on p. 155)

Crow Pose can be approached from Garland Pose or Tripod Headstand. Garland Pose is easier and safer for people who have difficulty with the Headstand. People with stiff hips often find the approach from Headstand easier.

From Garland Pose

- From Garland Pose, place your hands on the floor as close to your feet as possible. The back of your arms will press against your shins and your elbows will be outside your legs.
- Shift your weight *forward* from your feet to your hands, until your feet come off the floor easily. Then, with a strong exhalation, press down with your wrists to come up.
- When you are in the pose, the action is the same as Cat Pose, but much stronger. Relax and let your weight rest on your arms as you inhale. As you exhale, take your abdomen well back, press down with your wrists, straighten your arms and round your back.
- To come down, roll your feet down to the floor.

From Tripod Headstand

- Start in Tripod Headstand or the Tripod Headstand preparation position.
- Bend your knees and place your shins on your upper arms. Bring your knees as far forward into your armpits as possible.
- Exhaling, drop your hips until there is no weight on your head.
- When the weight is centred on your wrists, exhale and press down strongly to come into the pose.
- When you are in the pose, the action is the same as Cat Pose, but much stronger. Relax and let your weight rest on your arms as you inhale. As you exhale, take your abdomen well back, press down with your wrists, straighten your arms and round your back.
- To come down, tuck your chin in and slowly roll back down until you are in the tuck position with your head on the floor. Exhaling, place your feet back on the floor or come back up into Headstand.

Finding the balance point for Crow Pose takes time and practice. Sometimes it is helpful to practise rocking back and forth from squatting into the Headstand tuck. When the movement is clear, work on finding the balance point in the middle.

Variation

Lotus in Crow (Urdhva Kukkutasana)
You can also do Crow Pose in Lotus.

- Start in Tripod Headstand. Cross your legs into Lotus.
- Continue as if you were doing Crow Pose from Headstand. Like many of the Lotus variations upside down, this pose is much easier for some people than the basic pose, because it is more compact and holds together better.
- Come back into Tripod Headstand and straighten your legs.
- Repeat with your legs crossed the other way.

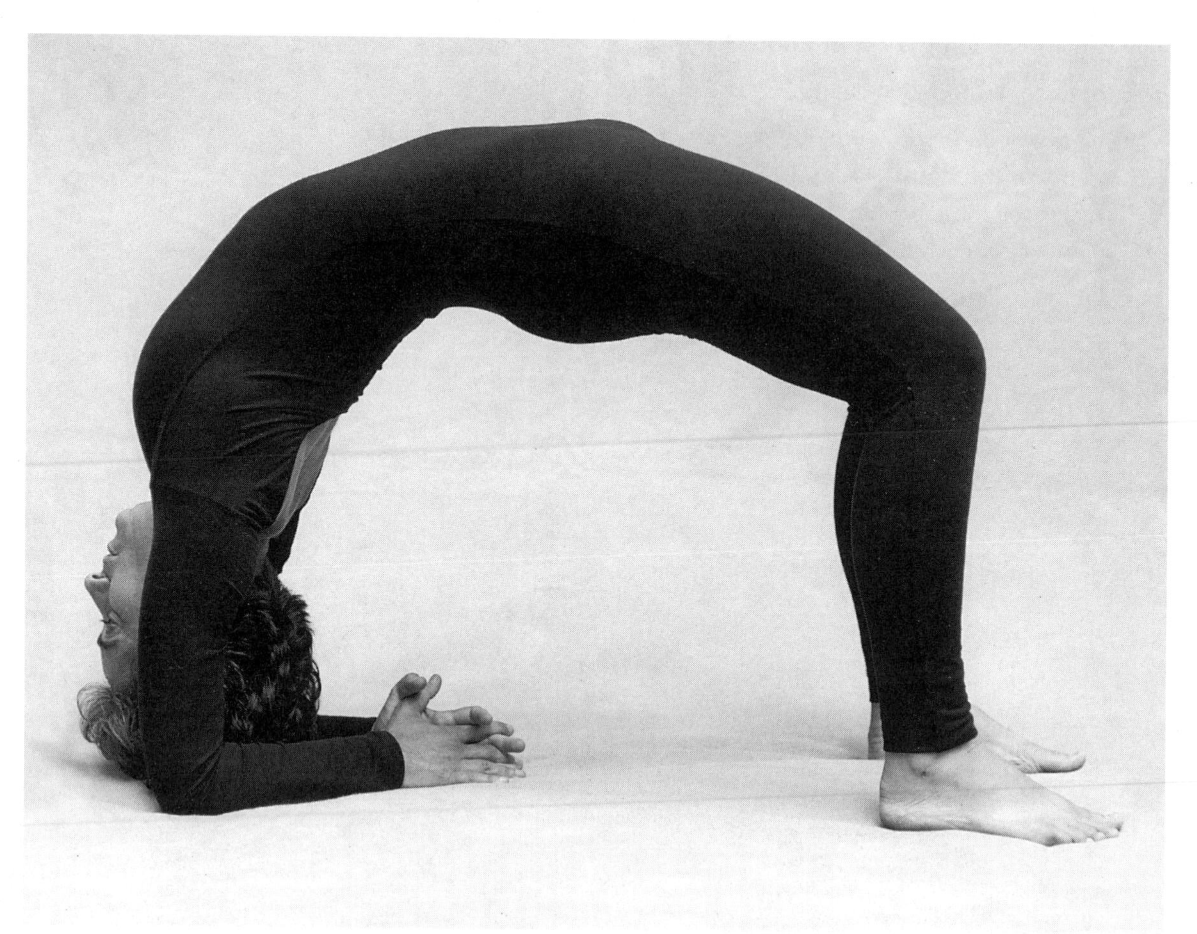

Head Balance Back Arch

CHAPTER 12

Backbends

BACKBENDS ARE DYNAMIC, energizing and joyous poses. They are extroverted and stimulating. The front of your body opens as your whole spine lengthens and expands, integrated and moving with your breath.

Backbends stimulate the nervous system and powerfully move the upper body. This new movement expands breathing capacity by allowing the back of the rib cage to move freely with the breath. The heart centre or chakra opens, bringing a powerful emotional release. Because they are so energizing, it is better to do backbends early in the day. Some people have trouble sleeping if they do them later.

In order to do backbends well and safely, you will need to apply everything you have learned about breathing, being grounded and lengthening your spine. There should be no pain or discomfort in your lower back during or after backbends. The back of the waist and the neck bend backward easily, and the upper back is usually stiff and unmoving. If you do backbends without consciously moving your whole spine, you can injure yourself. Done poorly, backbends can damage your back and make you feel frenzied, anxious and irritable.

To keep the back of your waist long in backbends, you will need flexibility in the front of your thighs. Practise the Standing Warrior Pose and Lunge Pose to develop this elasticity. The strong pelvic tilt, which is essential in backbends, stabilizes the lower back and benefits people with lower back problems. Cobra Pose is especially beneficial for people with herniated disks.

Guidelines

- *In preparing for any of the backbends, take a long time breathing, taking your belly back until you feel your spine lengthen.*
- *Let your buttocks release.*
  Wait until you can feel movement in your tailbone, sitting bones and back thighs as you breathe. This connection is exactly the same as when you are sitting. The awareness is the same although the positions and action are different.
- *When you can feel this release and extension, draw your tailbone and sitting bones under, using your back thighs more than your buttock muscles.*
  The thigh muscles are connected to the sitting bones. Lengthening your back thighs away from your pelvis will draw your pelvis under. Make sure that the back of your pelvis remains wide. Just contracting your buttocks to tilt your pelvis adds tension to muscles which are generally already under stress.
- *Follow the backbends with forward bends to lengthen your lower back, and to correct any accidental compression.*
  Forward bends are calming, introverted poses which counter-balance the stimulating effect of the backbends.
- *Do some twists after the forward bends.*
  Twists are corrective poses for misalignment of the spine. (Chiropractors frequently use twists to adjust the spine.) Since there are usually slight imbalances in your spine which can be aggravated in backbends, the twist at the end is a good precaution.

Bridge and Wheel Poses

These are basic backbends. In my opinion, they are the simplest and the safest of all of the backbends. They are a continuation of the Lying Release Pose that you practised at the very beginning to learn to deepen your breath.

Bridge Pose, Pelvic Tilt (Setu Bandha Sarvangasana)

Take a long time practising the Bridge Pose. When the action is clear and easy, you will be ready to start Wheel Pose. This is a classic exercise for people with lower back problems.

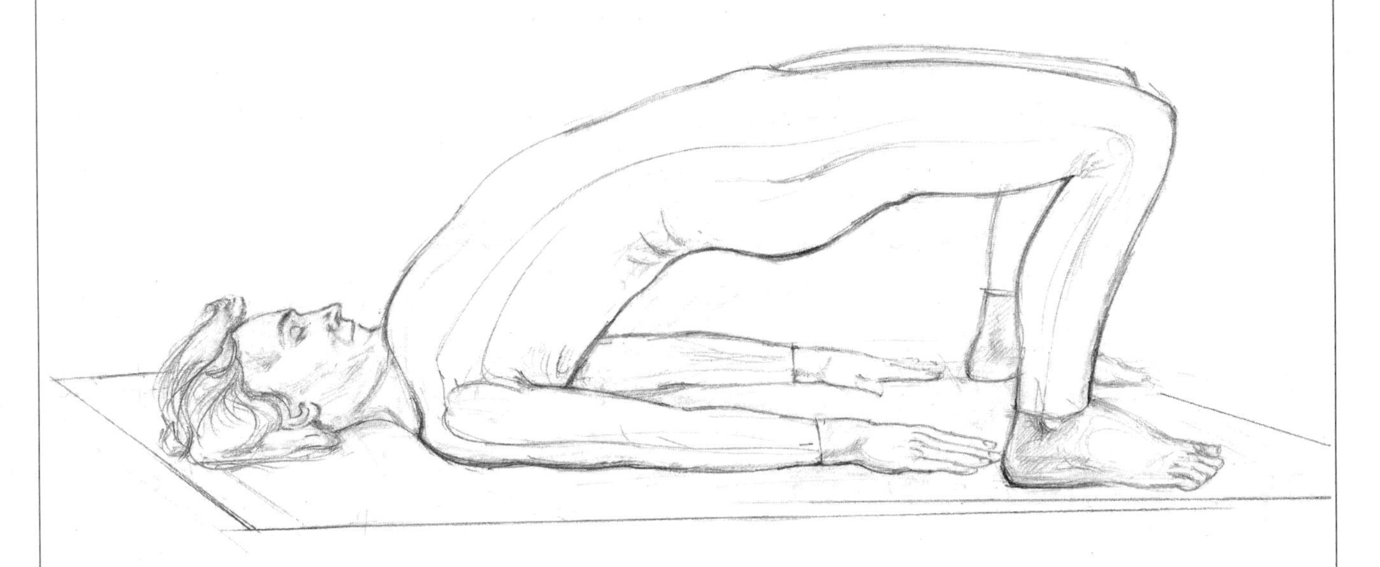

- Start by lying on your back with your knees bent and feet on the floor. Place your feet hip-width apart and as close to your sitting bones as possible. In this position, the back of your waist should be in contact with the floor.
- Be conscious of the contact of your feet with the floor. As you exhale and the back of your waist rests back, release the soles of your feet into the floor.

- Deepen your breath by drawing your abdominal wall further and further back as you exhale, pressing the back of your waist into the floor. Think of your breath moving right back to massage the front of your spine. When your spine releases you will feel a ripple go through your body. Your head and neck will move by themselves. This is the beginning of the "wave."
- When you feel your spine lengthening with your breath, press down with your feet to rock your pelvis slightly. Notice that the back of your waist goes down even more and that your tailbone and sitting bones curl up. Your buttocks are pulled under *as a result* of the action of your feet. There is a scooping movement of your pelvis and your hip bones roll toward you.
- Relax as you inhale.
- As the action and movement become familiar, gradually make the scoops bigger so that your pelvis lifts off the floor.
- Come up as far as you can, with the back of your waist resting back.
- Eventually you will be up on your shoulders in Bridge Pose.
- Stay in the pose, breathing and lengthening.
- Exhaling, roll down slowly, lengthening your spine as you come down.

You can tell when the back of your waist is shortened, because your belly and lower ribs push up to the ceiling. When this happens, come back down to the floor and start again.

If your knees splay out as you come up, your lower back and pelvis are tightening and narrowing. If necessary, you can loop a belt around your legs above your knees to keep them hip-width apart.

When you are finished the Bridge Pose, hug your knees to your chest (Little Boat Pose) to release and lengthen your lower back. (If you have done the backbend well, your back will be long and you won't need this release, but it is a lovely counterpose and a good precaution.)

Wheel (Urdhva Dhanurasana)

Wheel Pose continues from the Bridge Pose and is closely connected to the standing poses because your feet are the roots. Wheel Pose also prepares you for dropping back from standing. Coming up into the full backbend from the floor requires a combination of absolute solidity of your feet on the floor, and the elongation of your entire spine. The action of the pose is initiated by your feet. Your buttocks and back thighs will become strong and active as a result of the action of your feet, but do not initiate the movement. It is essential to be strong and grounded in the pose to support your spine and remain centred through the emotional release as your chest opens.

The stability of the lower body allows your upper back and shoulders to release. This release enables you to come up into the pose freely and easily. You may find that you are not able to come all the way up at first. Be patient. It can take a long time for your upper body to let go. Come as far as you can with ease. Remember, when you are ready to do a pose it takes very little effort. Pushing to get up before you are ready is liable to cause injuries and makes the pose more difficult.

It is very common for people to breathe and release beautifully while they are lying on the floor and then become tense the minute they decide to come up. As a result, their backs tighten and their feet turn out. If this happens, come down and start again. You must learn to remain relaxed and conscious as you come up into Wheel.

You may feel as if you need stronger arms to do the pose. However, trying to push with your arms will only tighten your shoulders and block the movement. Drop your solar plexus and diaphragm back as you exhale to release your upper back and shoulders. Eventually you will be able to straighten your arms. When you discover the "wave" and go up with the release of your spine and breath, you will be amazed at the ease and joy of the position.

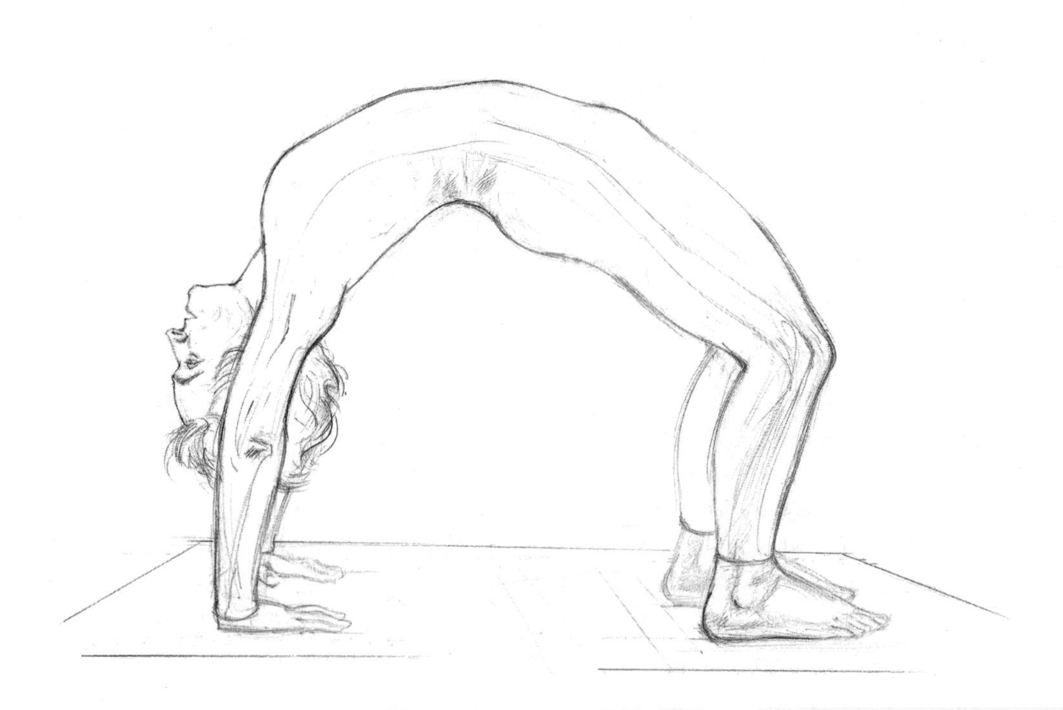

- Start in Bridge Pose, but place your hands on the floor behind your shoulders with your fingers pointing toward your toes.
- When your whole body has lifted off the floor, the weight will shift onto your hands. At that point, stretch your arms from your wrists to complete the pose.
- Remain in the pose for as long as you can continue to breathe and lengthen. Struggling to push higher is futile. When you can release while in the pose, you will be able to come up further by pressing down with your wrists and heels as you exhale.
- When you are comfortable in the pose, try lifting your head to lengthen your neck and release your upper back. When you drop your head again, shake your neck loose to release any tension.
- Bend your elbows to come down slowly, exhaling. Keep your feet securely planted until you are resting on the floor.
- When you are finished, hug your knees to your chest.

Prone Backbends

The prone backbends, Head Up Dog Pose, Cobra and Bow, are often taught as introductory poses. However, I think they are among the most difficult to do without compressing the back of the waist. I don't know why, but it is very hard to feel your breath moving down to your tailbone, sitting bones and back thighs when you are lying on your stomach. This lack of sensation makes you more likely to do the poses with contraction and muscular effort.

Learning to lift our heads while lying on our stomach is one of the very first movements that we discover. Babies can do Cobra brilliantly. If you are around a baby of six to nine months, try supporting its pelvis and wait for it to lengthen and lift. It is quite wonderful to watch, and teaches us that the wave of elongation of the spine is actually in our bodies, naturally and instinctively. We do not have to create it, but rather clear away the layers of tension which have blocked it.

Head Up Dog Pose (Urdhva Mukha Svanasana)

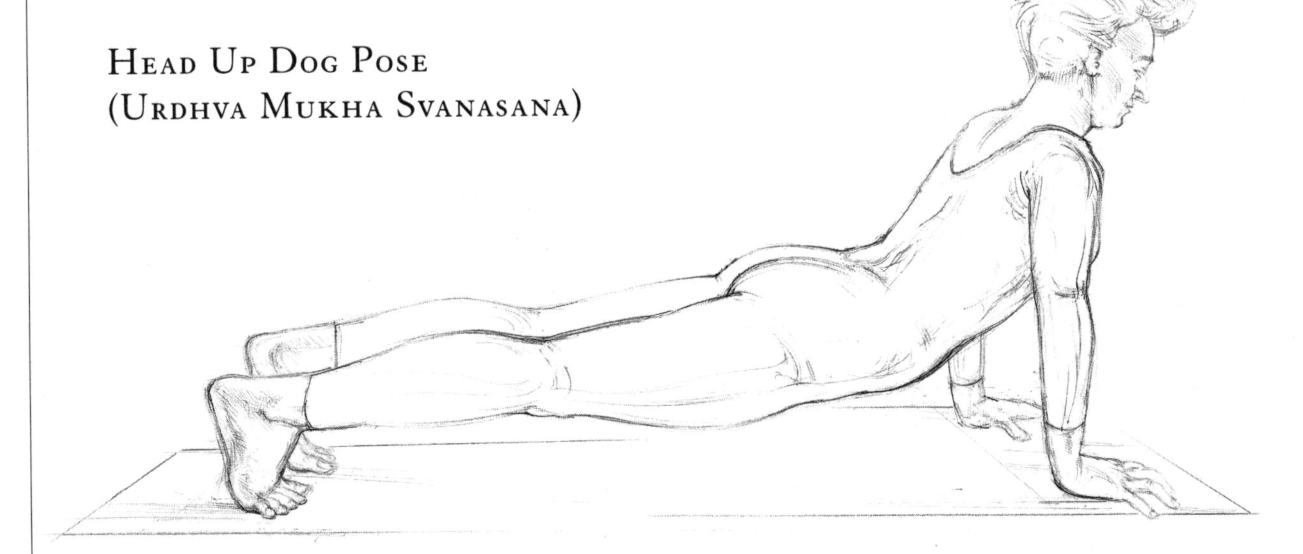

Before you start to come up, practise lying on your stomach feeling the movement of your exhalation down your back and into your legs. If you can take your hands into Prayer Position behind your back, it will help you to feel for movement in the back of your rib cage as you breathe.

In Sun Salutation, Head Up Dog Pose or Cobra follow from Child's Pose and Cat Pose. You can practise them like that or you can begin from the floor as described on the next page.

- Begin by lying on your stomach with your hands on the floor beside your ribs (as if you are going to do a push-up).
- Relax as you inhale, feeling the expansion of the back of your rib cage as you breathe.
- Focus on the movement of your breath down the back of your spine and through the back of your legs to your heels.
- Follow your exhalation down your back until you can feel your tailbone lengthen away. Then, draw your tailbone and sitting bones under. If you are doing the pose correctly, your back thighs will feel long and strong, and the back of your pelvis will broaden.
- At the end of your exhalation, when your spine has lengthened and your back thighs are strong, press down with your wrists to lift your upper body.
- When your spine is long and arching, use a stronger pressure on your wrists to bring your whole body off the floor.
- Drop your shoulders and shoulder blades. It is more important to have your shoulders low and wide than to have your arms straight.
- In the pose, continue to lengthen your spine as you exhale and press down with your wrists, stretching the back of your legs.
- When you are ready, exhale, and bend your elbows to come down.

This pose is classically done with the head bent back so you are looking at the ceiling. I rarely teach it this way because it is easy to damage your neck. To protect your neck, keep the back of your head in line with your upper back, so your neck follows the movement of your upper back in a smooth, even curve.

Cobra (Bhujangasana)

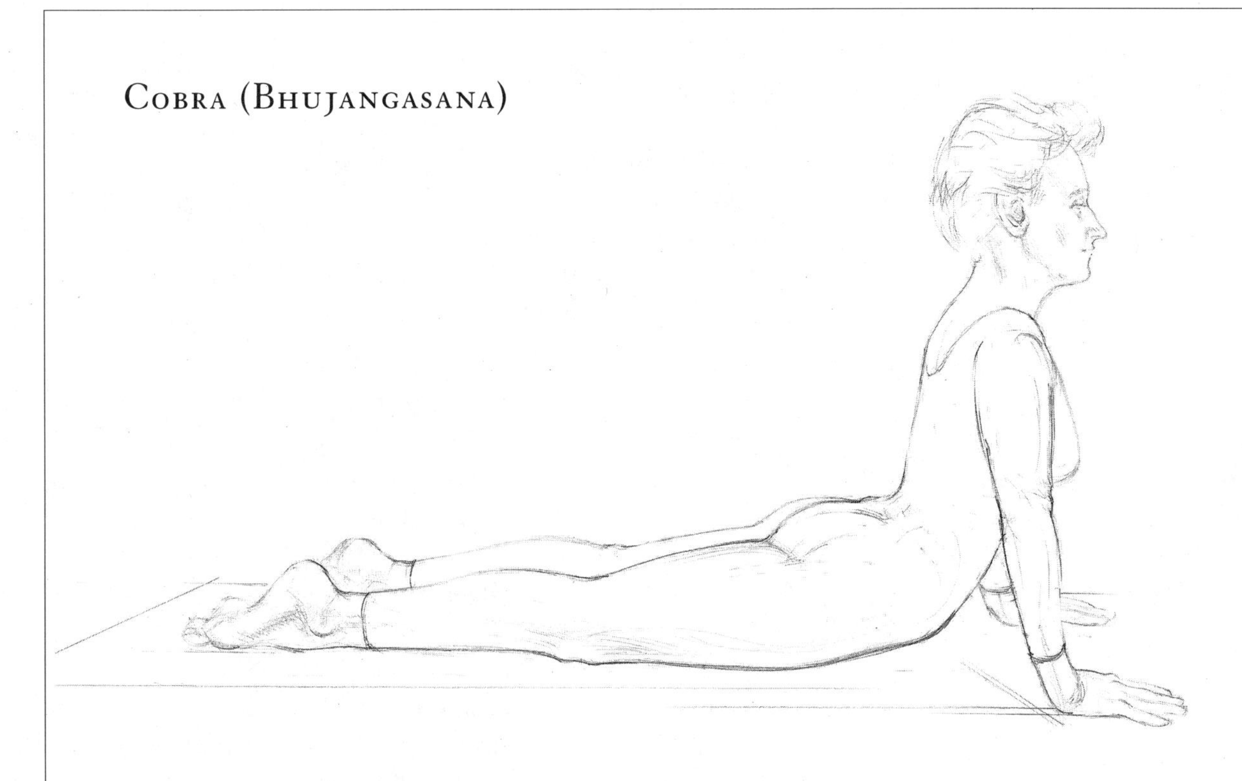

This pose is similar to Head Up Dog Pose except that the legs and pubic bone remain on the floor as the upper body lifts. You are much more likely to compress your lower back unless you are very careful, and can already do Head Up Dog Pose easily and well.

Physiotherapists use Cobra as an exercise for people with weak lower backs and herniated (slipped) disks to strengthen the back muscles and give greater support to a weak structure. The result is a band of strong muscle at the back of the waist which acts as a back brace, often relieving acute and chronic pain. However, our goal is an integrated action of the whole spine which brings span and freedom as well as strength.

Bow Pose (Dhanurasana)

Bow Pose is good for opening the upper chest and the front of the shoulders. Catching your feet creates a very nice connection through your body and integrates the posture. However, it is easy to compress your back in this pose. Only practise it when you are able to lengthen your spine with your breath, while lying on your stomach.

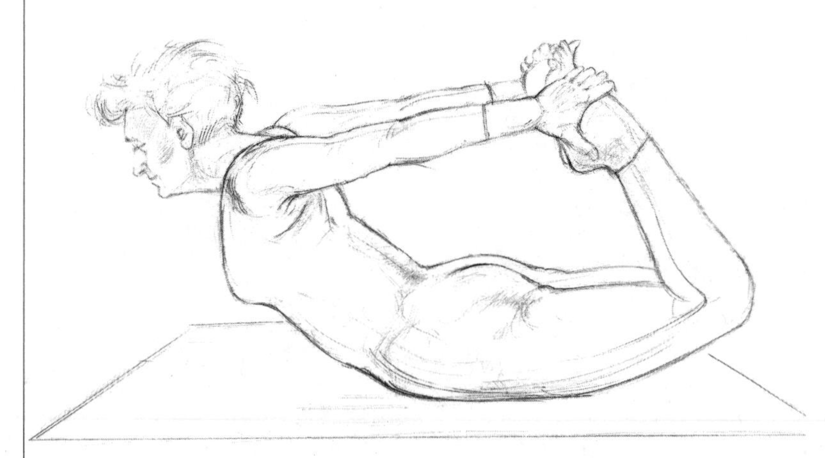

- Start by lying on your stomach.
- Reach back and catch your ankles.
- Follow your exhalation down your back until you can feel your tailbone lengthen away. Then, draw your tailbone and sitting bones under. If you are doing the pose correctly, your back thighs will feel long and strong, and the back of your pelvis will broaden.
- To come up, stretch your feet away from you.
- Let your head follow the movement of your spine.
- Relax your elbows and feel the back of your rib cage widen as you inhale.
- Continue in the pose as long as you can lengthen your spine with your breath, and then relax and come down.

Variations

You can create variations in Bow Pose by doing one side at a time, or by stretching diagonally (right arm, left leg). You can also lie on your side in the pose, opening the upper chest.

- To intensify the pose, stretch your arms over your head to catch your feet. You will probably need to use a belt. This version of the pose is an intense stretch of the shoulders and upper body, but is actually safer for the lower back.

Dropping into Backbends

In these poses, we start to explore the wave directly. You need to be very grounded, secure and relaxed in the poses for the release to take place. Otherwise, you are liable to tighten and compress out of fear as you move into them.

At first, these poses are intimidating because you cannot see the ground, and have no sense of the distance to drop. As they become familiar and you develop better control, they will become less frightening.

Bridge Pose from Shoulderstand (Setu Bandhasana from Sarvangasana)

Going into Bridge Pose from Shoulderstand is the easiest dropping pose (see photograph on p. 30). You can start leading with one leg until you have the confidence and control to drop back with your legs together.

If your upper back is stiff, you will need to let your elbows slide apart as you drop, to relieve the pressure on your wrists. You should be on a blanket rather than on a sticky mat, so your arms can slide apart easily. If you are using a belt around your arms in Shoulderstand, take it off before you start to drop back.

This backbend is a good counterbalance to Shoulderstand since it frees the upper chest and throat.

The action of dropping back is a continuation of the movement of Shoulderstand itself. Remain passive as you inhale. As you exhale, press down with your elbows to create lift in the pose. Wait until you feel the wave of your breath through your spine. This movement will lengthen the back of your waist and lift your knees up. Practise in this position until your body is in a straight line from your shoulders to your knees. It is much more difficult to be vertical in Shoulderstand when your knees are bent than when they are straight.

As you start to arch back, remember that in this pose, like all backbends, the bend is in the upper back and not in the waist. In an optimal Shoulderstand, your hands would be touching your shoulder blades, providing a fulcrum for the bend.

- From Shoulderstand bend your knees so they are pointing up to the ceiling and your feet drop behind you.
- Lengthen your spine as you exhale, lifting your knees toward the ceiling.
- Gradually start to drop back. Continue to lengthen your spine with each breath.
- Continue breathing and lengthening for as long as you can before finally allowing your feet to drop to the floor. Eventually you will be able to control the movement all the way down.
- In Bridge Pose, press down with your heels as you exhale to lengthen your spine and lift your pelvis.
- To come out of the pose, let your elbows slide out, then lower your back to the floor or jump back into Shoulderstand.

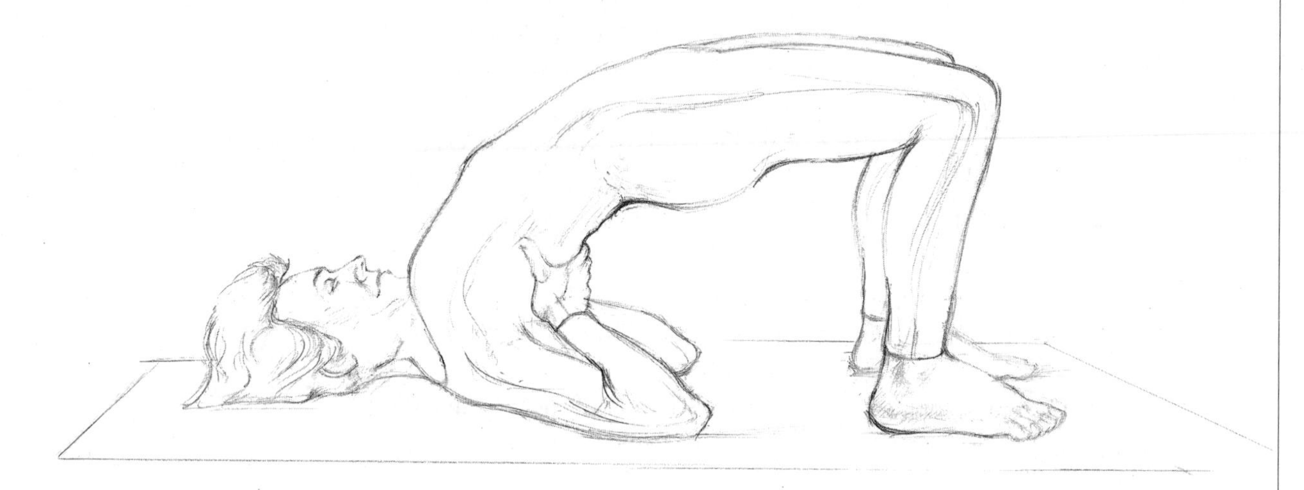

Variation

Single Leg Bridge Pose (Eka Pada Setu Bandhasana)
This variation on Bridge Pose is a wonderful opening of the whole front of the body.

- From Bridge, bend one knee to your chest. The foot on the floor needs to be secure and stable, and your knee in line with the foot.
- Exhaling, press down on the floor with your heel, and straighten the bent leg, so the foot is pointing up to the ceiling.
- To come down, exhale, bend your knee back to your chest, and then put the foot on the floor.
- Repeat on the other side.

Head Balance Back Arch (Dwi Pada Viparita Dandasana)

Before you start to practise dropping back from Headstand, you need to be stable in Headstand, able to do Wheel with ease, and confident dropping back from Shoulderstand.

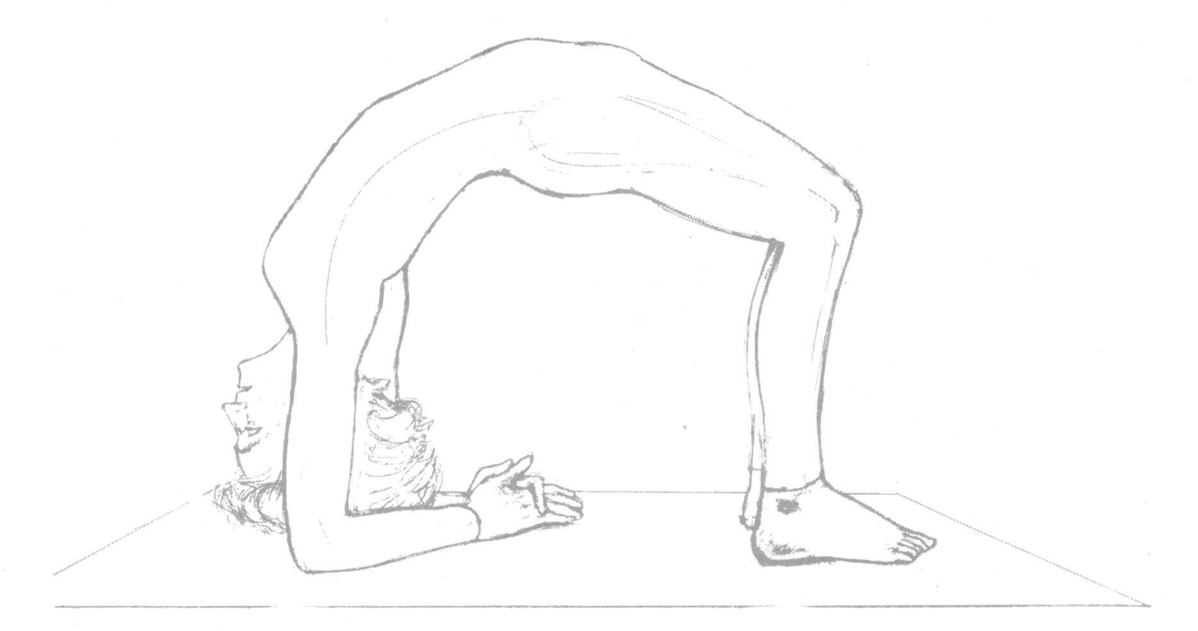

From Wheel

The pose is a more intense opening of the shoulders and upper back than Wheel.

- From Wheel, bend your elbows and come down until your head is resting on the floor.
- Switch your arms into Headstand position.
- In Head Balance Back Arch, press down with your elbows as you exhale, and lift your head off the floor.
- Plant your heels to lift your hips and lengthen your spine.
- To come down, bend your knees and slowly roll down.

Dropping Back from Headstand

The fear at the beginning of this pose is similar to Shoulderstand because you cannot see the ground and have no sense of the distance to drop. You can start by dropping onto a table or a bed, where the drop is slight, until you get used to the feeling. Or start about two feet away from a wall and practise dropping back to the wall. You can gradually move further and further from the wall and walk your feet down the wall until you are in the final pose. As always, once the pose becomes familiar, it will be less frightening.

The action is exactly the same as in Shoulderstand, and is a continuation of the movement of Headstand itself.

- From Headstand, bend your knees.
- As you exhale, press down with your elbows. Feel the wave of your breath through your spine, lengthening the back of your waist and lifting your knees up.
- Gradually start to drop back. Continue to lengthen your spine with each breath.
- Continue breathing and lengthening for as long as you can before finally allowing your feet to drop to the floor.

It is possible to control the movement all the way down and to spring back into Headstand.

Variation

Single Leg Variation (Eka Pada Viparita Dandasana)
This pose is a wonderful opening of the whole front of the body. It is a striking and beautiful pose.

- From Head Balance Back Arch, bend one knee to your chest.
- Exhaling, press down on the floor with your heel, and straighten the bent leg, so your foot is pointing up to the ceiling. The foot on the floor needs to be secure and stable, with your knee in line with the foot.
- To come down, exhale, bend your knee back to your chest, and then put your foot on the floor.
- Repeat on the other side.

Wheel from Standing

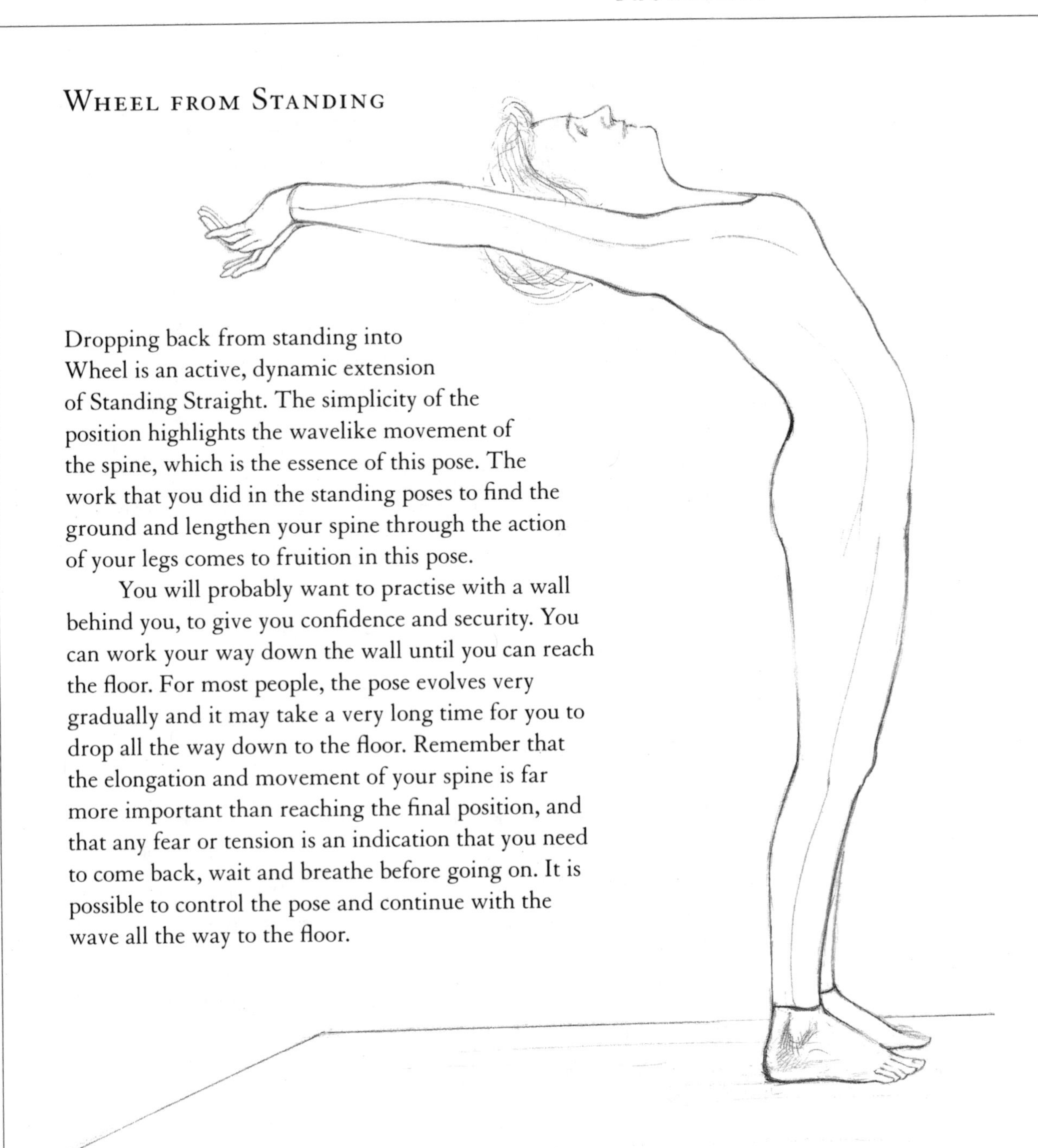

Dropping back from standing into Wheel is an active, dynamic extension of Standing Straight. The simplicity of the position highlights the wavelike movement of the spine, which is the essence of this pose. The work that you did in the standing poses to find the ground and lengthen your spine through the action of your legs comes to fruition in this pose.

You will probably want to practise with a wall behind you, to give you confidence and security. You can work your way down the wall until you can reach the floor. For most people, the pose evolves very gradually and it may take a very long time for you to drop all the way down to the floor. Remember that the elongation and movement of your spine is far more important than reaching the final position, and that any fear or tension is an indication that you need to come back, wait and breathe before going on. It is possible to control the pose and continue with the wave all the way to the floor.

- Start by standing straight, with your arms up over your head. Leave your shoulders dropped and your arms loose and free.
- Take time to ground and drop weight from the back of your waist, down the back of your legs to your heels. Wait until you feel that your lower body from the waist down is grounded and strong and that your upper body is light and free.
- On an exhalation, press your heels into the floor. The movement rebounds from the ground like a ball bouncing. Stretch your ankles, knees and then your back thighs. The more you stretch your legs, the more your spine will lengthen and the more powerful the "wave" will be.
- Let the wave carry your upper body up.
- When your upper back lengthens and lifts, stretch your arms and let your head go back, following the movement of your spine.
- As you inhale, bring your head forward again and let your knees bend slightly.
- When you understand the action of your legs and pelvis, your upper back will release and lengthen spontaneously. Continue practising this way until you can feel the elongation of your body from your heels to the crown of your head. Then, start to bend back.
- As you start to go back in the pose, shift your pelvis forward to counterbalance the weight of your body. But keep the back of your waist long and your heels absolutely rooted.
- As you go back, continue to expand and explore the wave-motion. See how long you can continue breathing and lengthening.
- Come up on an exhalation, pressing down strongly with your feet.

Be careful to keep your tailbone and sitting bones pulled down through the entire exhalation. Use the strength of your back thighs to pull the back of your pelvis down strongly, otherwise the back of your waist will tend to shorten as your upper back lengthens and lifts.

Try practising with your hands behind your back in Prayer Position, so you can be sure there is movement in your upper back.

Be careful when you take your head back, because it is easy to compress the back of your neck. There is a balanced place in which both the front and back of the neck are free, and the curve of your neck follows from the movement of your upper back.

Camel Pose (Ustrasana) and Pigeon Pose (Kapotasana)

These poses are similar to Wheel from standing, except that you start with kneeling, and the roots are in the knees. Some people find it easier and less frightening to work from the kneeling position, since they are closer to the ground.

Your back thighs need to be strong and anchored, since they do not have the support of the heels. Keep your thighs as vertical as you can while you go back. The stretch on your front thighs will be intense.

- In Camel Pose, drop your arms back from your shoulders to catch your heels. Arch your head back only when your upper back is flexible and you can keep the back of your neck long.

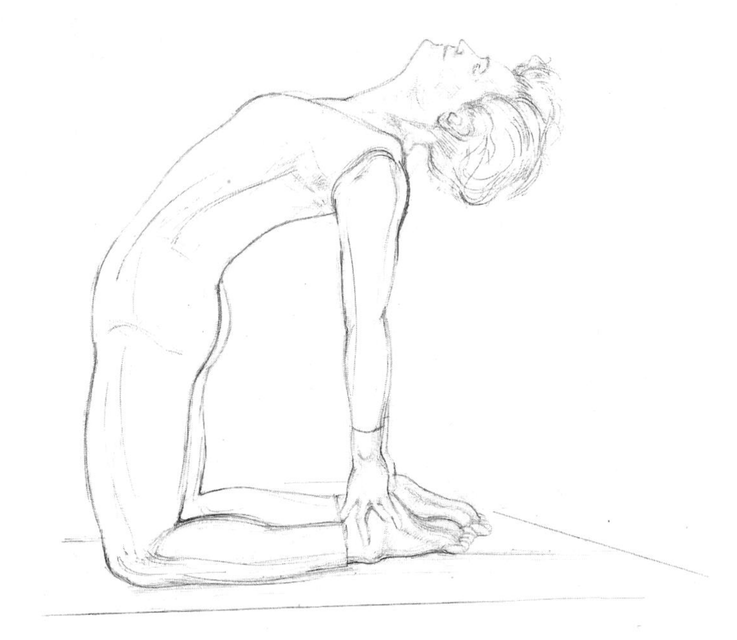

- In Pigeon Pose, take your arms over your head. When you can put your hands on the floor, bend your elbows, so your arms will be in a loose Headstand position. This is a very intense backbend.

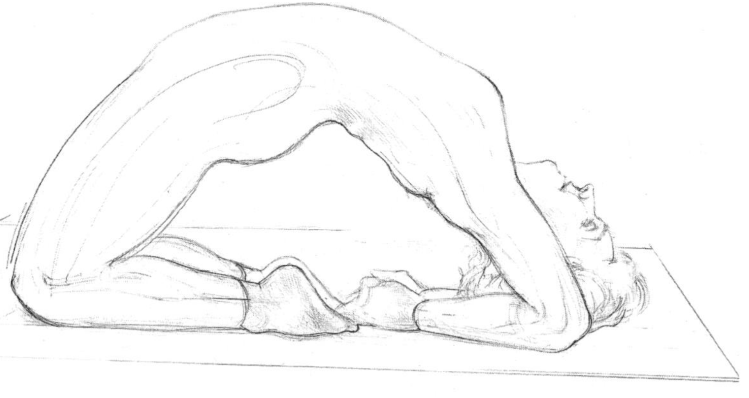

Other Advanced Backbends

Try these poses when you are ready for a more powerful extension and release. The cautions in these poses are the same as any other backbends, namely that the back of your waist and neck must be long and lengthening, and your upper back should move freely and easily.

One Leg King Pigeon Poses (Eka Pada Raja Kapotasana)

This name is given to a series of variations on Pigeon Pose, in which one leg is bent as in the basic sitting poses and one leg is stretched back.

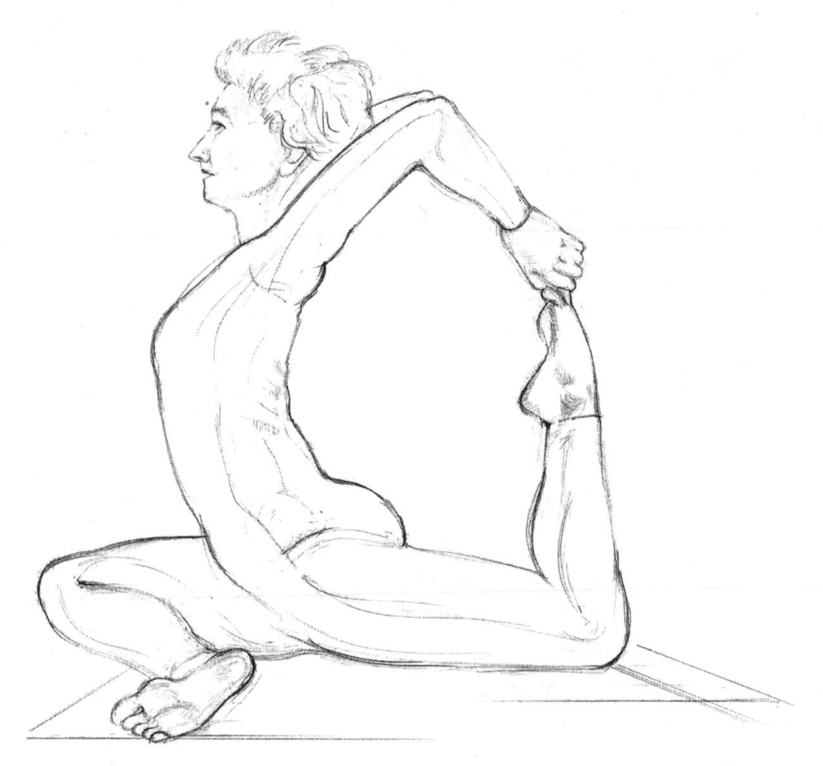

The full poses are powerful backbends which should only be attempted by experienced students; however, the Lunge Pose and the Pigeon Preparation Stretch are basic and safe preparations. Start to move more deeply into these poses only when you have the flexibility in the hips and shoulders, and the length in the lower back to do so safely. The instructions for all of the positions is the same. The position of your front leg will vary.

- Start in the preparation position.
- Keeping your hands on the floor in front of you for balance, come up lengthening your spine with your breath as you do in Cobra.
- When your body is upright, bend your back leg and catch your foot with one hand.
- When you are ready, reach back and catch your foot with the other hand.
- Focus on the movement of your breath down the back of your spine and through the back of your legs.
- When your breath reaches your sitting bones and tailbone, draw them under. Activate your back thighs to anchor your pelvis, leaving your sacrum wide and free. The movement of your spine must come entirely from your breath, your back thighs and your spine, since you do not have the support of your arms as you did in Cobra.
- As your spine lengthens and your upper back releases, stretch your back foot away from you.
- When your upper back is free and lifted, take your head back, keeping the back of your neck long.
- Continue to breathe, drop and lengthen while you are in the pose.
- Release and repeat on the other side.

When you are starting, catch your foot as in Bow Pose. For a more intense stretch, reach over your head to catch your foot. If you are unable to catch your foot, use a belt. The stretch on the front thigh of your back leg will increase considerably.

Variation I

- The front leg is bent as in Half Bound Angle Pose as illustrated.

Variation II

- The front leg is bent back as in Half Hero's Pose, and rests partially under the buttock (p.192).

Variation III

- The front leg remains in the Lunge Position.

Splits (Hanumanasana)

This pose stretches the front and back thighs intensely.

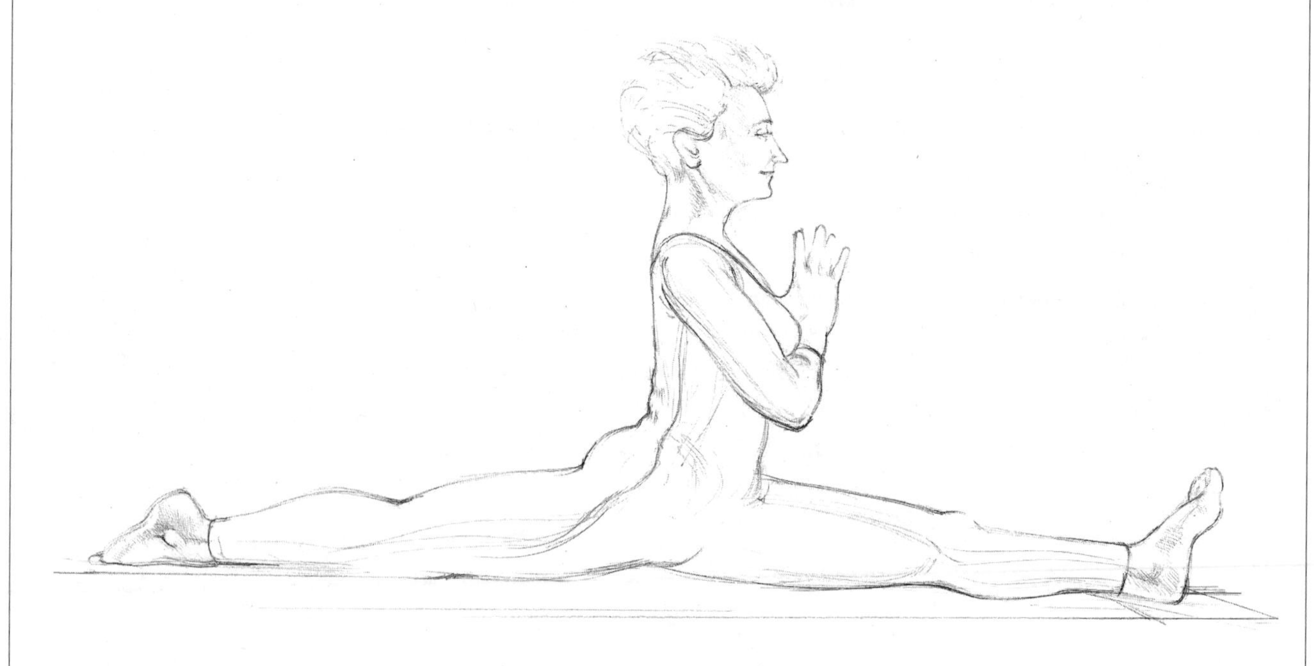

- Start in the Lunge Pose.
- Using your hands for balance and support, slowly straighten your front leg out in front of you.
- As you exhale, drop your pelvis toward the floor.
- When your front leg is straight and you are sitting on the floor, bring your hands into Prayer Position.
- Repeat on the other side.

The Dancer (Natarajasana)

This pose is both a backbend and a standing balance. The action is the same as Wheel from standing.

- Start by standing straight.
- Bend one knee and catch your foot behind you.
- Let the weight of the bent leg drop from your pelvis, stretching your front thigh.
- Remain passive as you inhale. As you exhale, drop your awareness into your foot, then stretch your standing leg to lengthen your spine.
- As your upper back releases, let your shoulders drop.
- Keeping the back of your waist long and your pelvis vertical, gradually stretch your back foot away from you at the end of your exhalation.
- When you are able to balance, bring your other arm up to catch your foot. Keep your arms loose and relaxed.
- Repeat on the other side.

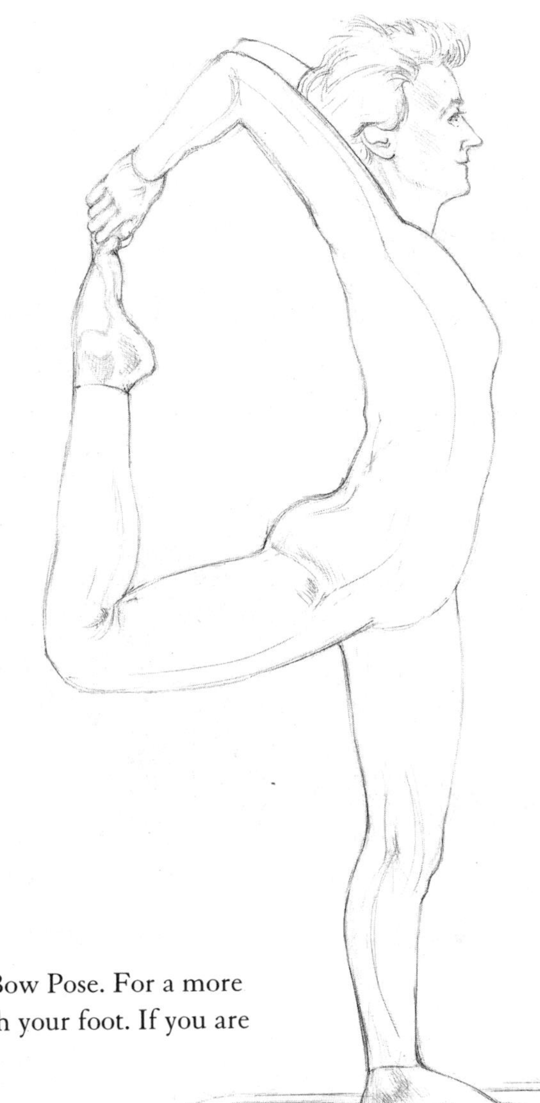

When you start, catch your foot as in Bow Pose. For a more intense stretch, reach over your head to catch your foot. If you are unable to catch your foot, use a belt.

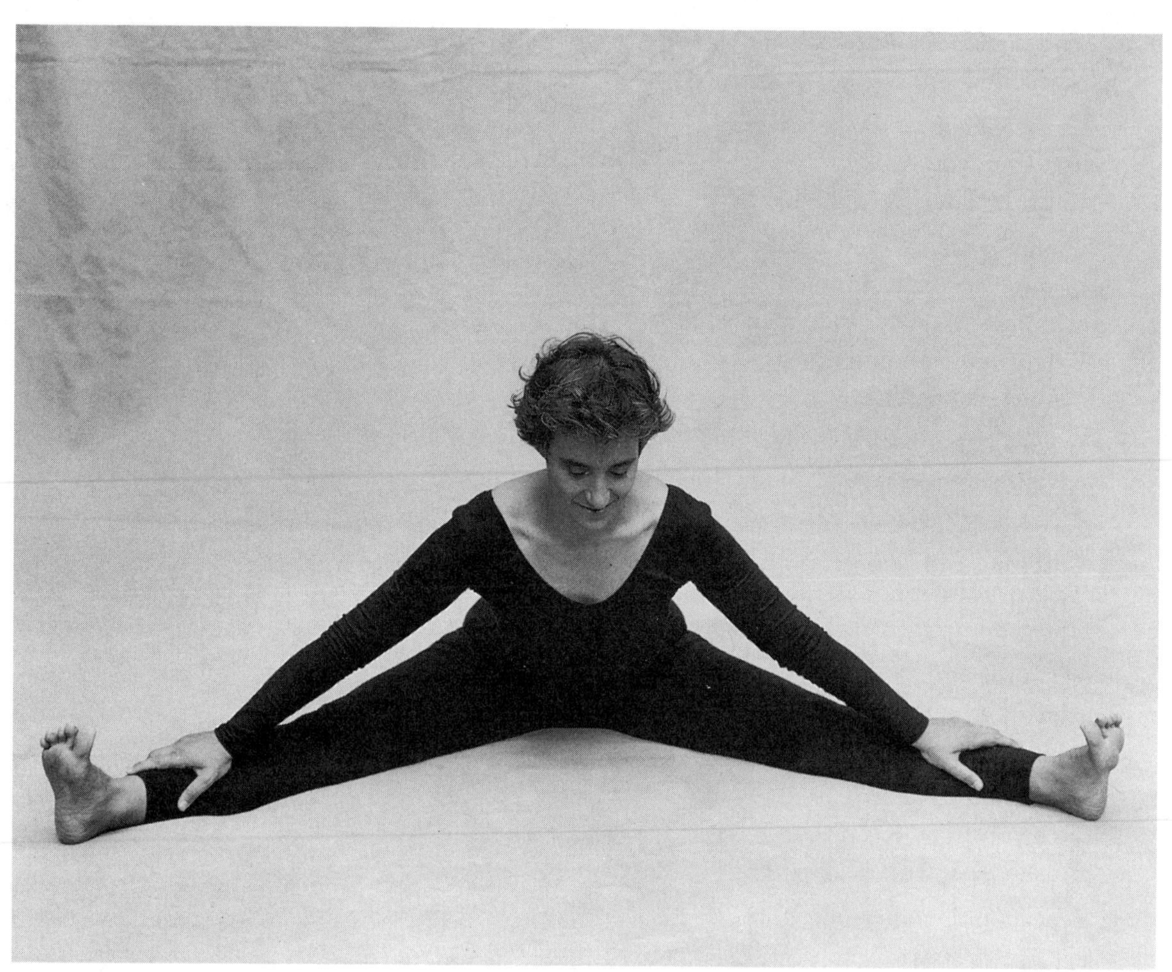

Wide Angle Pose

CHAPTER 13

Sitting Poses and Forward Bends

LIKE THE STANDING POSES, sitting poses promote freedom and balance in the hips and pelvis, and flexibility in the legs, knees, ankles and feet. There are many sitting poses; as a group they use the hip joint in all possible ways. You can be very flexible in one type of movement and very stiff in another, or stiff on one side and flexible on the other. Some people have loose hip joints and can do the bent leg positions with ease, but are limited when they straighten their legs.

In all sitting poses, the roots are in the tailbone and sitting bones. The back of the pelvis drops to lengthen your spine. Sitting poses bring your pelvis into direct contact with the ground and will gradually develop the flexibility in your hips and pelvis that you need to sit straight easily, whether you are at a desk or for your breathing practice. Openness and support in your pelvis and lower back free your arms and shoulders, and reduce the chance of repetitive stress injuries.

Guidelines

Caution: Do not bend forward if you have a herniated (slipped) disc; it may feel good at the time but can damage you in the long run.

Pregnant women should not bend forward after the first trimester, since the forward movement may compress the uterus and put pressure on the baby.

You can bend forward in all of the sitting poses. Bending forward is calming, restorative and introverted. You can practise forward bends when you are ill or exhausted.

One of Vanda's favourite sayings is: "In this way of working we have infinite time, and no ambition." There are no poses where this is truer than in forward bends, especially for men. Unless you have unusually flexible hips, you will probably find progress in these poses extremely slow.

To develop flexibility in your hips and hamstrings, practise standing poses, Standing Forward Bends and Plough variations. You can stretch your legs while you are lying on the floor, or lie on your back with your legs up against a wall. In this position, you can spread your legs wide apart and let gravity stretch them for you, and then bend your knees and bring your feet together in the Bound Angle Pose.

The focus in forward bends is back and down — the opposite of what you would expect from looking at the poses. Focus on your breathing to find a quiet centre in the pose. Use the awareness of your breath to bring energy and movement to the postures. The forward bends open the back of your body, just like Child's Pose. Pay attention to your back as you breathe. Be aware of your back opening and filling as you inhale, releasing and lengthening as you exhale. Notice where you can feel movement and where you can't.

At first, you may need to lean backwards and support yourself with your arms. Focus dropping your weight down into your pelvis, rather than trying to *sit up straight*. When you can sit easily, bring your arms forward and rest your hands on your legs. As we discussed in the chapter on breathing, it takes time, patience and perseverance for your breath to reach the base of your pelvis and the large muscles of your thighs, which need to release to allow you to go forward. If you feel stuck, try Rapid Abdominal Breathing.

As you start to go forward, resist the temptation to pull with your arms. Let your arms and shoulders remain relaxed and passive. Every once in a while, gently shake your head and shoulders to keep your upper body loose and relaxed.

Once you can go forward easily, focus on lengthening your spine and broadening the back of your pelvis as you breathe. You can stay in the forward bends for a very long time, 5–10 minutes in each pose. Let your breath move through your entire body. Let your body lengthen forward. Let your legs release away from your hips as you exhale. The process of expansion, extension and elongation continues, especially when you are fully forward. There is never a final pose, and there is no limit to how much you can release and lengthen with your breath. Feel the wave of release moving through your spine. Let gravity take over as you surrender further and further to the ground.

To get a sense of the wave movement, practise the Cat Pose action while you are going forward. As you exhale, take your abdomen well back and make a big round shape with your back to release your spine and drop your pelvis. As your pelvis drops, you will be pulled back up toward sitting. Go with this pull. At the end of your exhalation, release your spine and drop forward. Relax and remain passive as you inhale.

Forward bends open and expand the back of the body. Be careful not to strain your knees or lower back when you practise extended forward bends. If your back gets tired, lie down and bend your knees to your chest between the poses. Use the pelvic tilt to counterbalance the forward bends, and to strengthen and stabilize your lower back.

Practise forward bends after backbends to lengthen your lower back, and stretch your buttocks and back thighs.

Simple Sitting Poses

Any of the simple poses described below can be used for breathing and meditation. Use the one(s) that you find most comfortable. You can go forward in any of them.

The last three, Wide Angle Pose, Bound Angle Pose, and Basic Sitting Forward Bend, are commonly done going forward, but you can use them for sitting and breathing as well.

Simple Crossed Legs (Sukhasana)

Sitting with your legs crossed is a comfortable position for beginning students. As you become more flexible, take your knees further apart, and bring your feet closer to your pelvis.

If your hips are very stiff, you can sit on a firm cushion or pile of blankets to allow your knees to drop. This will enable you to sit straight with ease. As you become more flexible, lower the support until you are able to sit on the floor.

Perfect Posture, Posture of the Adept (Siddhasana)

This pose is a classic pose for meditation, and is a preparation for Half Lotus. If you are using this pose for breathing practice, be sure to alternate the position of your legs.

- Bend your right leg and bring your right foot as close as possible to your pubic bone.
- Bend your left leg, and place your left foot on your right shin, so the left ankle rests on top of your right one.

Thunderbolt Pose (Vajrasana)

Thunderbolt Pose, sitting on your heels, is one of the easiest sitting poses. It gives a gentle stretch to the front thighs, the shins, the ankles and the top of the feet. It is easy to keep the pelvis vertical and the spine straight, so the upper body is relaxed and free. You can feel your sitting bones going down, as they drop over the back of your heels.

- Start by kneeling with your knees hip-width apart.
- Bend your knees and sit down on your heels.

If your heels tend to roll apart, loop a belt around them to bring them in line with each other. If you have stiff ankles or your feet cramp, put a rolled blanket under your ankles. If you have knee problems, you can put a rolled blanket on your heels to reduce the stretch on your knees.

Variation

Toes Turned Under

This pose intensely stretches the balls of the feet and the toes, and tones the soles of the feet. Some people find this position excruciating, while others are able to sit in it quite comfortably.

- Turn your toes under so the balls of your feet are on the floor.

Hero's Pose (Virasana)

Caution: Do not do this pose if you have torn the meniscus (cartilage) or ligaments of your inner knee.

Hero's Pose, sitting between the heels, is a more intense pose than simply kneeling. It stretches the front thighs and the joints of the legs more. Be careful to avoid any strain on your knees. Your thighs should be parallel.

- Start by kneeling with your knees hip-width apart, and your feet wider apart than your hips.
- Bend your knees and sit down between your heels.

If you are unable to sit with your hips on the floor, sit on the end of a folded blanket.

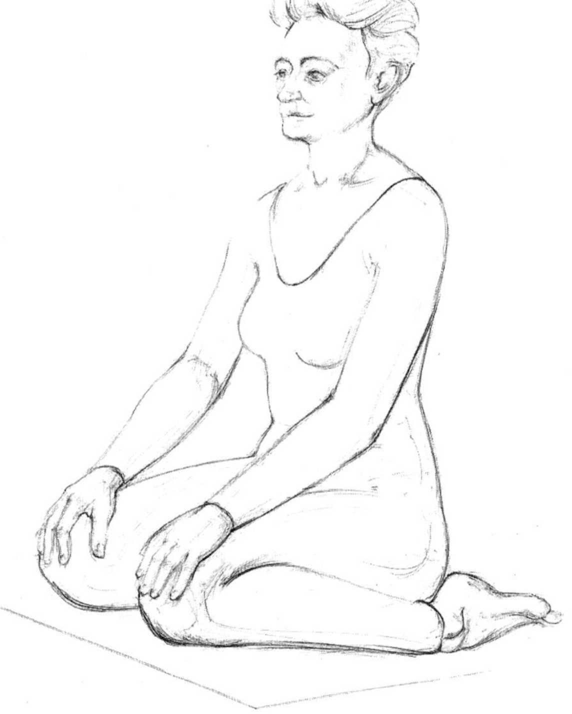

Cow's Head Pose (Gomukhasana)

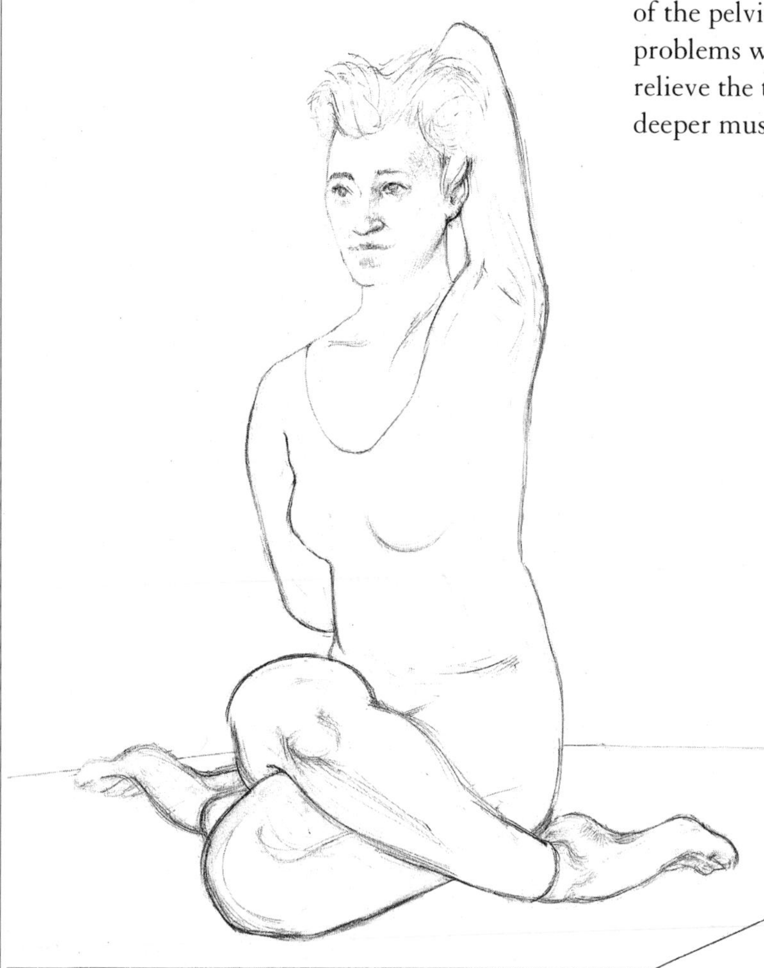

Cow's Head Pose stretches the back of the pelvis and the outer hips. If you have had problems with your lower back, this pose will relieve the tension in your buttocks and the deeper muscles at the back of your pelvis.

- Start by sitting with your legs straight.
- Cross your right leg over your left, so that your right knee is resting on your left one, and your right foot is beside your left hip.
- Bend your left leg, so that your left foot is beside your right hip.
- Then, take your right arm behind you and bend your elbow so the back of your hand is resting on your back.
- Exhaling, stretch your left arm up over your head, bend your elbow and drop your hand behind your neck.
- If you can, catch your hands. Leave your shoulders relaxed and dropped.
- Release and repeat on the other side.

If your hips are stiff, leave the bottom leg straight.

If you cannot catch your hands, use a belt. Be careful not to hunch your shoulders or twist your wrists to catch your hands.

Wide Angle Pose, Star Pose (Upavista Konasana)

This pose stretches the inner thighs and the hamstrings. If you have knee or ankle injuries which prevent you from doing any of the other sitting postures, you can use this pose for breathing and meditation.

- Sit with your legs wide apart.

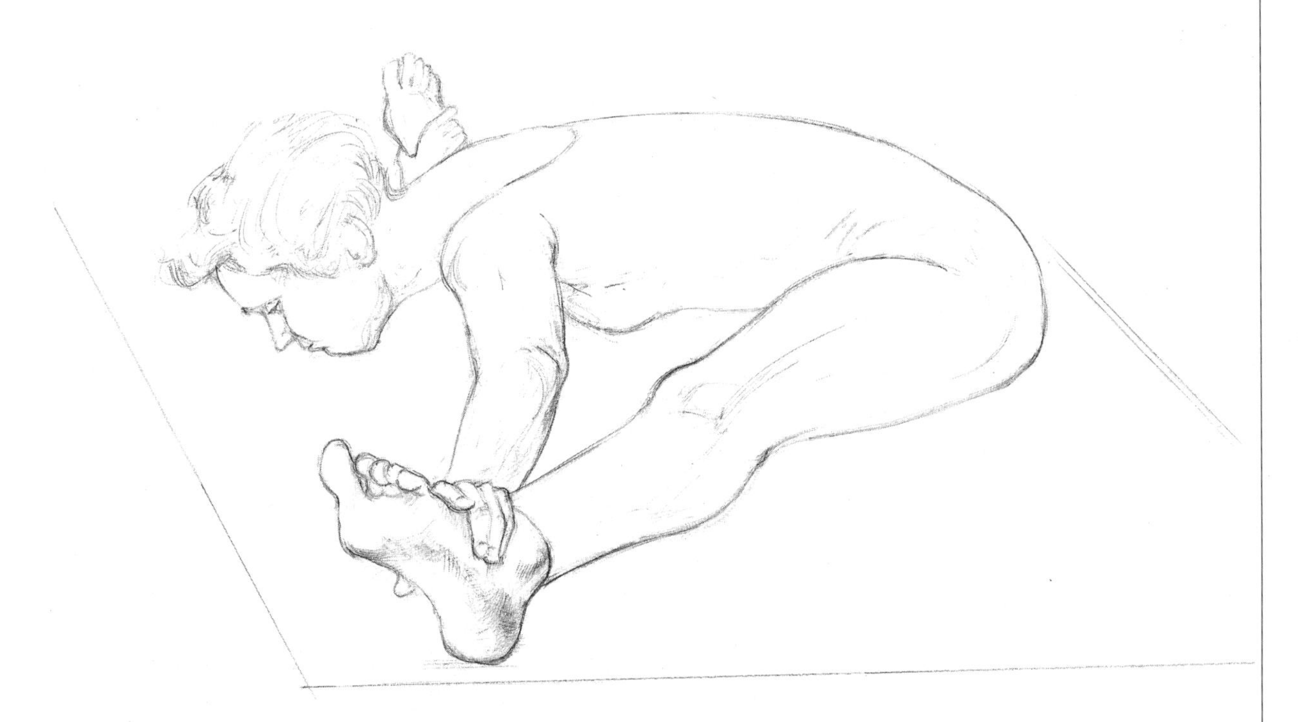

Variations

There are a number of ways to vary this pose.

- Turn to the right.
- Stretch forward over your right leg leaving your left sitting bone down.
- Stay forward as long as you are comfortable and then release and repeat on the other side.

Once you are able to stretch over each leg you can also turn as in the Half Bound Angle Twist (see p. 201).

Bound Angle Pose, Butterfly Pose, Cobbler's Pose (Baddha Konasana)

- Sit in the Wide Angle Pose.
- Bend your knees and bring the soles of your feet together.

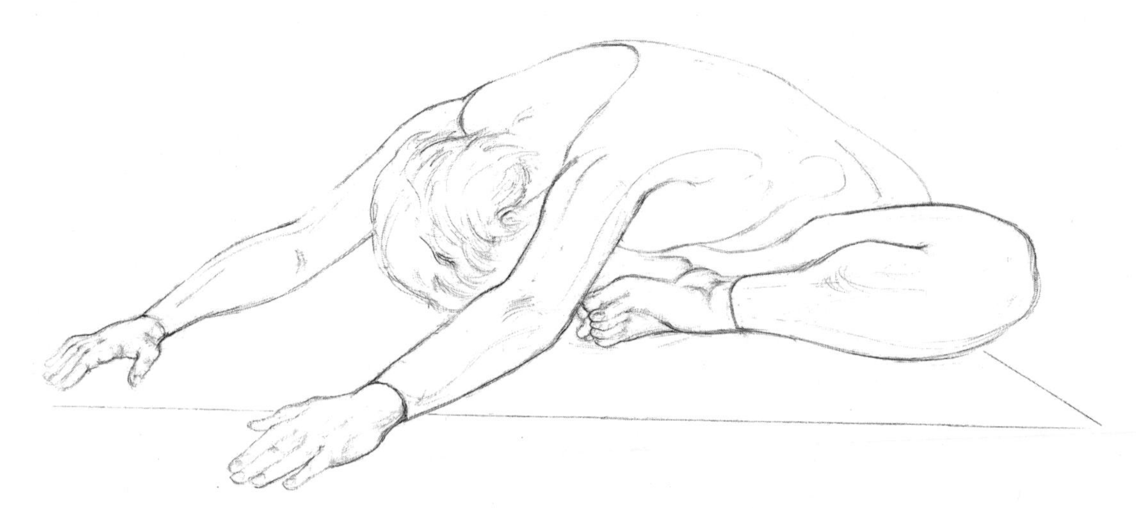

Adjust the position of your feet so you can sit comfortably with the weight forward of your sitting bones. As your hips become more flexible, bring your feet closer to your pubic bone. If your hips are very stiff, support your knees with rolled blankets or cushions. The support helps your hips and legs to release. When you remove it, your hips drop easily.

In this position, you can massage your feet so they open like a book, with the soles facing the ceiling. This gives you the stretch on your outer ankles, which you will need for Lotus Pose. It also allows your knees to drop.

Both Wide Angle Pose and Bound Angle Pose open the interior pelvis. They are classic pre-natal exercises and are good for menstrual or bladder problems.

Lotus Pose (Padmasana)

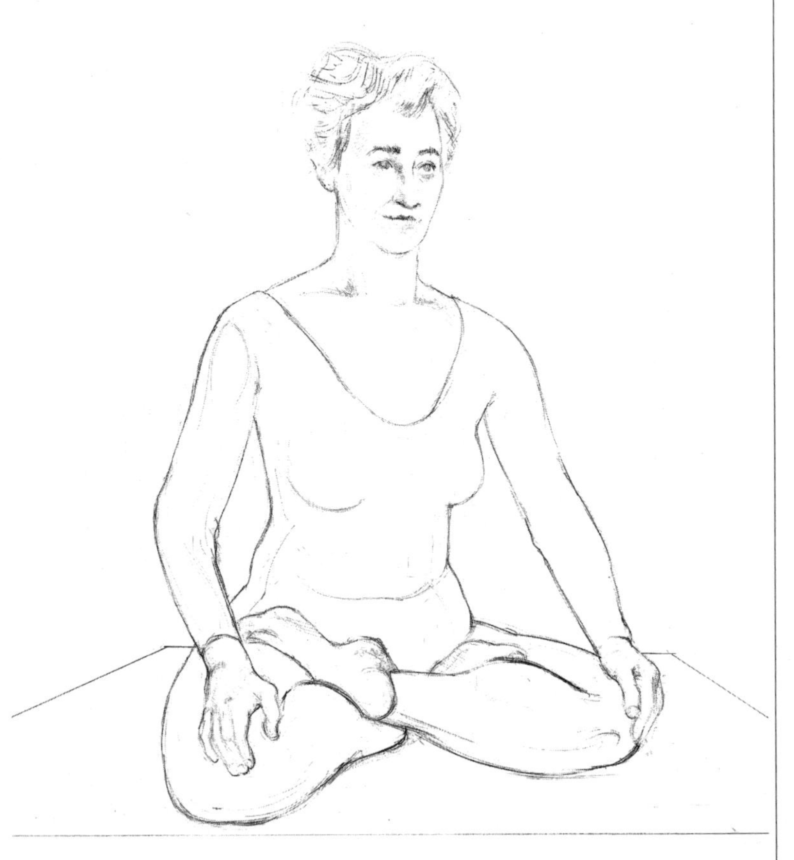

In this pose, both hips are weighted. As a result, the pose is extremely stable and grounded. Because the position is so stable, it is easy to sit straight and breathe easily in this pose. Concentration is also improved.

Lotus Pose is one of the classical poses associated with yoga practice. As I mentioned earlier, I have injured my knees a number of times because I felt I ought to be able to do this pose better. I can only advise you not to repeat my mistake. It may take you a long time to develop the flexibility in your hips to do this pose easily, but it should never strain your knees. If you have trouble sitting in Lotus, practice the Pigeon Preparation Pose, Wide Angle Pose, the Bound Angle Pose, and the Half Lotus Forward Bend.

- Bend your right leg and place your right foot on your left thigh, as close to your left hip as possible.
- Then, place your left foot on your right thigh, as close to your hip as possible.
- Release and repeat on other side.

If you are using this pose for breathing practice, be sure to alternate the position of your legs. It is better to have your knees wide and on the floor than to have them close together but off the ground.

Variation

Half Lotus Pose (Ardha Padmasana)

- If you are unable to do the full Lotus Pose, you can start with one foot resting on the opposite thigh and the other leg tucked underneath you.

Basic Sitting Forward Bend (Paschimottanasana)

Going forward with both legs straight out in front of you is one of the more difficult forward bends. Start with this pose and then come back to it again when you have done the bent leg variations and see if you can go forward more easily.

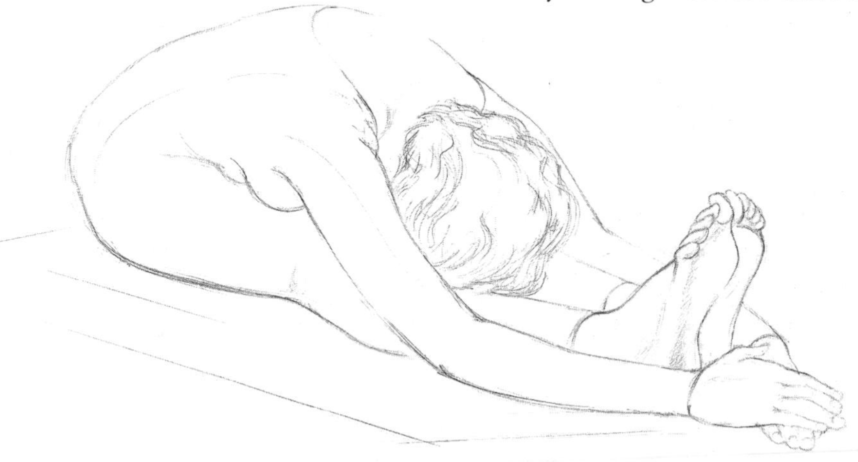

- Start by sitting on the floor with both legs straight out in front of you, together or hip-width apart, and catch your feet or place your hands on your legs.
- As you exhale, drop the back of your pelvis and lengthen your spine to go forward.
- Stay forward as long as you want, and then come up exhaling.

Variations

Reclining Forward Bend (Urdhva Mukha Paschimottanasana I)

- Do the pose lying on your back. It is safer for your lower back than sitting.
- Release the weight of your hips to the ground.

  If you are unable to catch your feet, use a belt.

Upright Forward Bend (Urdhva Mukha Paschimottanasana II)
For more challenge, try this pose sitting upright.

- Bend your knees and catch the outer edges of your feet.
- Exhaling, straighten your legs toward the ceiling. Your body and legs will form a "V." If necessary, lean against a wall for support.

One Leg Straight, One Leg Bent

In all of the following variations, you will need to give more focus to the bent leg side in order to balance your pelvis. The aim is to be centred and balanced, with equal weight on either side of the pelvis.

To relieve your knees and ankles, you can do the Basic Sitting Forward Bend between the bent leg poses.

Half Bound Angle Pose (Janu Sirsasana)

The Sanskrit name for this pose means "head to knee pose." This is very misleading. When you are able to go forward fully, your head will go past your knee. Focus on dropping the back of your pelvis and lengthening your spine and legs, rather than pulling your head down.

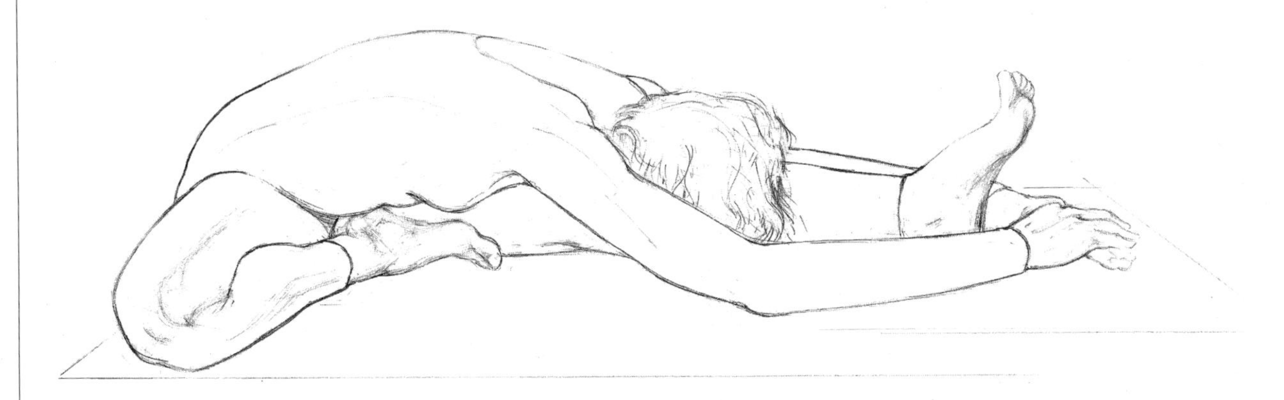

- Start sitting with your legs straight.
- Bend one leg and place your heel on the inside of your thigh as close to your pubic bone as possible.
- As you exhale, let your bent leg release away from your hip and drop toward the floor.
- From this position, go forward, breathing and lengthening.
- As you go forward, keep your spine centred, not curving toward the straight leg.
- Stay in the pose for as long as you want, and then come up and repeat on the other side.

As you become more flexible, move your bent knee further away from your straight leg.

Half Hero's Pose (Triang Mukhaikapada Paschimottanasana)

In this pose, the bent leg side of the pelvis is often off the ground and is difficult to feel. Leaning into your hip will compress your waist more and does not release the pelvis. If you are very tilted, sit with the straight leg side of your pelvis on a blanket, to make your hips level.

Remain as centred as possible, and drop your pelvis from within as you exhale. Aim to feel the movement of your breath right down to your sitting bone.

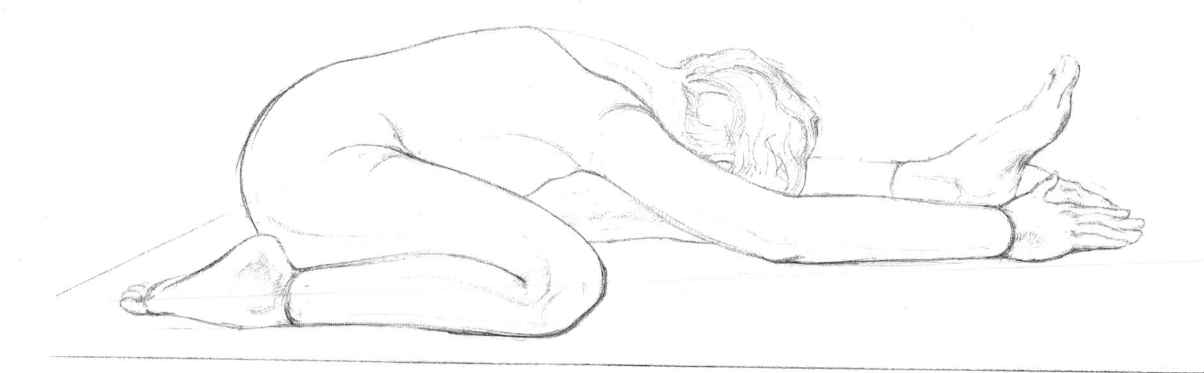

- Start by sitting with your legs straight.
- Bend one leg back as in Hero's Pose.
- From this position, go forward, breathing and lengthening.
- Stay in the pose for as long as you want, and then come up and repeat on the other side.

Variation

Heron Pose (Krounchasana)

- Instead of leaving your straight leg on the floor, bend it and catch your foot.
- Slowly straighten your lifted leg up toward the ceiling. Your leg and spine form a "V." As you exhale, both your spine and the lifted leg lengthen.
- Keep your shoulders dropped and your arms loose.
- Wait for your leg to release before bringing it toward you. Do not round your back in order to bring your head to your leg.

Half Lotus Forward Bend (Ardha Padma Paschimottanasana)

This pose is an important preparation for Full Lotus Pose. The weight of your bent leg anchors the straight leg and powerfully roots the pose. When you are able to place your foot at the very top of your thigh, the outer edge of your foot will be right in your hip joint. As you go forward your foot will slide back creating a secure base from which it is easy to lengthen and extend.

If you have difficulty with this pose, practice the Bound Angle Pose, the Wide Angle Pose, Half Bound Angle Pose and the Pigeon Pose Preparation stretch. You can work on this pose lying on your back or in Shoulderstand. It is easier to do when the weight is not on your hips.

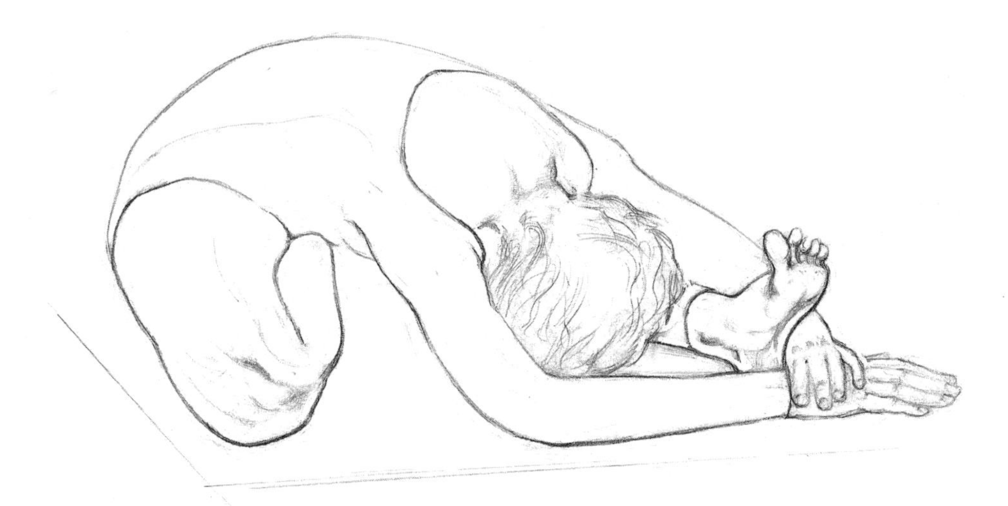

- Start by sitting with your legs straight.
- Bend one leg and place your foot on the opposite thigh.
- From this position, go forward, breathing and lengthening.
- Stay in the pose for as long as you want, and then come up and repeat on the other side.

Be very careful not to strain your knee or overstretch your ankle to get into the position. If you feel any strain, or your foot puts uncomfortable pressure on your thigh muscle, move it down toward your knee.

Sage's Forward Bend (Marichyasana I)

This pose can be done as a twist or as a forward bend. It is an easy twist but more awkward as a forward bend. The action is similar to Garland Pose and Crow Pose and prepares you for both of them. The bent leg hugs in toward the body, so it is a counter-balance to Half Bound Angle Pose and Half Lotus, in which the leg is turned out.

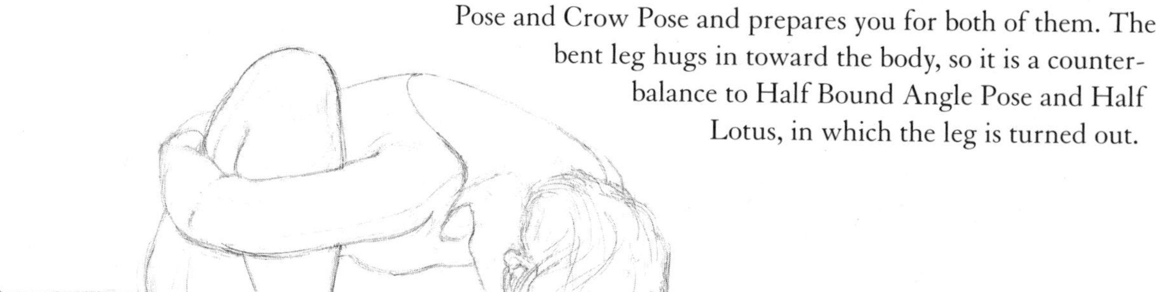

- Start by sitting with your legs straight.
- Bend your right leg and place your right foot on the floor as close to the sitting bone as possible.
- Take time to lengthen from your right hip out toward your fingertips. Then wrap your right arm around your right leg. Reach your left hand behind your back and catch your left wrist with your right hand.
- From this position, go forward, breathing and lengthening. Press your right foot on the floor as you exhale, to bring your sitting bone down and lengthen your spine.
- Bring your bent knee as close to your side ribs as possible. If your right foot slides in toward your left leg, then your knee will fall away from your body.
- Stay in the pose for as long as you want, and then come up and repeat on the other side.

If you can't catch your hands behind your back, bring your arms forward as you do in the other sitting poses. The use of your heel in this pose will give you the feeling of the action in the sitting bones that is needed in all of the forward bends.

Advanced Forward Bends

These poses are an intense stretch of the back thighs and the back of the pelvis. Approach them with extreme caution if you have lower back problems.

Tortoise Pose (Kurmasana)

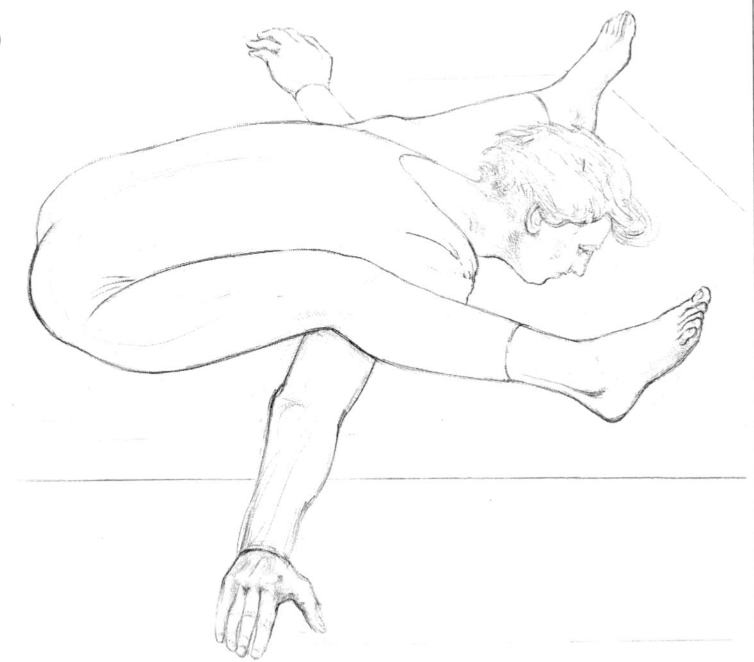

Tortoise Pose is an intensification of Wide Angle Pose and resembles a tortoise in its shell. It is for people who can stretch forward completely on the floor and want to go on further.

- Start by sitting with your legs wide apart.
- Bend your knees and put your feet on the floor.
- Drop your body between your legs, as you did in Garland Pose.
- When your shoulders are below your knees, wriggle your arms underneath your legs.
- Bring your knees as close to your shoulders as possible.
- Exhaling, slowly straighten your legs and go forward.
- Stay in the pose, and continue to lengthen your spine as you breathe.
- When you are ready, release your legs and come back to sitting.

In the full pose, the torso is flat on the floor with the arms and legs straight. Your arms can either be stretched out to the side, or beside you reaching back. It is possible to place the chin and the chest on the floor.

"When, again as a tortoise draws its limbs in on all sides, he [the yogi] withdraws his senses from the objects of sense, and then his understanding is well-poised."
— *Bhagavad Gita*

Sleeping Tortoise (Supta Kurmasana)

This pose is similar to Tortoise Pose, except that your ankles are crossed. Wrap your arms around your back as in Garland Pose.

- Begin as you did in Tortoise Pose.
- When your arms are underneath your legs, cross your ankles. Drop your head in front of your ankles.
- Reach your arms behind you and then catch your hands behind your back.
- Stay in the pose for a while, and then cross your ankles the other way.

As your spine and shoulders release, you will be able to catch higher on your back. If you cannot reach your hands, use a belt.

One Leg Behind the Head (Eka Pada Sirsasana)

Babies do this movement easily and naturally when bringing their feet to their mouths. For most adults it is strange and unnatural. The pose is valuable because it stretches the back thighs intensely and gives you the rotation in your hips that you need to do Lotus. Once this position is achieved there are many variations.

- Start by lying down, with one leg bent and your foot on the floor.
- Take the other foot in your hands and circle it toward your head. Draw your foot up and toward your forehead as you exhale, and release it away as you inhale.
- Round your back and bring your head forward to slide your leg behind your head.
- When your foot is behind your head, bring your hands into Prayer Position.
- Repeat on the other side.

It is easier to bring your leg up if your back is rounded. Try resting your head on a pillow or folded blanket, or lean against a wall with your back very round.

Take your exhalation well back into the back of your waist to release your hip.

If the pose is easy for you, straighten the other leg.

Sleeping Pose (Yoga Nidrasana)

To do this pose you need to have mastered the previous one, but you can approximate the pose by lying with two pillows, one under your head and one under your hips. Bend your knees up beside your ribs. This is an extremely restful pose and a wonderful stretch on the back. Try it and you will understand why the full pose is called the "sleeping pose."

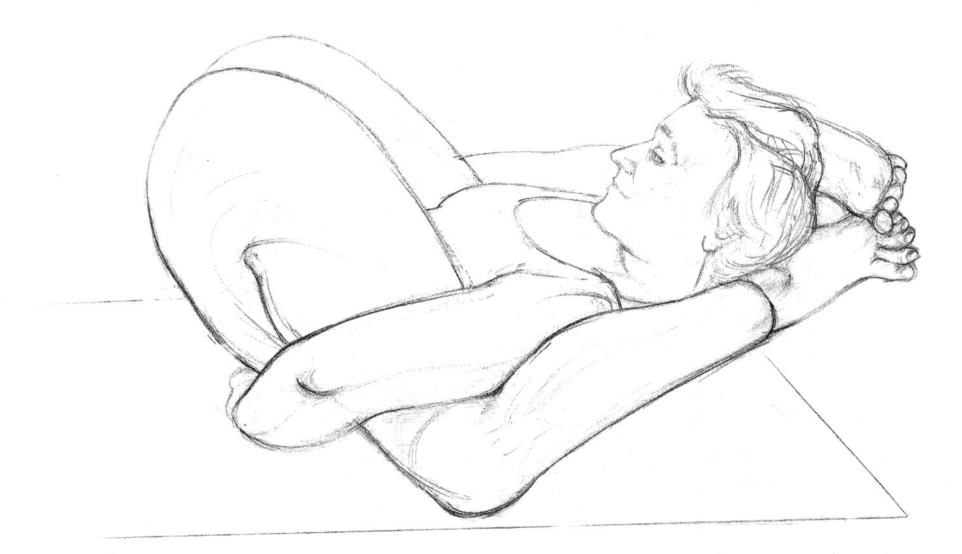

- Start by lying on your back.
- Take one foot behind your head.
- Take the other foot behind your head and cross your ankles. Rest back on your crossed ankles, like a hammock.
- Then catch your hands behind your back.
- When you are ready, release your legs and come back to sitting.
- Repeat with your ankles crossed the other way.

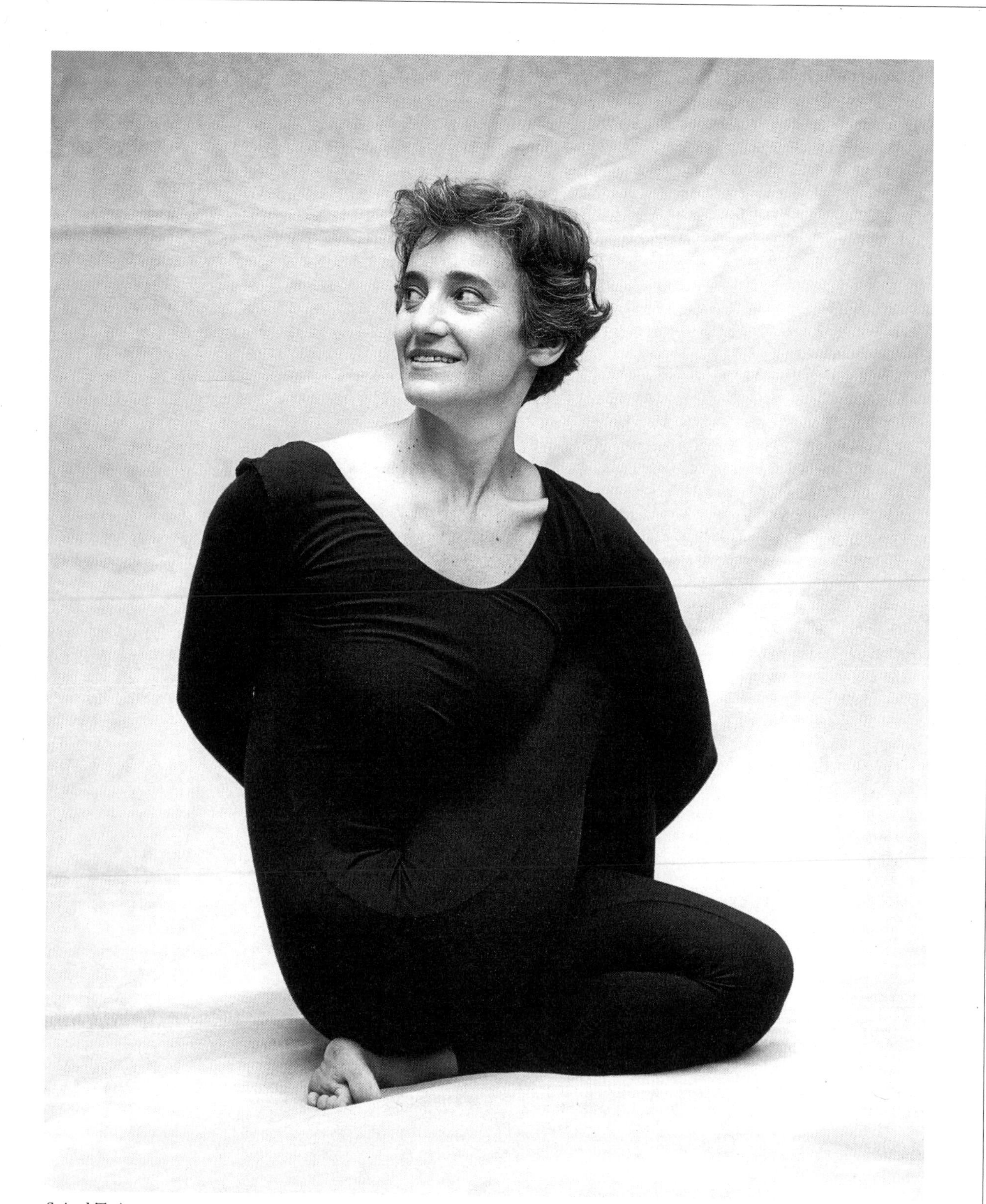

Spinal Twist

CHAPTER 14

Sitting Twists

Caution: Be careful doing twists if you have back problems. Do not do them if you have bruised, broken or dislocated ribs. Avoid twists during menstruation or if you are suffering from irritation or inflammation of your internal organs (cystitis, irritable bowel, colitis, etc.).

Pregnant women should only do gentle twisting in poses which are open and which provide space for the fetus.

TWISTS ARE FREEING, balancing and energizing. Sitting Twists are the most intense of the various kinds of twisting poses. They increase the range of movement of the spine and promote flexibility, especially in the hips and upper back.

Like all other sitting poses, the foundation of the sitting twists is in the pelvis. The anchoring point is on the side you are moving away from, so when you turn to the right, remember to focus your attention on your left sitting bone. It is easy to turn your head and upper body, but turning from the hips requires a deeper release and awareness. It is difficult to breathe deeply while in an intense twist, but you can still move your belly into the back of your waist with your breath. Intense twists massage and stimulate the internal organs. When you turn deeply inside, the twists will tone and stimulate your abdominal organs, benefit your digestion and relieve constipation.

Guidelines

Practise twists after the sitting poses, because your hips and spine will be released already. It is essential that you continue to lengthen, increasing the space between the vertebrae, as you rotate. It is like taking the cork out of a bottle, creating space and openness as you turn.

Twists use the limbs more actively than the forward bends do and are generally easier, once you are over the initial confusion of what goes where. Focus on the line of your spine as the central axis of the pose. When you are able to find this line, the confusion and awkwardness dissolves and the pose falls into place. Once you are in the pose, you will turn automatically as your spine lengthens.

We all have some rotation in our spines, because we do not use our bodies symmetrically and our internal organs are not symmetrical. Twisting counterbalances these long-standing rotations. When practising a twisting pose, do the more difficult side twice or hold it longer. If you are involved in a sport or other activity in which you are always turning to one side (e.g. playing the violin or flute, racquet sports, golf, etc.), be sure to do some twists the other way before and after.

Twists are easier for people with long limbs. If you have a wide body and short limbs, focus on the more open twists. You will find the ones where you have to reach around your leg more difficult. Take a long time to lengthen from your hip to your fingertips before you try to catch around. When you are able to bring your shoulders past the bent knee, your arms will be free to wrap easily. Focus on your breath and the elongation of your spine and don't struggle to get into the full pose until you are ready.

You can twist in almost all of the simple sitting poses discussed on pp. 184–190. These twists are all suitable and beneficial for pregnant women, since they keep the space in the abdomen.

Approach them all the same way.

- Focus on the "back" sitting bone and leg. Keep the back sitting bone anchored and let the back leg release away from the hip.
- Exhaling, lengthen your spine and turn.
- Release and repeat on the other side.

Half Bound Angle Twist (Parivrtta Janu Sirsasana)

This is a free and open twist. The twist is easiest when the angle between the bent and straight legs is wide.

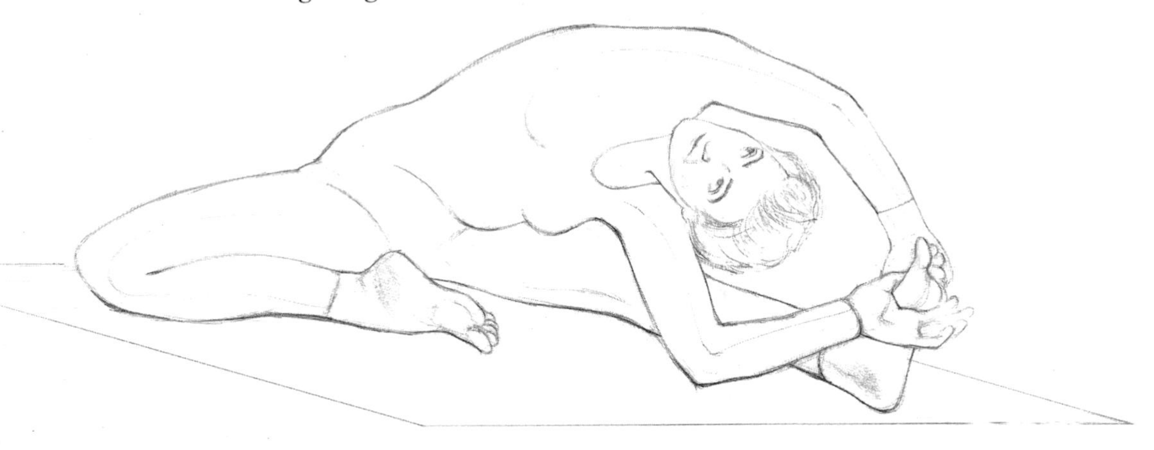

- Start by sitting with your legs straight.
- Bend your right leg and place your heel on the inside of your thigh. Move your knee as far back as you can.
- Turn to the right, exhaling, lengthen the left side of your body along your left leg. Place your left elbow on the floor and catch your left foot.
- Reach over with your right arm and catch your left foot.
- As you exhale, drop your right sitting bone, lengthen your spine and turn toward the ceiling.
- Release and repeat on the other side.

Your right sitting bone is the root in the pose. When your elbow is on the floor, it becomes part of the foundation. Use it to twist more as your spine lengthens.

The sides of your spine need to be stretched equally. Lengthen your left side and be careful not to overstretch your right ribs.

If you are unable to go into the pose, sit straight, with your left hand on your left leg, and your right hand on the floor outside your right leg. Press your right hand on the floor as you exhale, to lengthen and turn.

Variation

Try a similar pose with your legs straight in Wide Angle Pose.

Spinal Twist (Ardha Matsyendrasana)

Like Cow's Head Pose, this pose opens the back of the pelvis and stretches the outer thighs. As you proceed to the more advanced versions of this twist, your abdominal muscles and internal organs will also turn, toning and stimulating your digestive system.

Throughout this sequence remain aware of the line of your spine in the centre of the pose.

Preparation

This is a very easy introductory twist.

- Start by sitting on the floor with both legs straight.
- Bend your right leg and cross your right leg over your left. Place your right foot on the floor outside your left thigh, as close to your left hip as possible. Turn to the right.
- Hold your right knee with your left hand, and place your right hand on the floor beside your hip for support.
- As you exhale, drop your hips, deepening and releasing your right hip, and lengthening your spine.
- Continue to turn to the right, drawing your right leg toward you as you turn.
- When you are able, take your left elbow outside your right leg. Keeping your elbow bent, press it against the outer thigh to turn further as your spine lengthens.
- When you are fully turned, reach your left arm through the space between your right calf and the thigh. (You will have to wriggle a bit to get it through.) Then, catch your left hand with your right.
- Relax your shoulders and drop your elbows, as you exhale. Feel as if your left elbow is weighted, and your right shoulder light.
- Press down with your right foot as you exhale, to continue to lengthen and turn. This action deepens your hip joint and lengthens your spine. As your spine lengthens, the turn will continue by itself.
- Release and repeat on the other side.

Easy Version

- Start in the preparation position.
- Bend your left leg so that your left foot is beside your right hip.
- Continue as the preparation twist.
- Release and repeat on the other side.

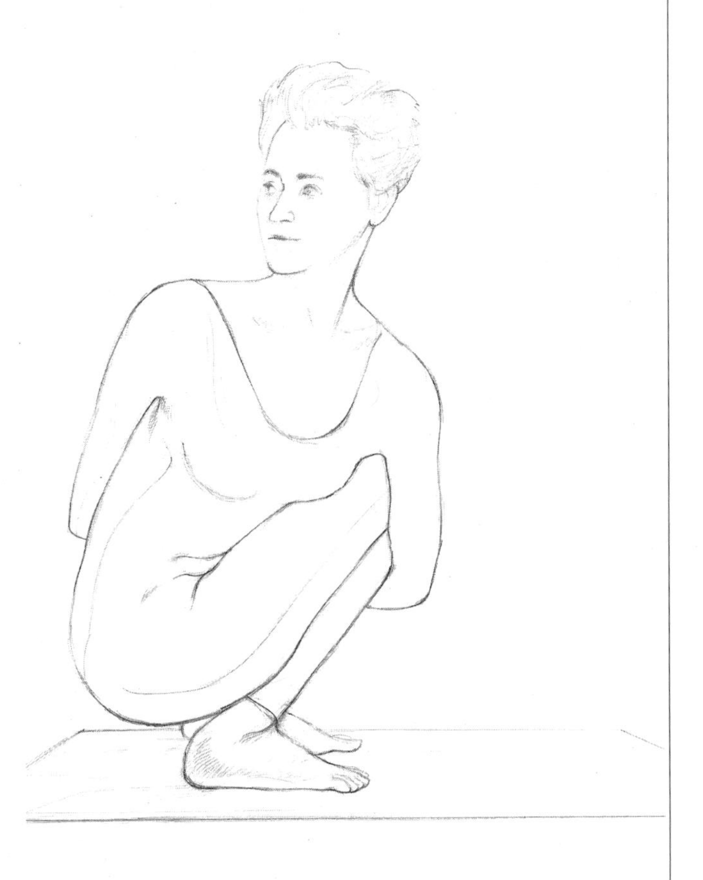

Full Pose

This pose (*illustrated*) is similar to the easy version, except that you sit on the lower foot.

- Flex your ankle and try to sit so that both cheeks are on your instep. The resulting pose is a more intense twist of the spine and the abdominal organs.
- When you can catch your arms easily, try wrapping your left arm around the outside of your right leg.
- Draw your abdominal muscles in as you exhale, to reach the roots of twist in your hips and deep inside your pelvis.
- Release and repeat on the other side.

Intense Spinal Twist (Paripurna Matsyendrasana)

This is an extremely intense twist. You need very flexible hips to get anywhere near it.

- Start by sitting on the floor with both legs straight.
- Bend your left leg, and place it on your right thigh in Half Lotus, as close to your right hip as possible.
- Bend your right leg and cross it over your left thigh. Place your right foot on the floor outside your left thigh, as close to your left hip as possible.
- Continue as in the previous twists.
- Release and repeat on the other side.

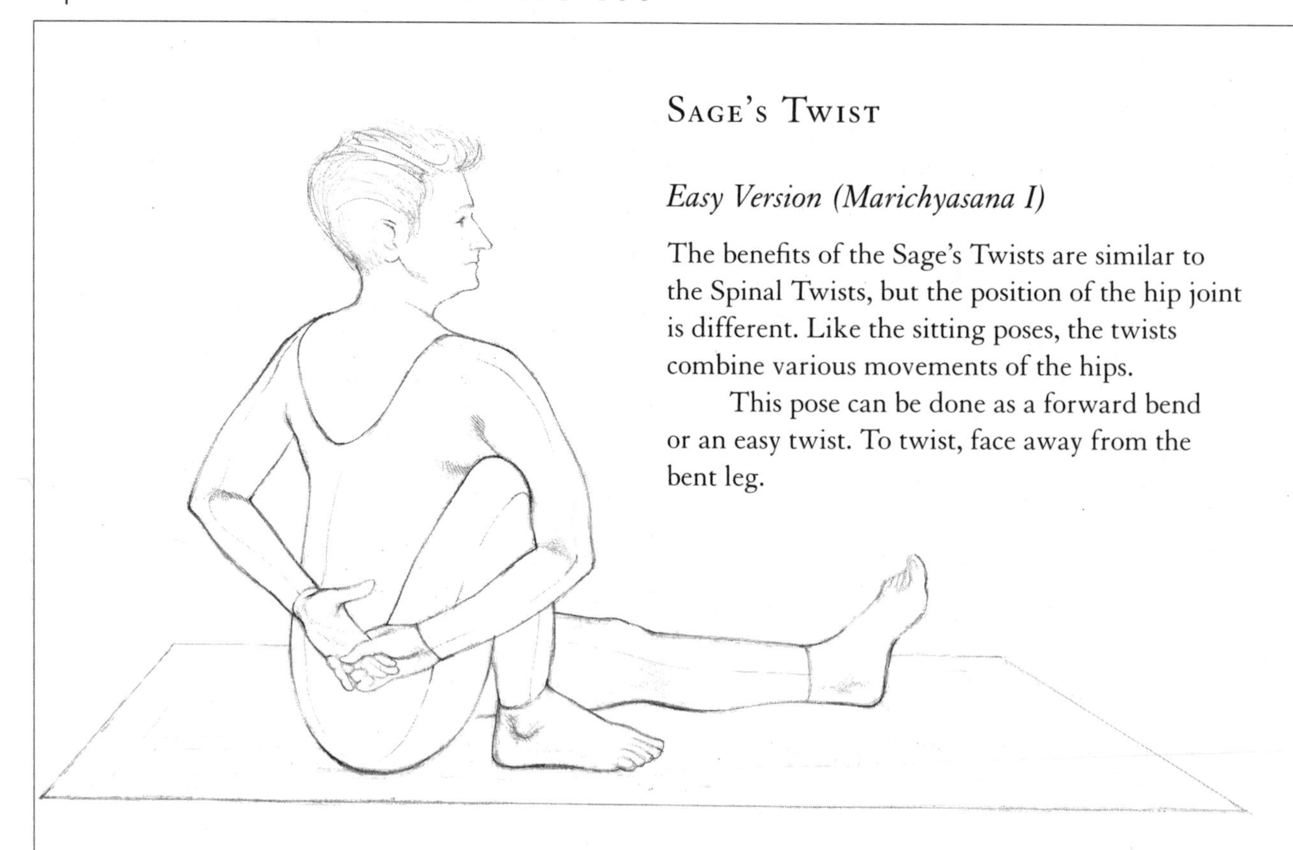

Sage's Twist

Easy Version (Marichyasana I)

The benefits of the Sage's Twists are similar to the Spinal Twists, but the position of the hip joint is different. Like the sitting poses, the twists combine various movements of the hips.

This pose can be done as a forward bend or an easy twist. To twist, face away from the bent leg.

- Start by sitting on the floor with both legs straight.
- Bend your right leg. Place your right foot on the floor, as close to your right sitting bone as possible.
- Turn to the left.
- Stretch your right arm away from you. Take time to breathe and lengthen from your right hip to your fingertips.
- Wrap your right arm around your right leg and then bend your left arm and catch your left hand with your right. Hug your right leg close your body, with as little space as possible between your thigh and your ribs. Bring the weight to the inner edge of your foot, to keep your shin vertical.
- As you exhale, drop your pelvis, deepening and releasing your right hip.
- As your spine lengthens, turn your head to the left.
- Let your left leg lengthen away from you.
- Release and repeat on the other side.

If you cannot catch around, place your right hand on your left shin, and place your left hand on the floor for support. If you can almost catch, use a belt.

To be more active in the pose, press down with your right foot as you exhale. As your spine lengthens, the turn will happen by itself. Using your foot will help you to find the action in the pose.

Variations

Instead of having your left leg straight, you can bend as you do in the Half Bound Angle Pose, Half Hero's Pose and Half Lotus sitting poses.

Full Pose (Marichyasana III)

In this pose, you turn toward the bent leg instead of away from it. In order to take your arm outside your leg, your straight leg, hips, abdominal muscles and internal organs all have to turn. Breathe deeply and take lots of time to lengthen. (*See instructions for the full pose on the next page*.)

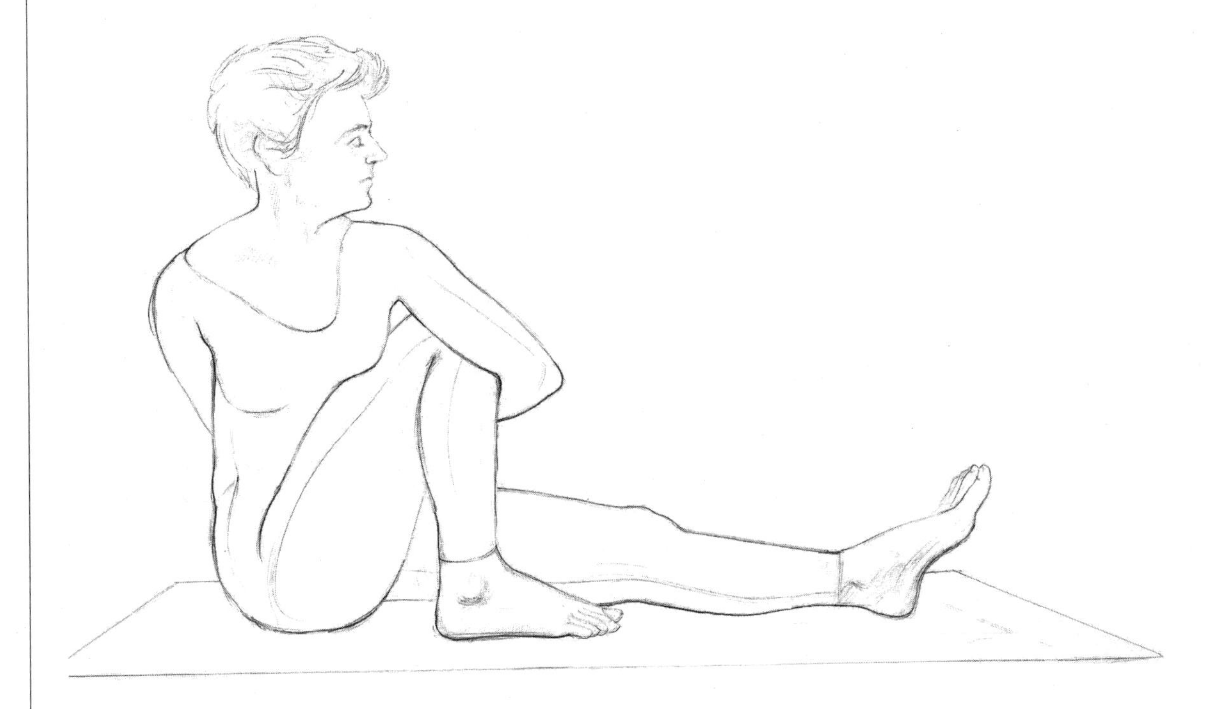

- Start by sitting on the floor with both legs straight.
- Bend your right leg. Place your right foot on the floor, as close to your right sitting bone as possible. Turn to the right.
- Stretch your left arm away from you. Take time to breathe and lengthen from your left hip to your fingertips.
- Take your left elbow outside your right leg. Then, wrap your left arm around your left leg, bend your right arm and catch your right hand with your left. Drop your left elbow as much as possible to keep your weight forward in the pose. If you can almost catch, use a belt.
- Keep your right shin vertical, with the weight on the outer edge of your foot.
- As you exhale, drop your pelvis, deepening and releasing your right hip.
- As your spine lengthens, turn your head to the right.
- Lengthen your left leg away from you.
- Release and repeat on the other side.

To be more active, press down with your right foot as you exhale to continue to lengthen and turn. As your spine lengthens, the turn will happen by itself. Being able to use your foot will help you to find the action in the pose.

Variations

You can do the same variations in this pose that you did in the easier version of Sage's Twist.

Squatting Twist (Pasasana)

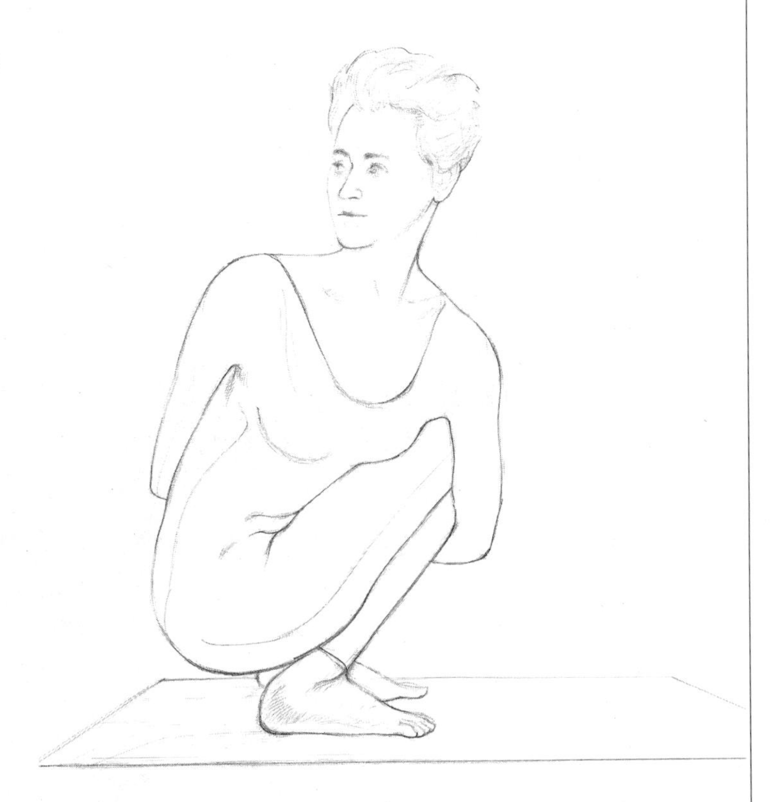

This twist releases the sacrum and flexes the hips and the ankles intensely.

- Start by squatting on the balls of your feet, with your feet and knees together.
- Turn to the right and stretch your left arm away, and lengthen from your left hip to your fingertips. Use your right hand for balance.
- When your spine has lengthened, drop your left arm outside your thighs.
- Continue to drop your left elbow and slowly take your heels down, keeping your knees as far forward over your toes as possible.
- Then, wrap your arms behind your back as in the Sage's Pose.
- As you exhale, press your heels toward the floor, lengthen your spine and turn your head to the right.
- Release and repeat on the other side.

If you cannot catch your hands, you can use a belt. Your weight has to be well forward, otherwise you will fall when you try to catch your hands.

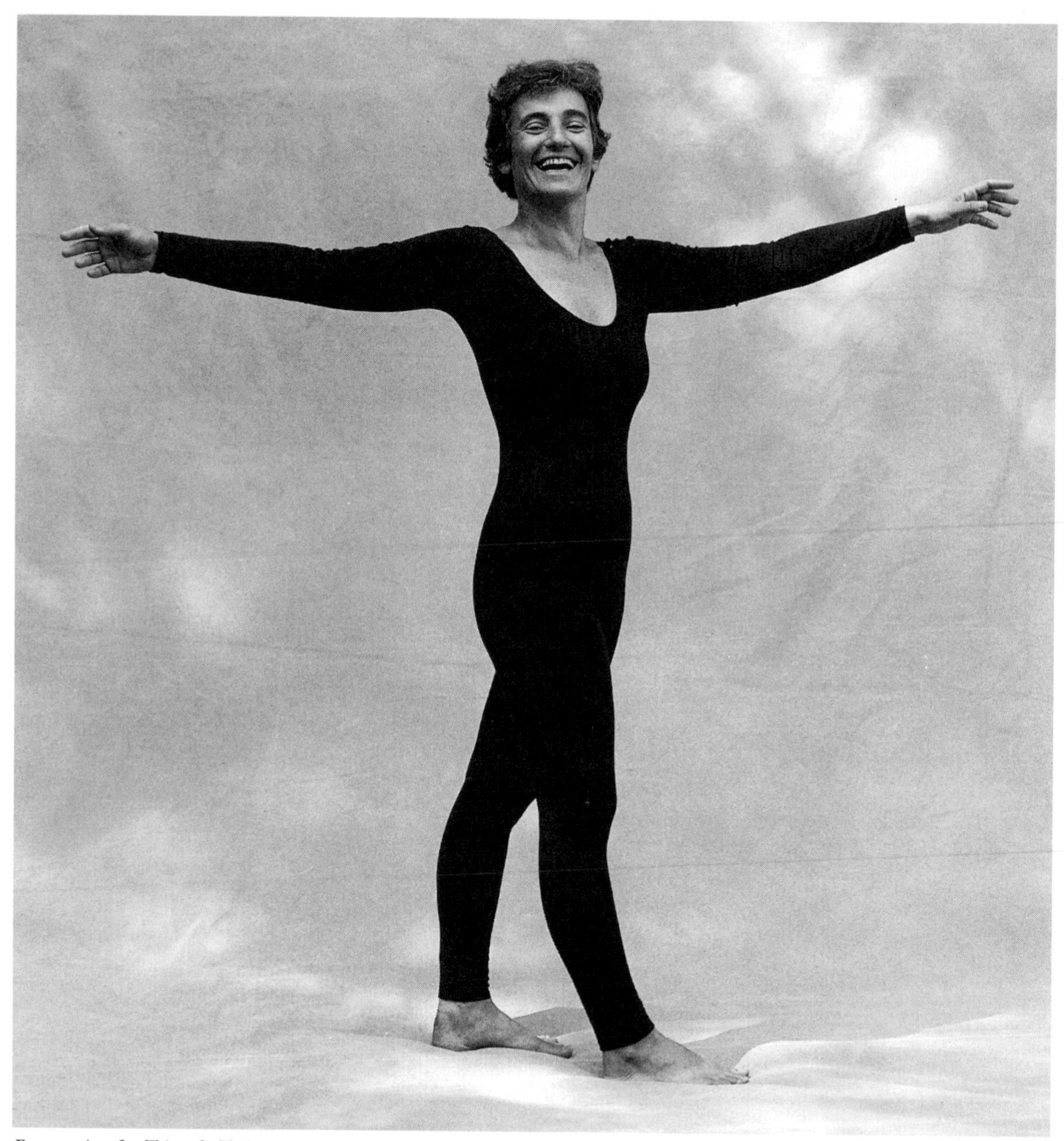

Preparation for Triangle Twist

CHAPTER 15

Suggested Practice Sequences

THE FOLLOWING practice routines are designed to help you establish your own practice. Numbers 1–3 are very basic sequences, 4–6 are intermediate and 7–10 build up to an advanced practice.

Before starting to practise, review the practice guidelines in Chapter 3. Start or end your practice with quiet centring poses, and include breathing as a regular part of your routine. If you want to focus on a particular type of pose, you can follow the sequences given in the text.

Beginner Series

#1 Basics

This practice teaches you to focus on your breath, work in simple poses with your breath and find the line of gravity through your spine when you are upright. It includes a variety of movements of your hips and spine, and promotes flexibility, strength and awareness in your legs.

Start in Relaxation with your legs bent and feet on the floor

Little Boat

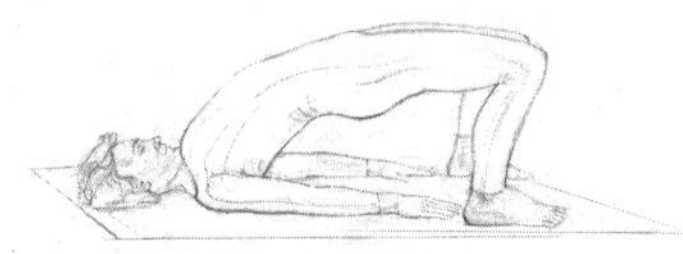

Bridge Pose

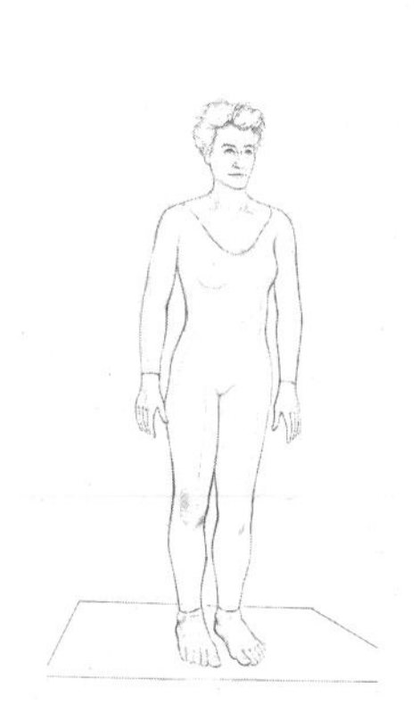

Standing Straight

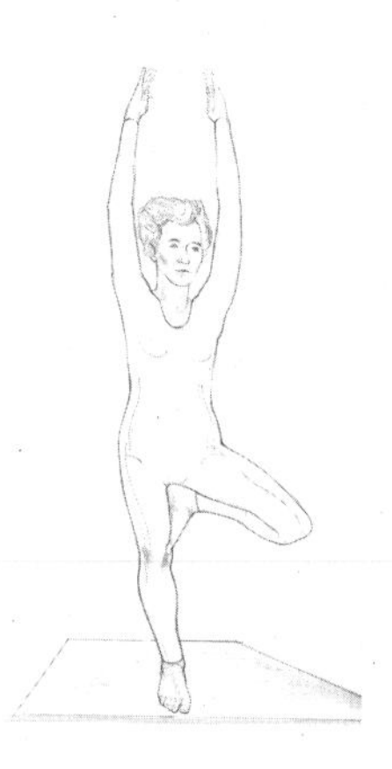

Tree Pose

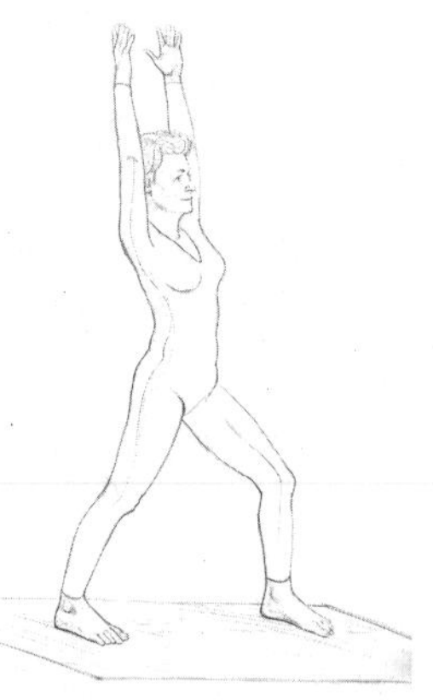

Warrior I

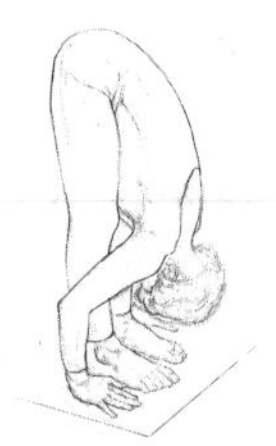

Standing Forward Bend

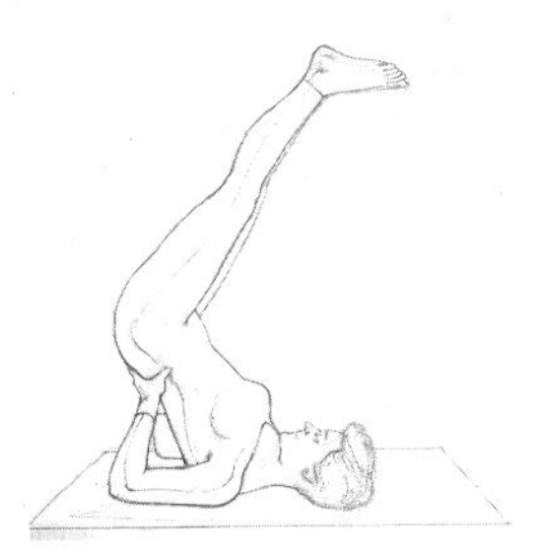
Half Shoulderstand

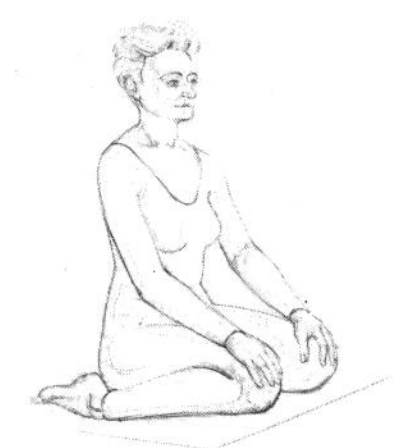
Hero's Pose

Simple Spinal Twist (see pp. 202–203)

Sit in any comfortable position and follow your breath for 5 minutes.
Deep Relaxation Pose

#2 Sun Salutation

This series builds from the basic poses into Sun Salutation. After you are warmed up from Sun Salutation, you will do a simple backbend preparation pose. Simple sitting poses and twists complement and counterbalance the energy of the Sun Salutation and backbends.

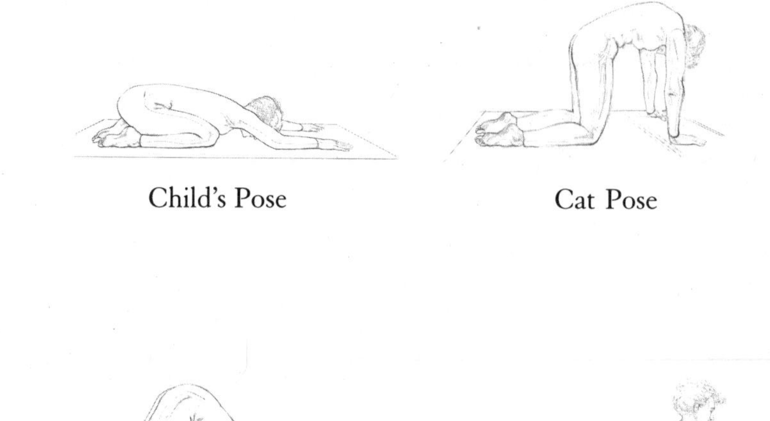

Child's Pose

Cat Pose

Dog Pose

Lunge Pose

Practise stepping forward from Dog Pose into the Lunge Pose and back again until you can move smoothly and easily.

Simplified Sun Salutation — 3x each side

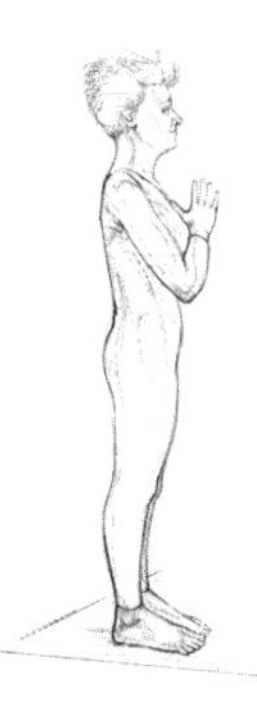

- Begin in Standing Straight with your hands in Prayer Position.
- Then take your arms over your head while Standing Straight.

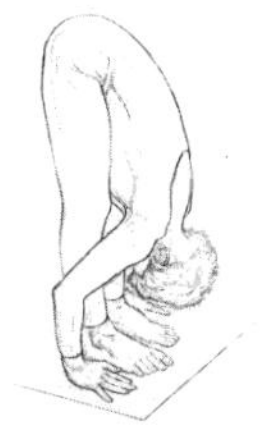

Standing Forward Bend

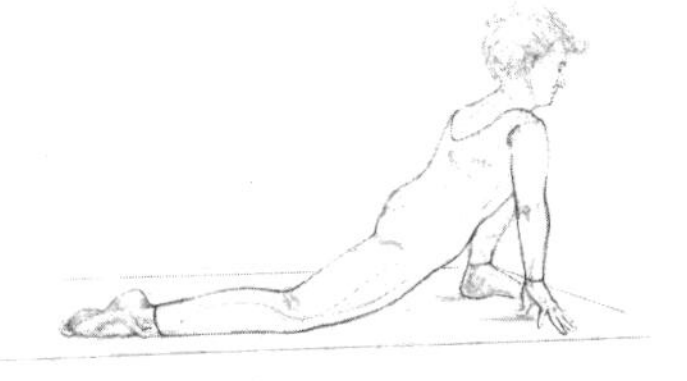

Lunge Pose

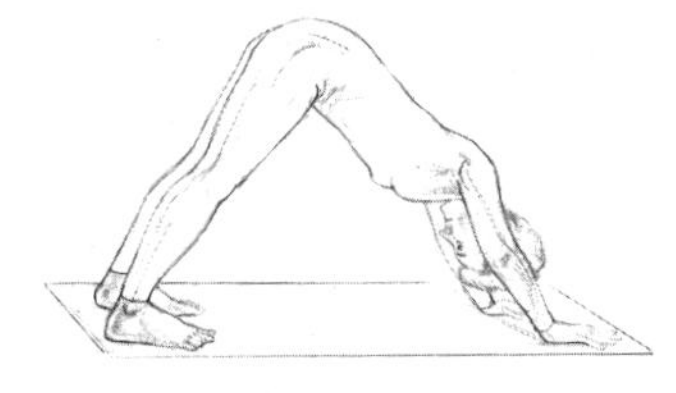

Dog Pose

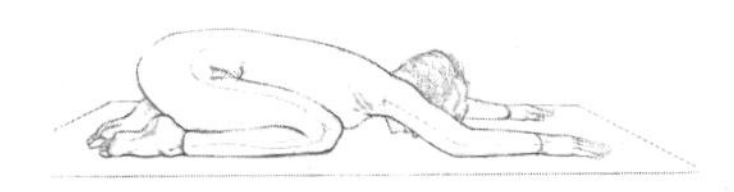

Child Pose

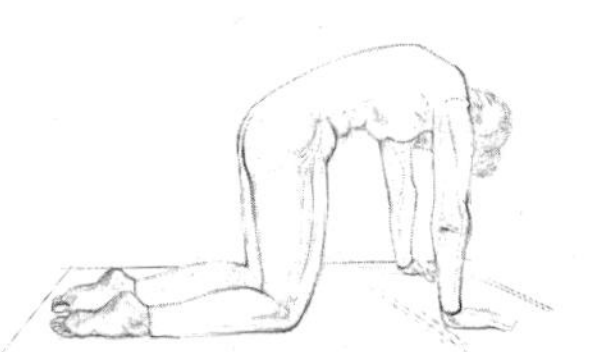

Cat Pose

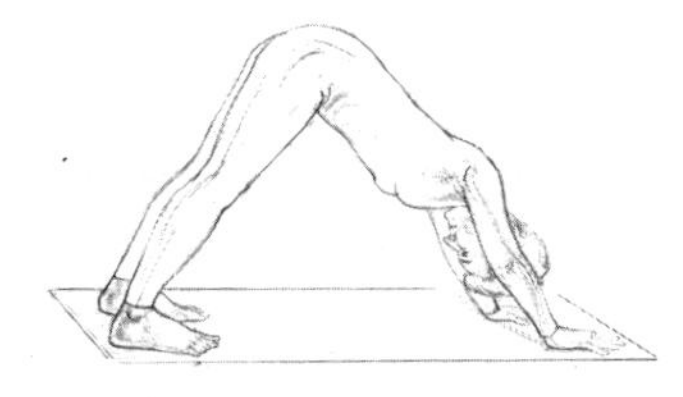

Dog Pose

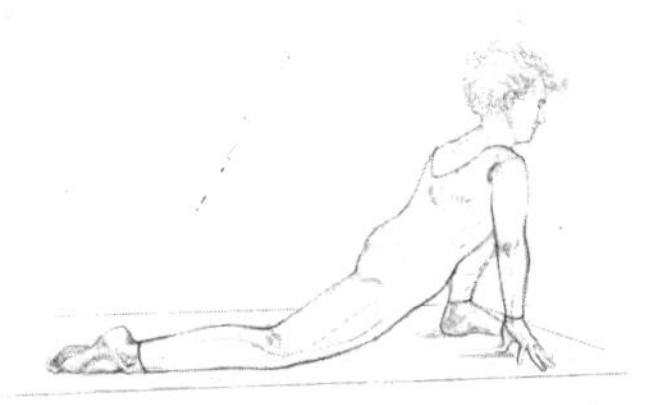

Lunge Pose

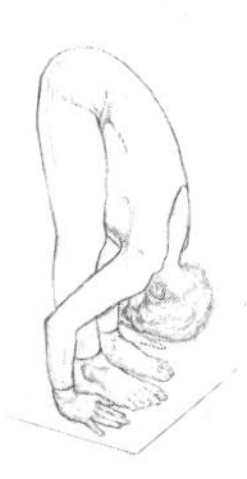

Standing
Forward Bend

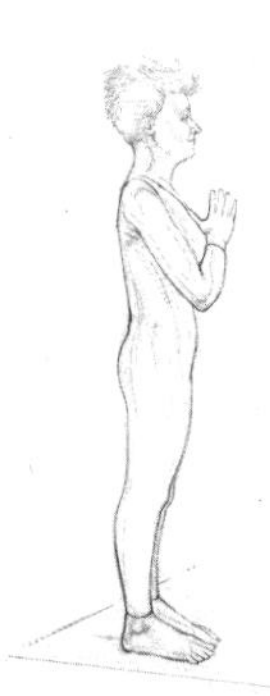

- Come up to Standing Straight with your arms over your head.
- Bring your hands into Prayer Position.

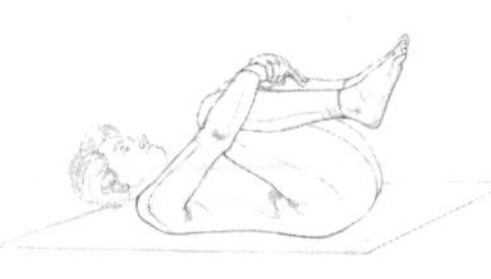

Bridge Pose

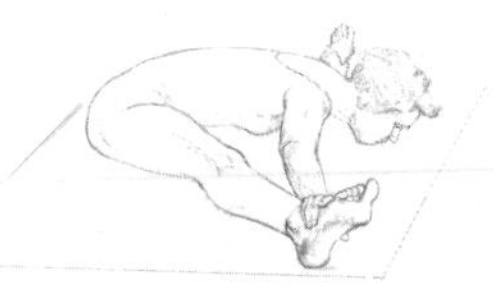

Little Boat

Wide Angle Pose

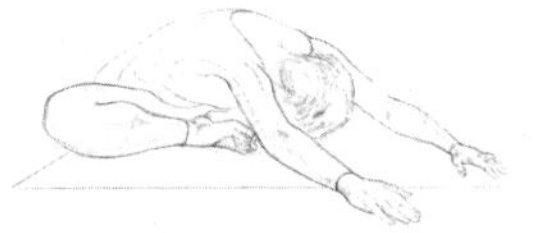

Bound Angle Pose

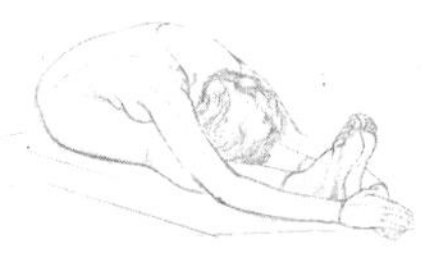

Basic Sitting
Forward Bend

Simple Spinal Twist (see pp. 202–203)

Sitting, follow your breath. When your breathing is smooth and steady, use a clock to time your basic rhythm. Try to equalize your inhalation and exhalation and maintain a steady rhythm for 3 minutes.
Deep Relaxation Pose

#3 Inversions

This sequence focuses on inversions. Inverted poses are usually intimidating because most people have very little confidence in their arms, and the poses themselves are disorienting. The preparation poses are to help you establish confidence in your arms. Handstand is the most intimidating inverted pose, but it is also one of the safest. Read the introduction to the chapter on inverted poses (p. 126) and pay special attention to the cautions.

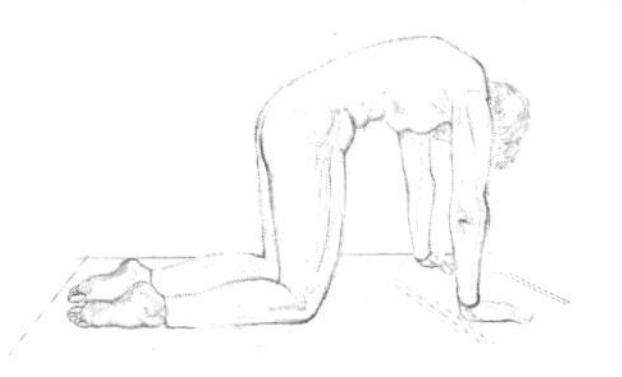

Cat Pose

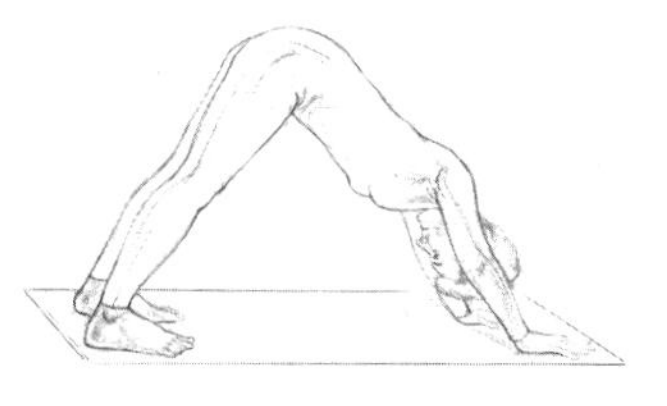

Dog Pose

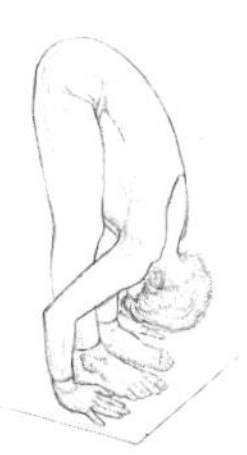

Standing Forward Bend

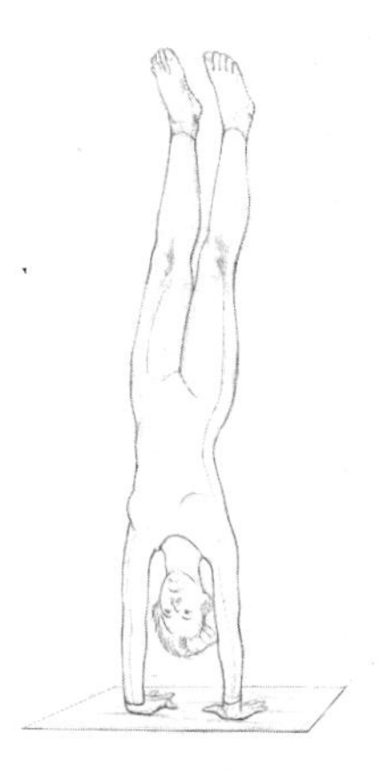

Handstand

Cat Pose Headstand Preparation (see p. 135)
Dog Pose Headstand Preparation (see p. 135)

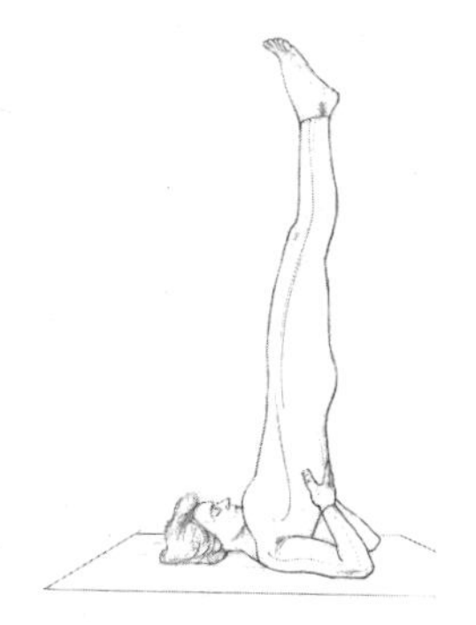
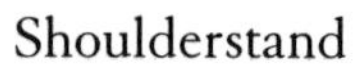
Shoulderstand

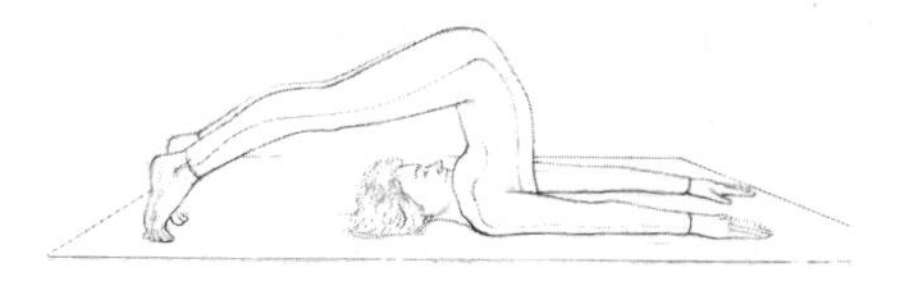
Plough Pose

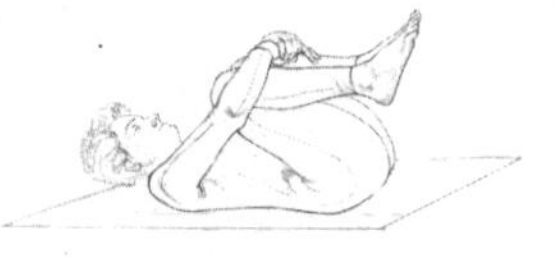
Little Boat

Sitting
Take time to see how it feels to be sitting upright after the inversions.
Lion Breath will help to relieve any residual tension in your neck and throat.
Follow your breath quietly for 10 minutes.
Deep Relaxation Pose

Intermediate Series

#4 Balanced Practice

This series covers standing, bending backwards, bending forwards and twisting.

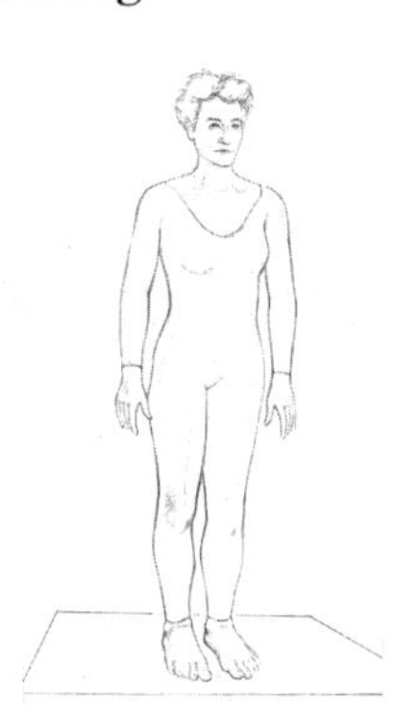

Standing Straight

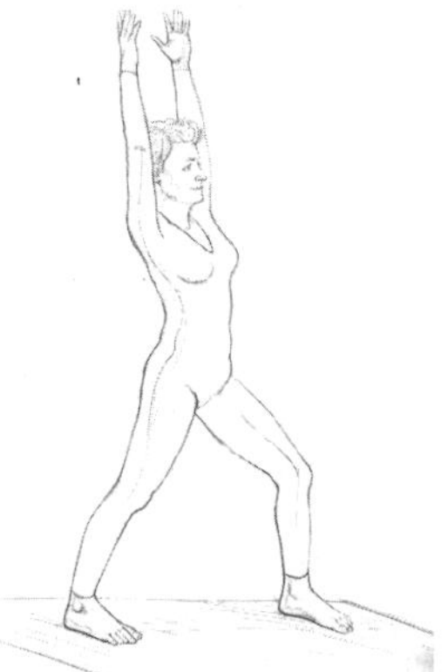

Warrior Pose I

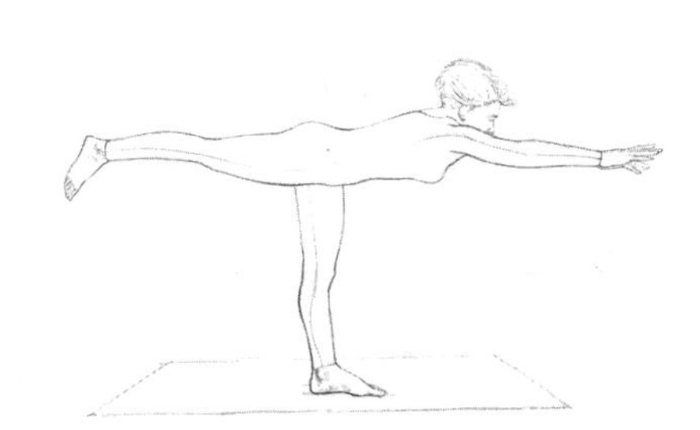

Warrior Balance

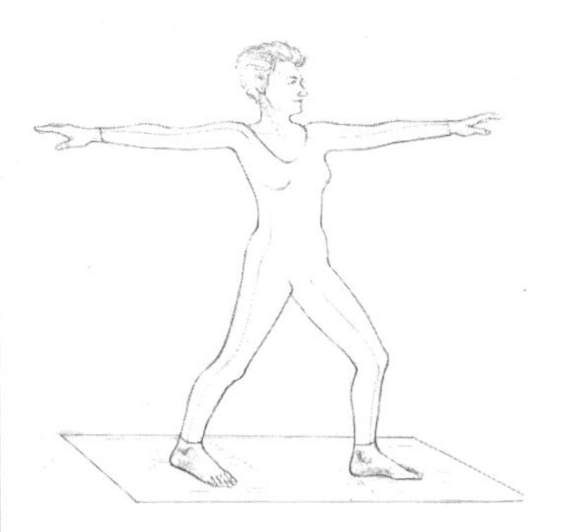

Warrior II

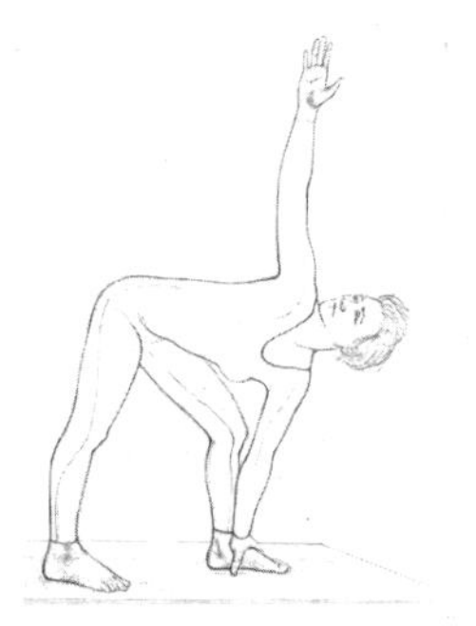

Side Angle Pose

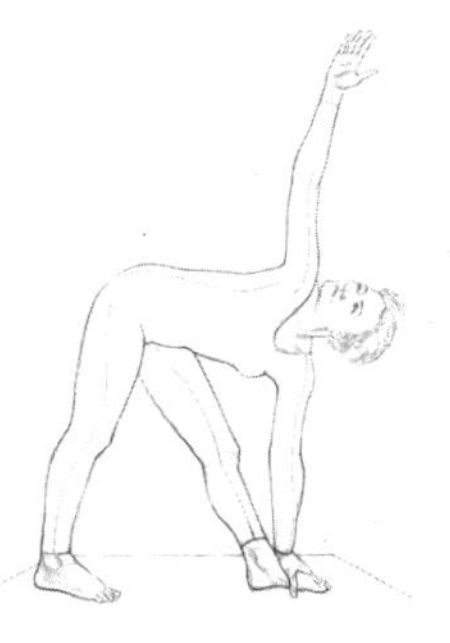

Triangle Pose

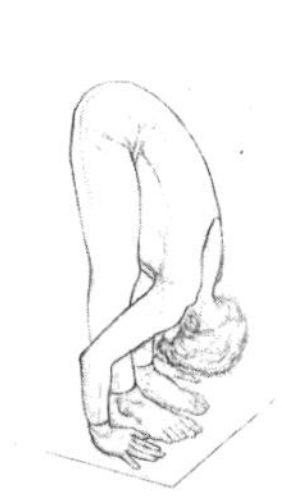

Standing Forward Bend

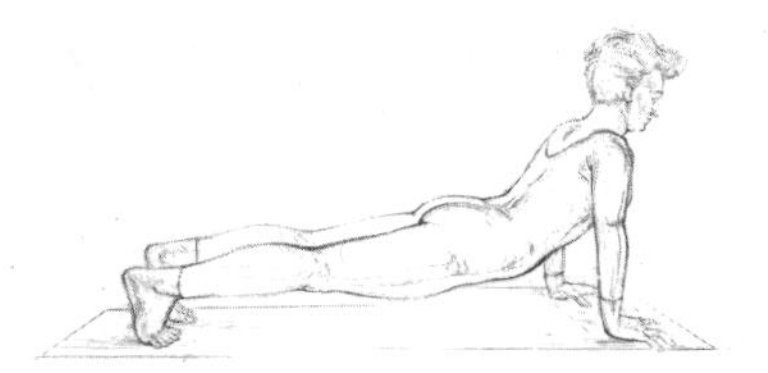

Head-Up Dog Pose

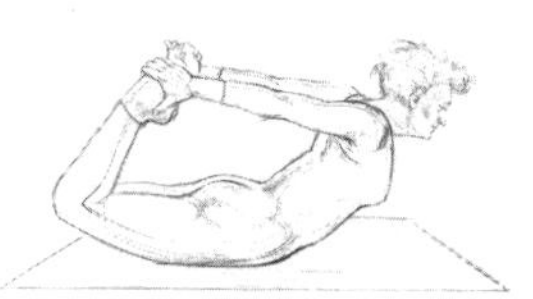

Bow Pose

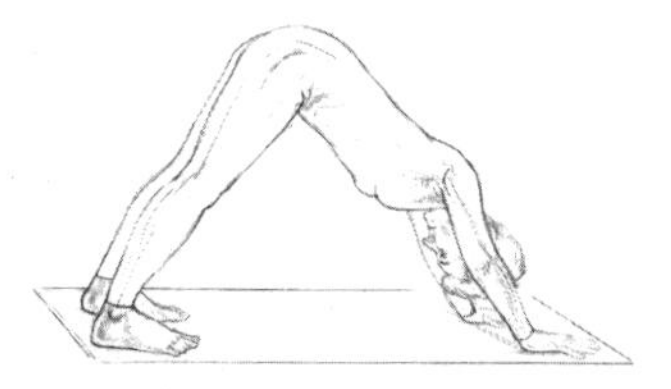

Head Down Dog Pose

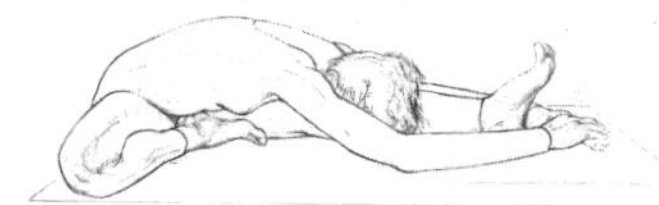
Half Bound
Angle Pose

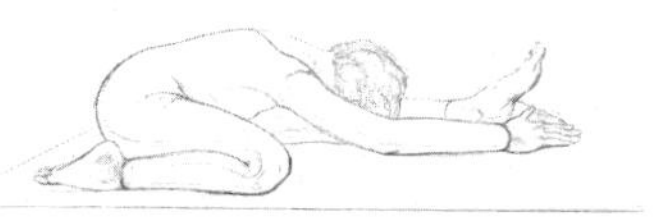
Half Hero's Pose

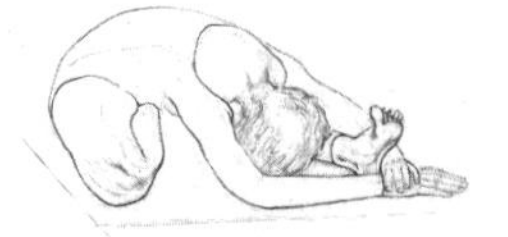
Half Lotus
Forward Bend

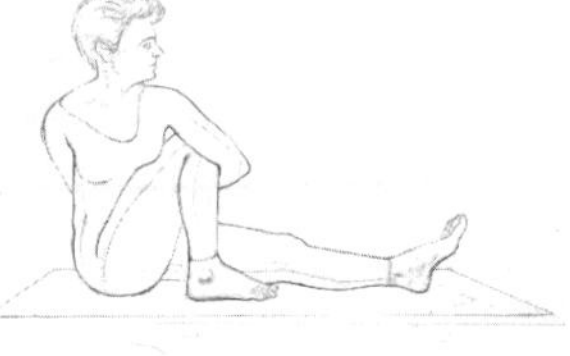
Sage's Twist

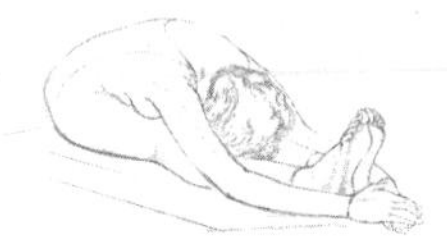
Basic Sitting
Forward Bend

Breathing
Follow your breath quietly and then lengthen every third exhalation.
Deep Relaxation Pose

#5 Active Practice

This heating and energizing series is best done in the morning.

Sun Salutation — 6x each side

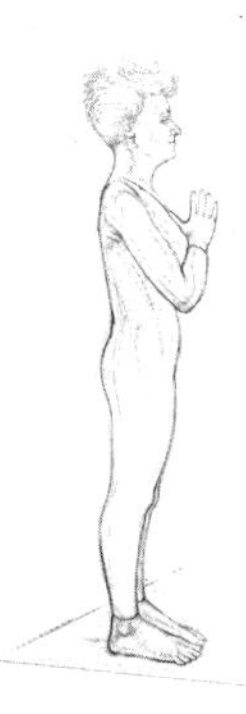

Standing Straight with hands in Prayer Position.

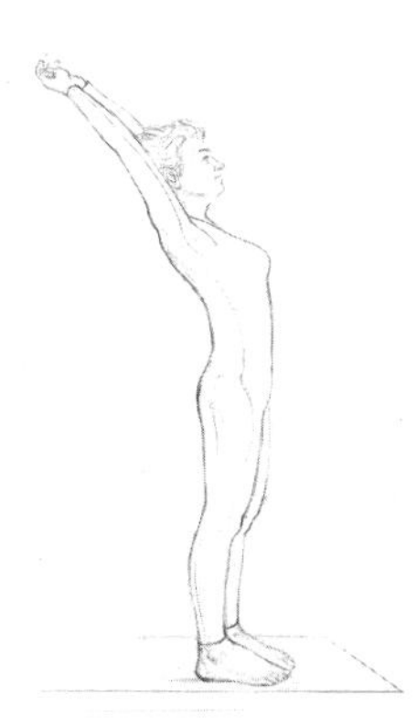

Standing Backbend

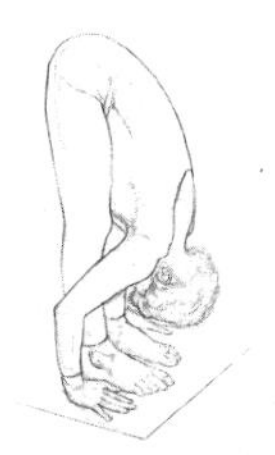

Standing Forward Bend

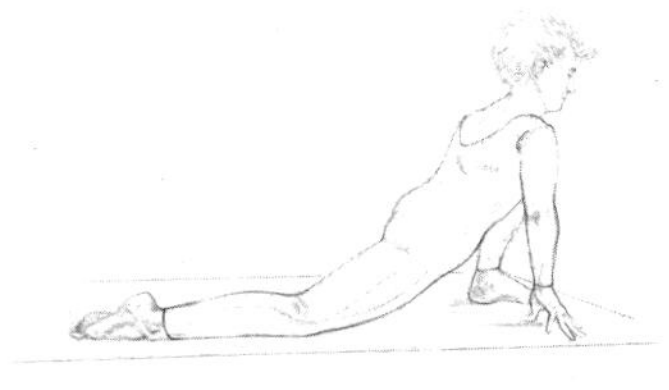

Lunge Pose

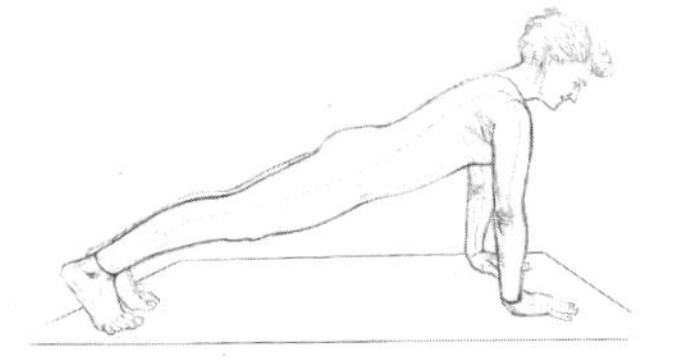

Plank Pose

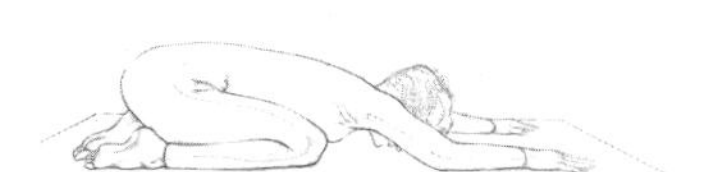

Child Pose

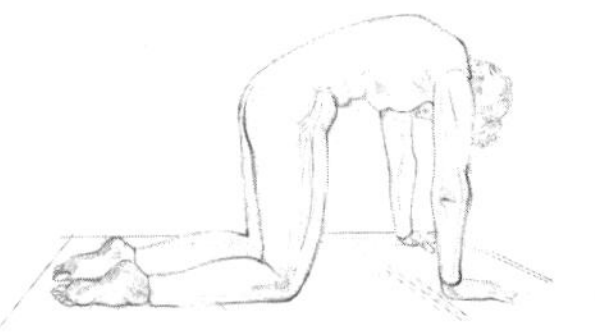

Cat Pose

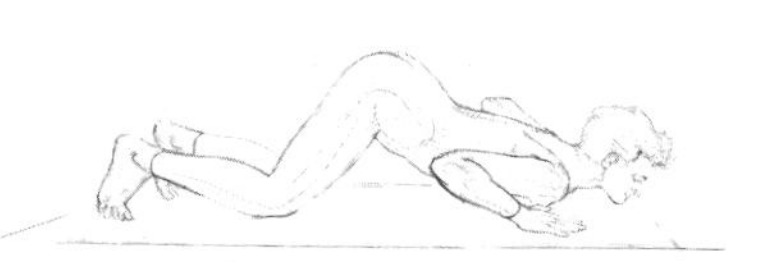

Dip Pose

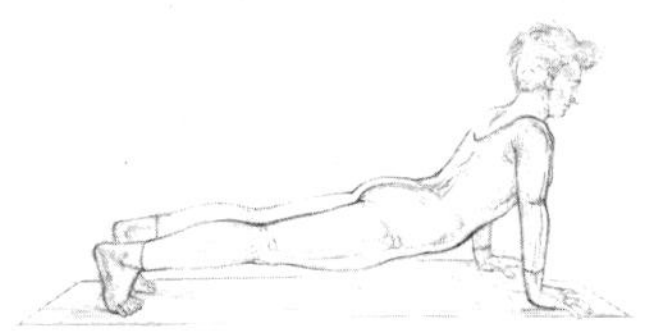

Head-Up Dog Pose or Cobra (see p. 167)

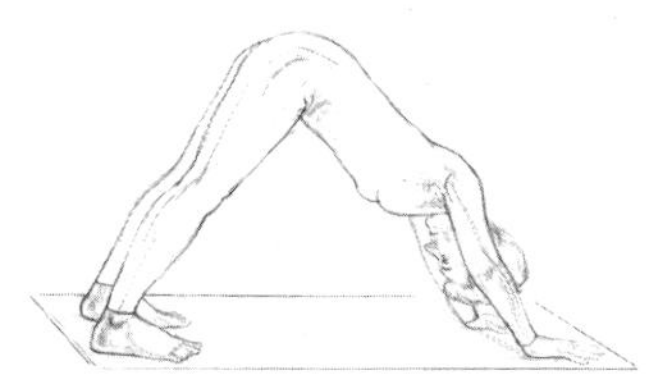

Head-Down Dog Pose

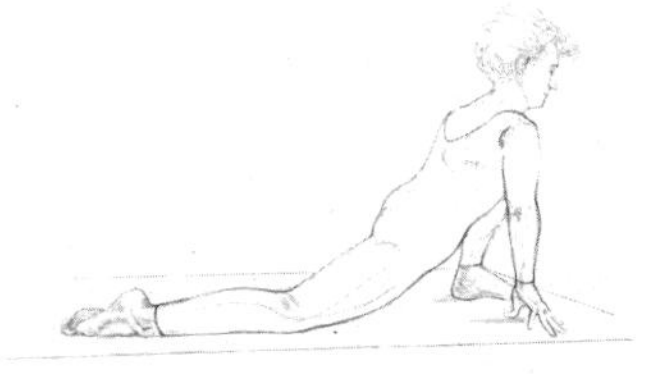

Lunge Pose

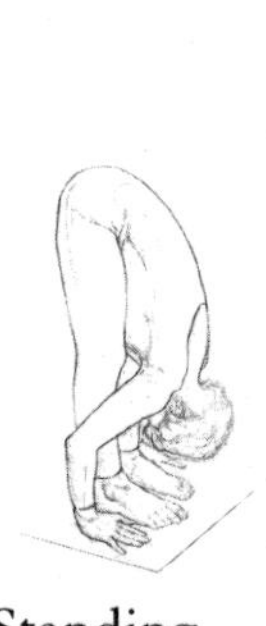

Standing
Forward Bend

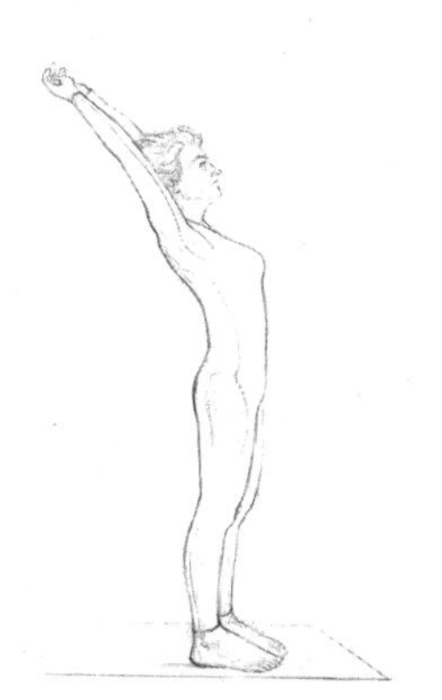

Standing Backbend

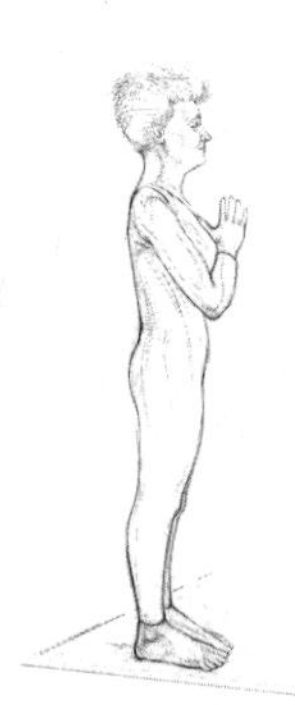

Standing Straight with
hands in Prayer Position

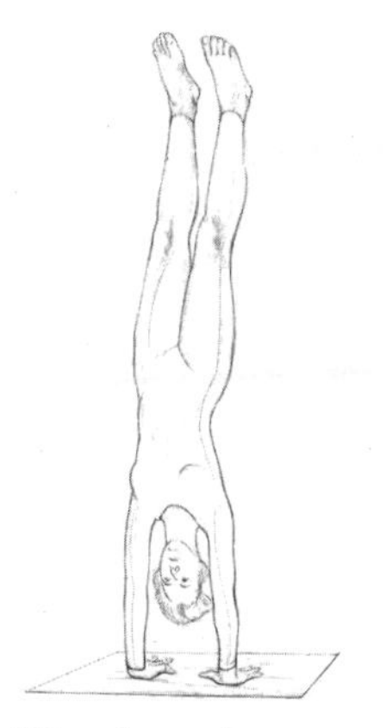

Handstand — 3x

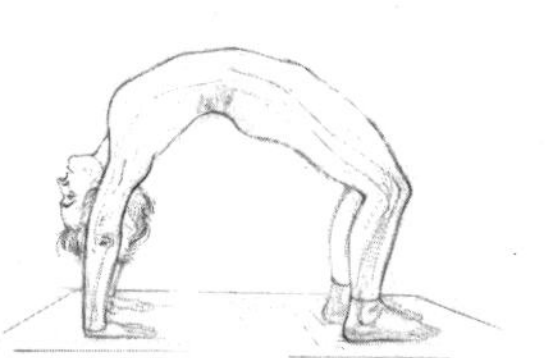

Wheel Pose

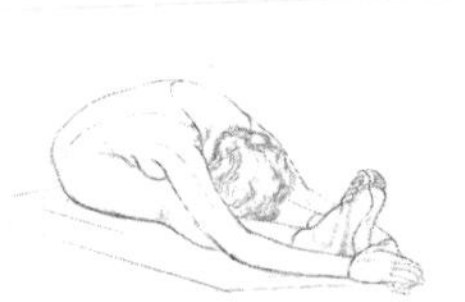

Basic Sitting Forward Bend

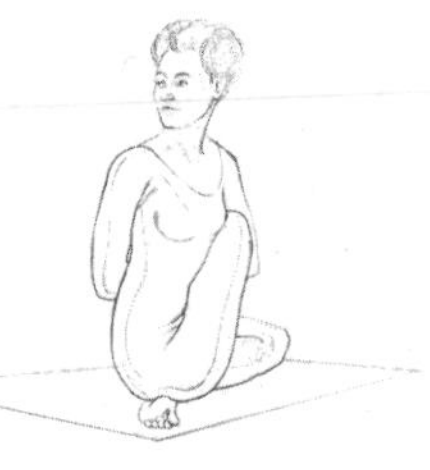

Spinal Twist

Breathing
Rapid Abdominal Breathing — Start with 3 rounds of 10 breaths each
and gradually build to 30 breaths per round.
Then sit quietly and follow your breath.
Deep Relaxation Pose

#6 Inversions

This series takes you into Handstand, Head and Shoulderstands, building up to each of these poses gradually. Add the Shoulderstand and Plough variations as you are ready.

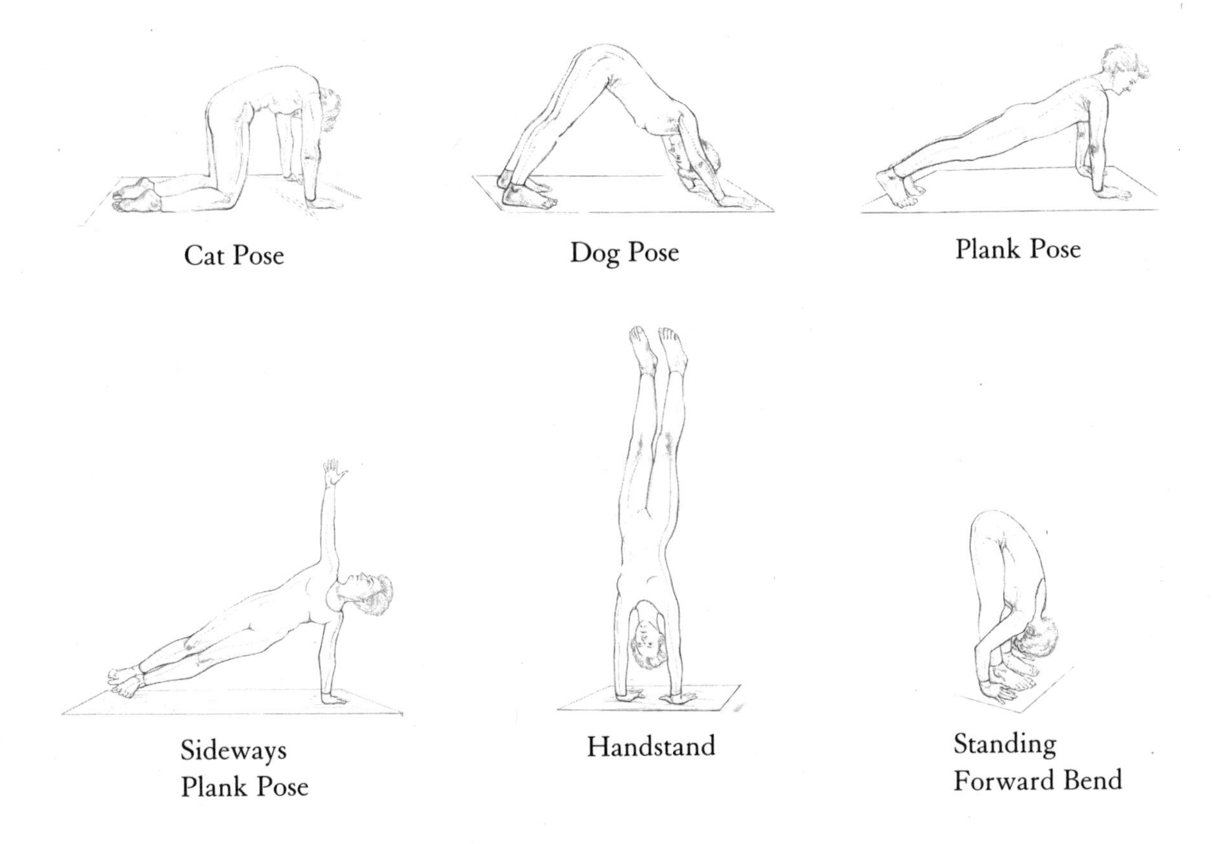

Cat Pose

Dog Pose

Plank Pose

Sideways Plank Pose

Handstand

Standing Forward Bend

Standing Straight, take some time to release your shoulders. Roll your shoulders, then do some neck rolls, and the arms from Eagle Pose, Cow's Head Pose, and Reverse Prayer Position (from the Triangle Forward Bend).

Cat Pose Headstand Preparation (see p. 135)
Dog Pose Headstand Preparation (see p. 135)

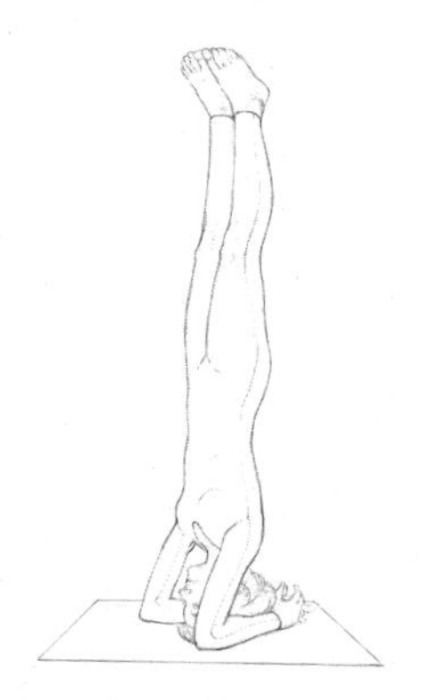

Headstand
near or against a wall

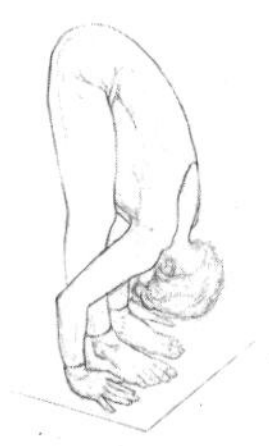

Standing
Forward Bend

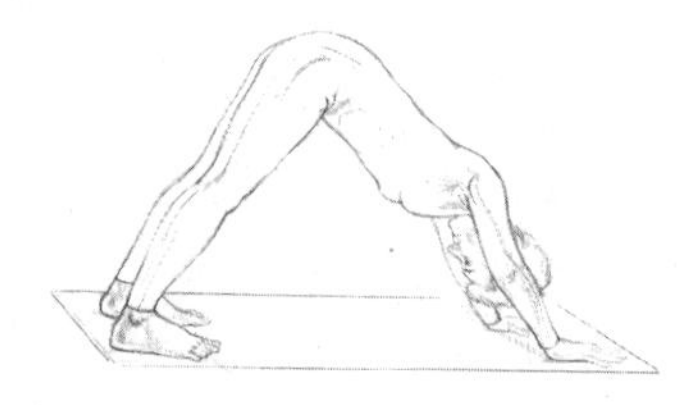

Dog Pose

Repeat the neck and shoulder stretches

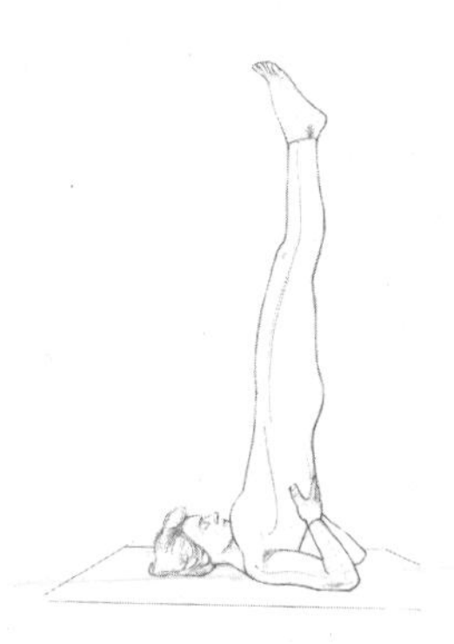

Shoulderstand

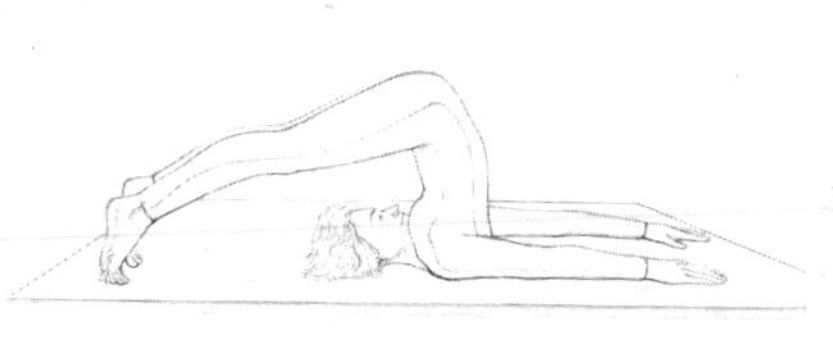

Plough

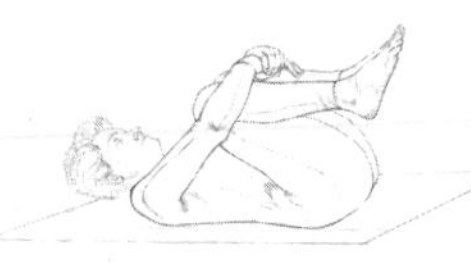

Little Boat Pose

Sitting
Establish a steady breathing rhythm. Pause at the end of the inhalation and the end of the exhalation.
Gradually build up to the Interval Breathing and the Square Breath.
Deep Relaxation Pose

Advanced

#7 Active Practice

Like the intermediate active practice, this series is warming and energizing, and should be done in the morning. For a more intense cardiovascular workout, do more Sun Salutations.

Sun Salutation — 12x each side (see p. 219 for illustrated sequence)

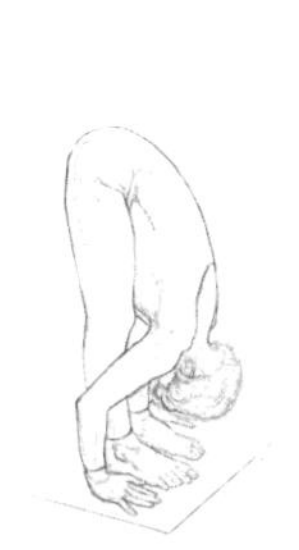

Standing Forward Bend

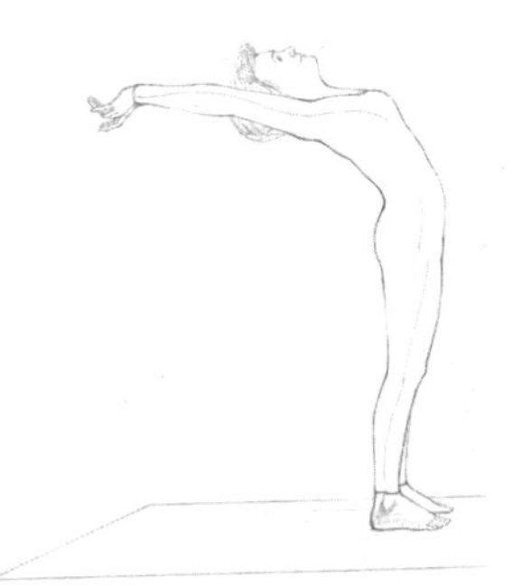

Wheel from Standing — Preparation

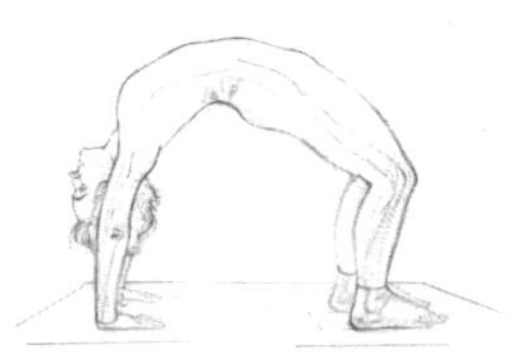

Wheel — pushing up from the floor 6x

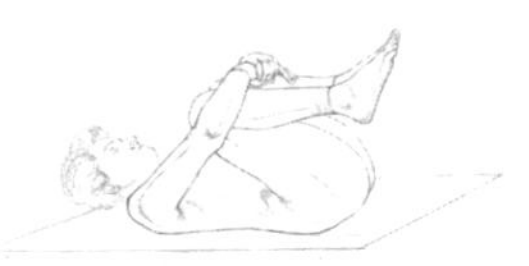

Little Boat

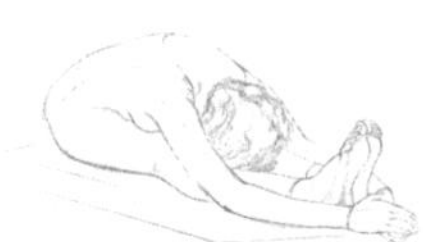

Basic Sitting Forward Bend

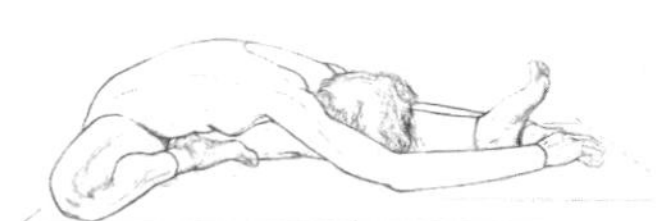

Half Bound Angle Pose

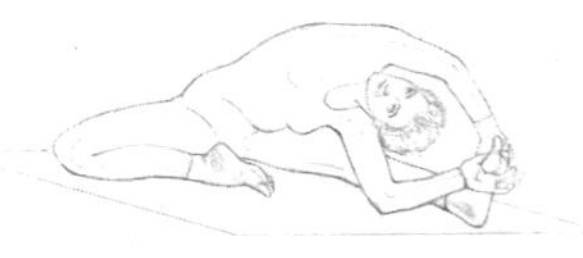

Half Bound Angle Twist

Rapid Abdominal Breathing — Start with 5 rounds of 30 breaths and gradually build up to 60 breaths per round. Follow with quiet breathing for 10 minutes.

Deep Relaxation Pose

#8 Focus on Backbends

This series uses Standing Poses to establish the ground and connection through the legs before coming up into backbends.

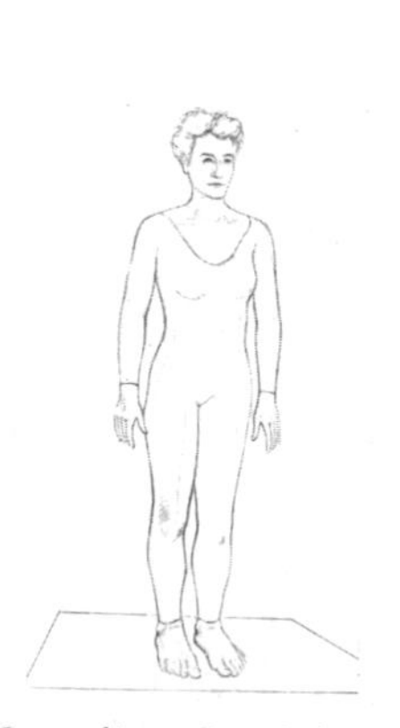
Standing Straight

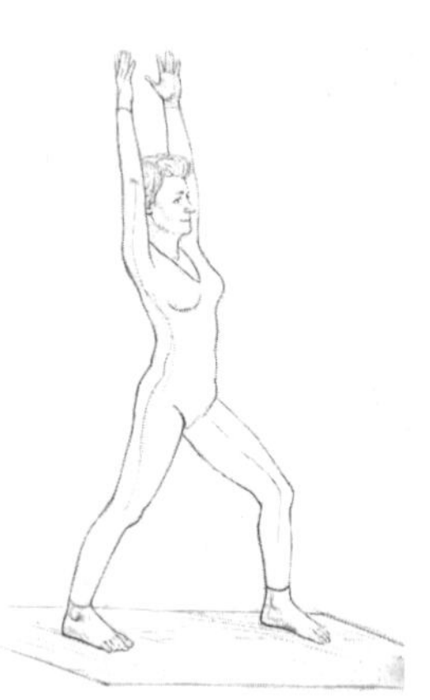
Warrior I

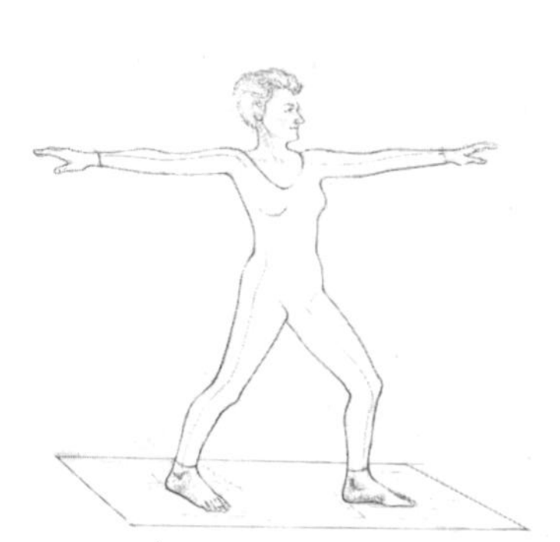
Warrior II

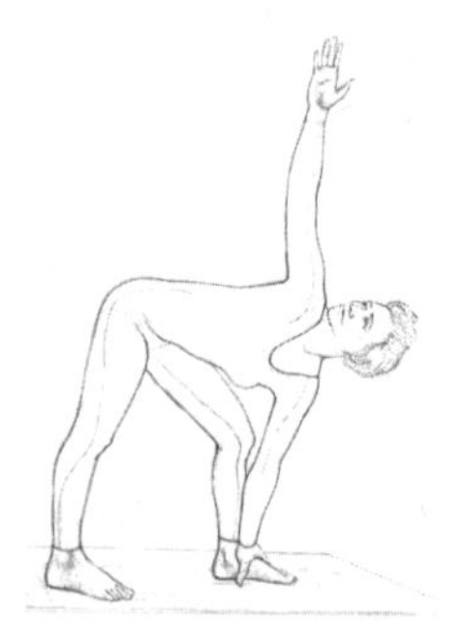
Side Angle Pose

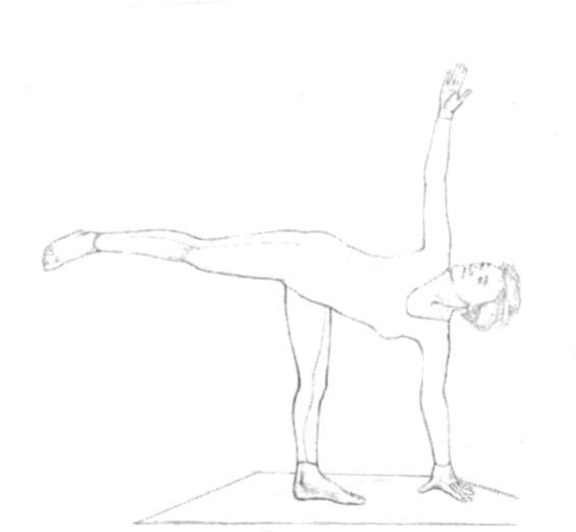
Half Moon Pose

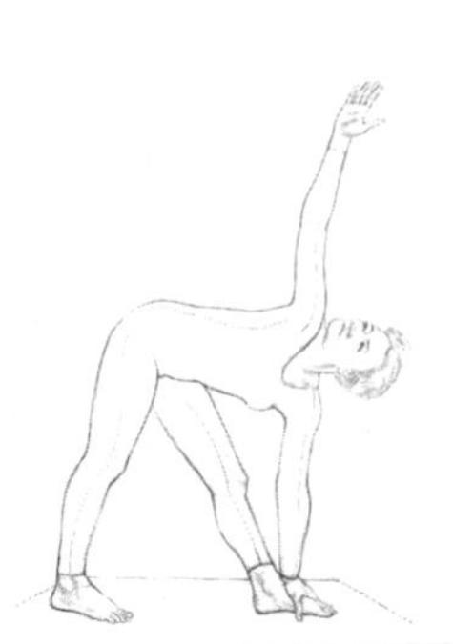
Triangle Pose

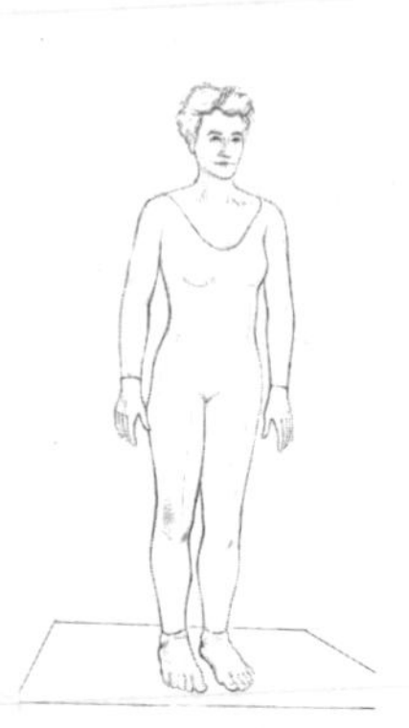
Standing Straight

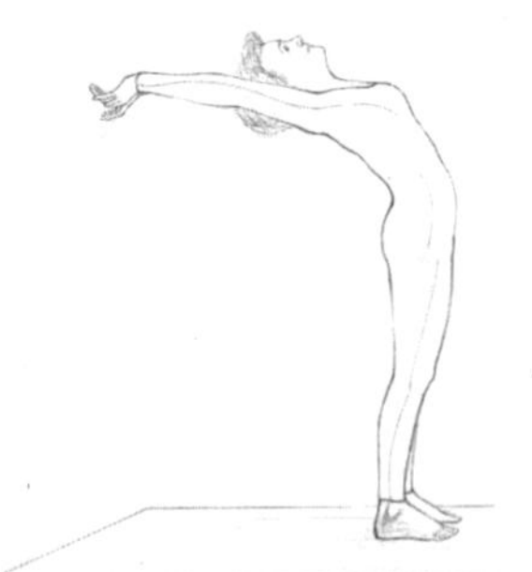
Wheel from Standing

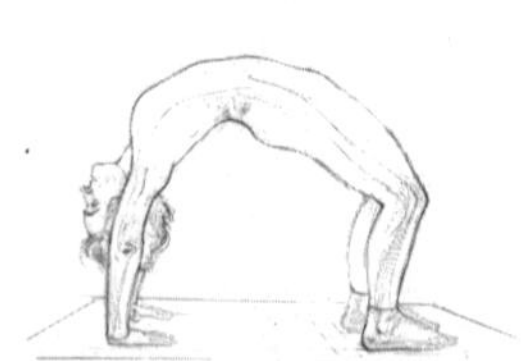
Wheel

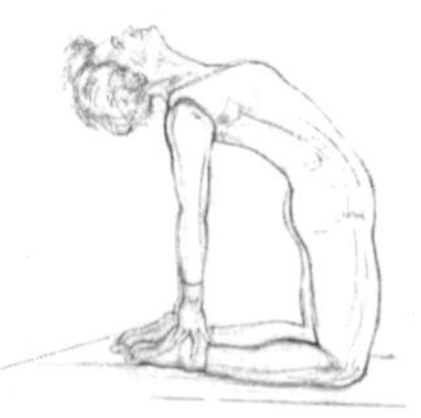
Camel Pose

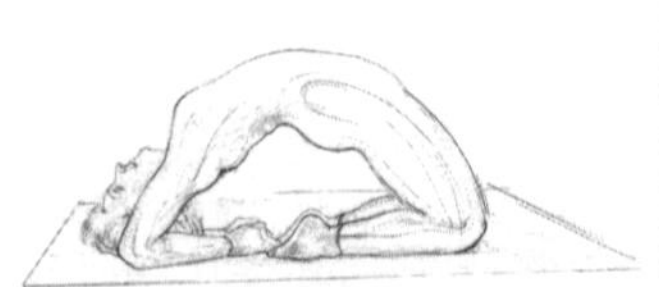
Pigeon Pose

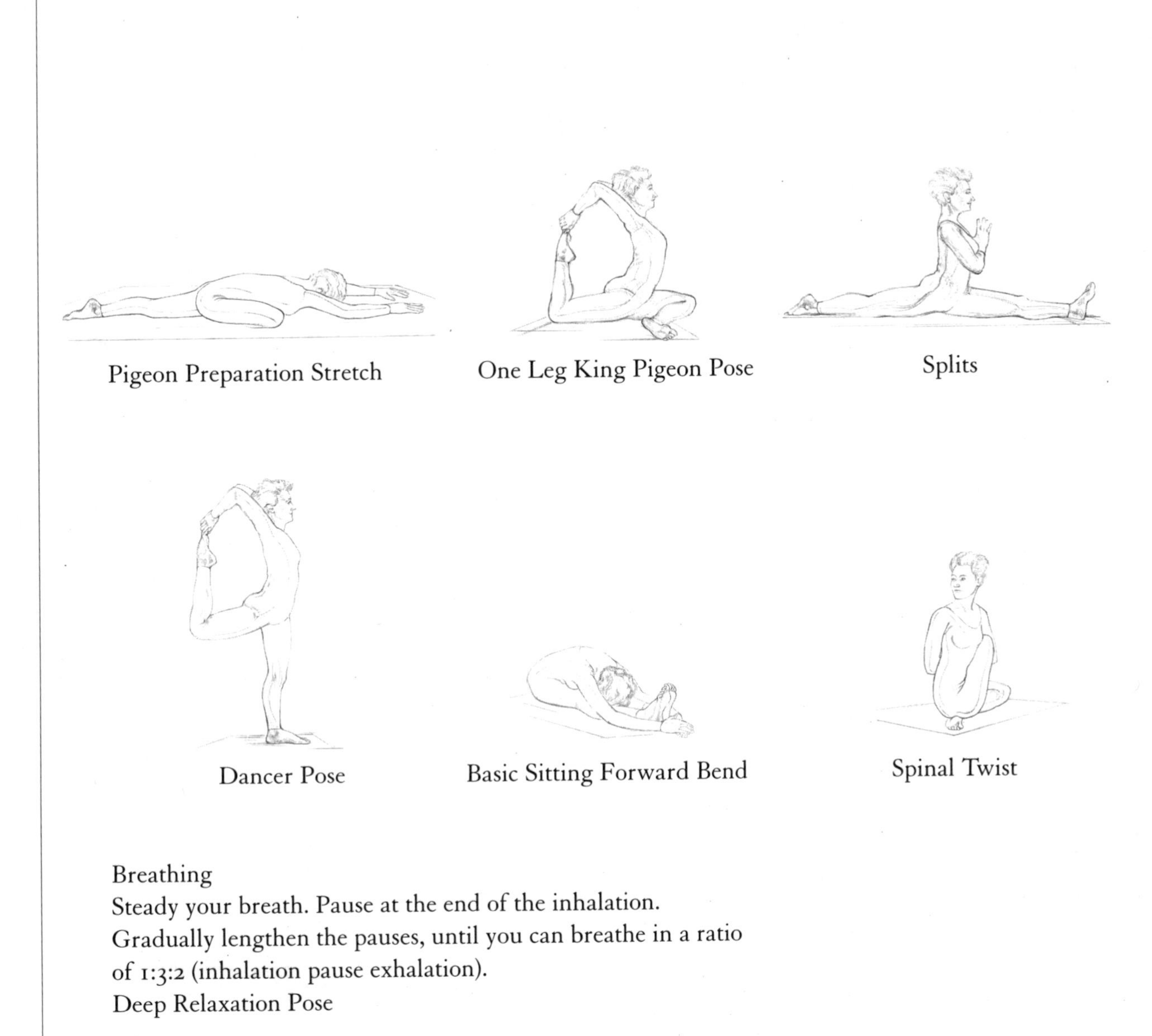

Pigeon Preparation Stretch
One Leg King Pigeon Pose
Splits
Dancer Pose
Basic Sitting Forward Bend
Spinal Twist

Breathing
Steady your breath. Pause at the end of the inhalation.
Gradually lengthen the pauses, until you can breathe in a ratio of 1:3:2 (inhalation pause exhalation).
Deep Relaxation Pose

#9 Inversions and Inverted Backbends

This strong and dynamic practice opens your upper body. Shoulderstand is done before Headstand in this series because it is much easier to drop back from Shoulderstand than from Headstand.

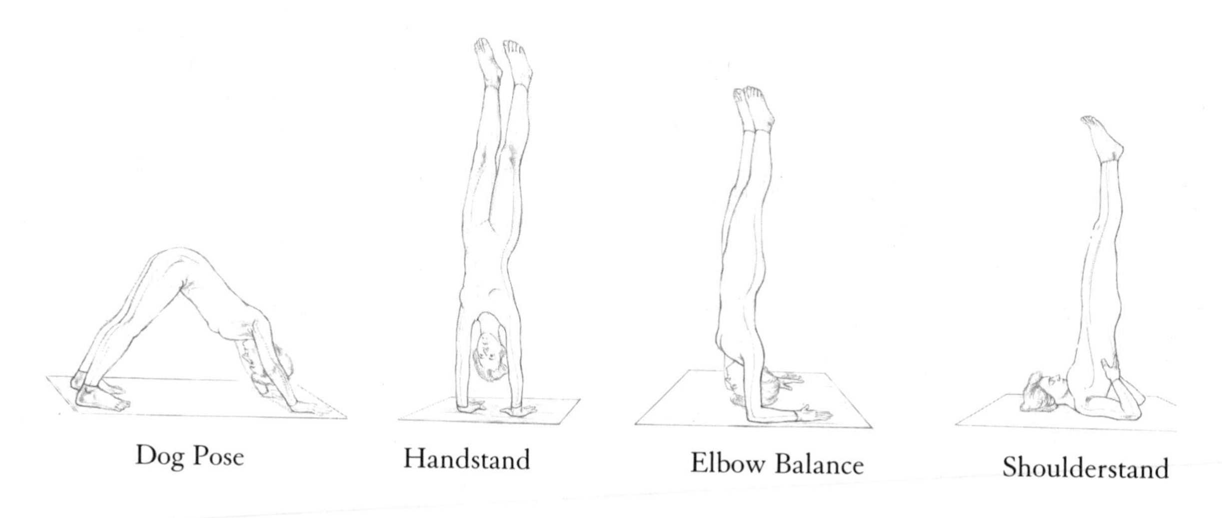

Dog Pose | Handstand | Elbow Balance | Shoulderstand

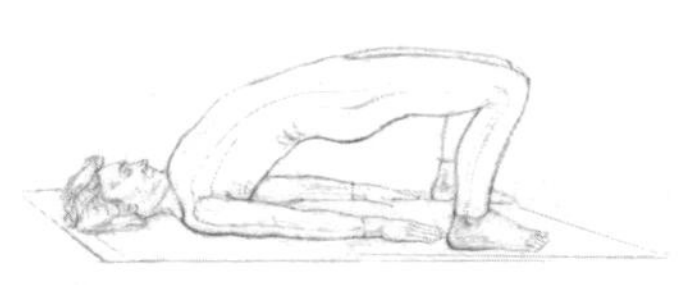

Drop from Shoulderstand into Bridge Pose.

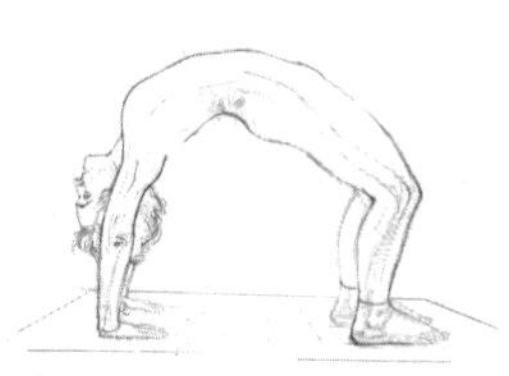

Wheel

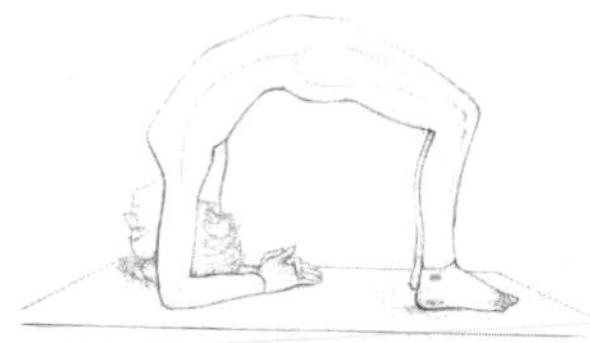

From Wheel, bend your arms and come into Head Balance Back Arch.

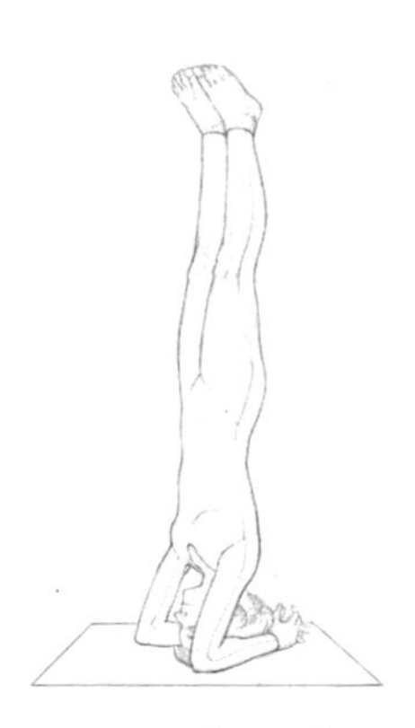

Headstand

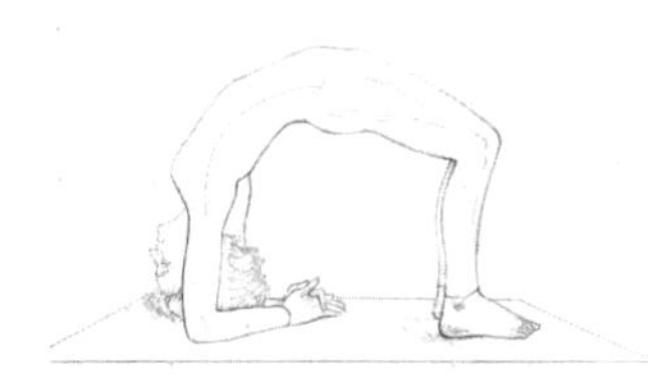

From Headstand start
to drop back into
Head Balance Back Arch.

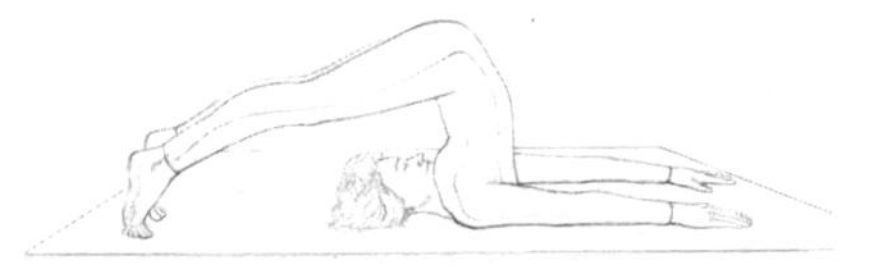

Plough

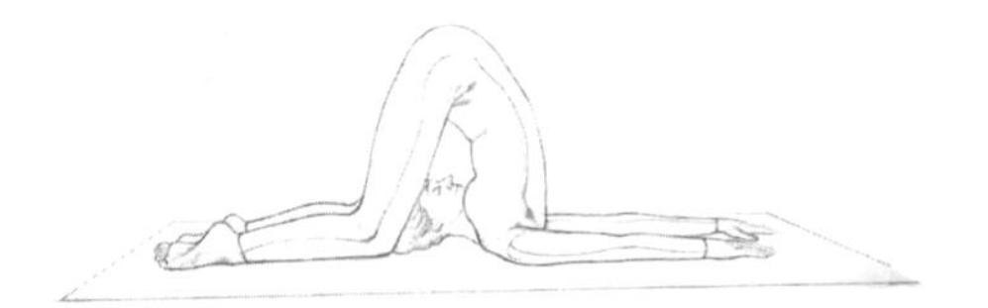

Plough with Knees Bent

Breathing
Steady your breathing. Then gradually increase the length of your exhalation until it is twice the length of your inhalation.
Deep Relaxation Pose

10 Crow Pose

These poses strengthen the arms and tone the abdominal organs. Remember that the weight is resting on your arms, which is a very different feeling than using your arms to hold you up. When you find the balance point, the amount of strength needed to do the pose decreases dramatically.

Usually, backbends are counterbalanced by forward bends. However, in this series, the intense forward bends are counterbalanced by backbends. If you do the Tripod Headstand, be sure to counterbalance it with Shoulderstand.

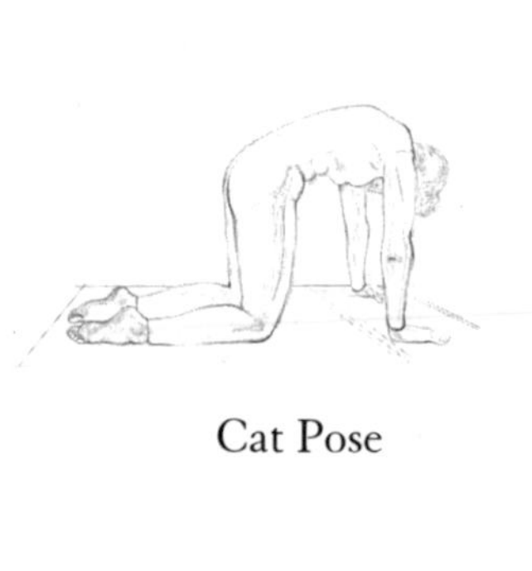

Cat Pose

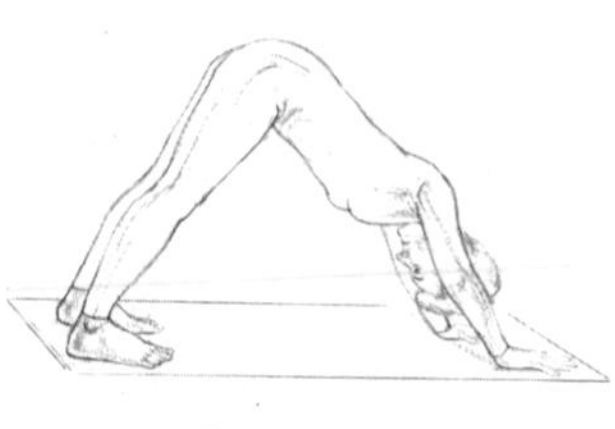

Dog Pose

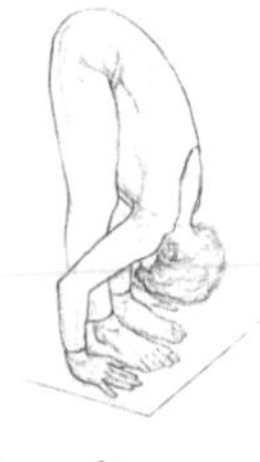

Standing Forward Bend

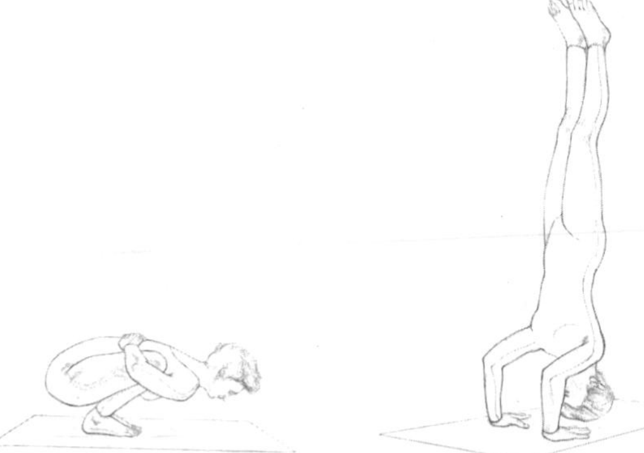

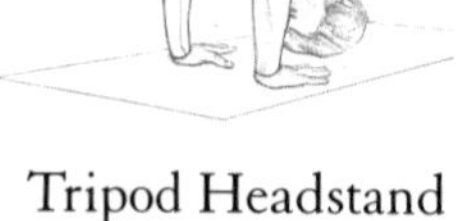

Garland Pose

Tripod Headstand

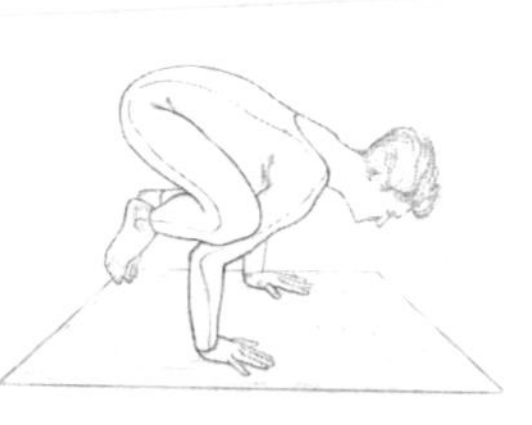

Crow Pose

Standing Forward Bend

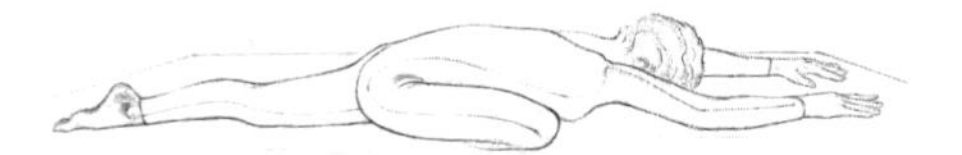

Pigeon Preparation Stretch

Lotus in Crow Pose (see p. 157)

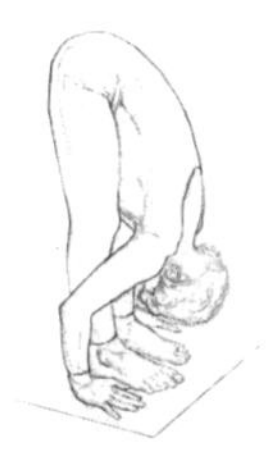

Standing
Forward Bend

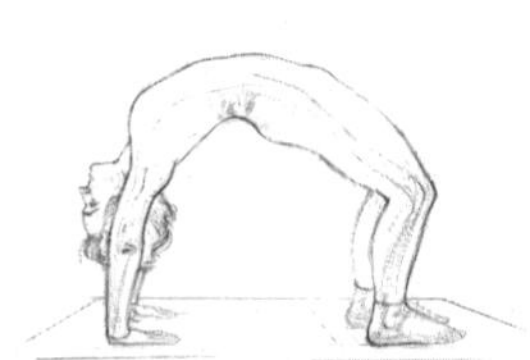

Wheel Pose

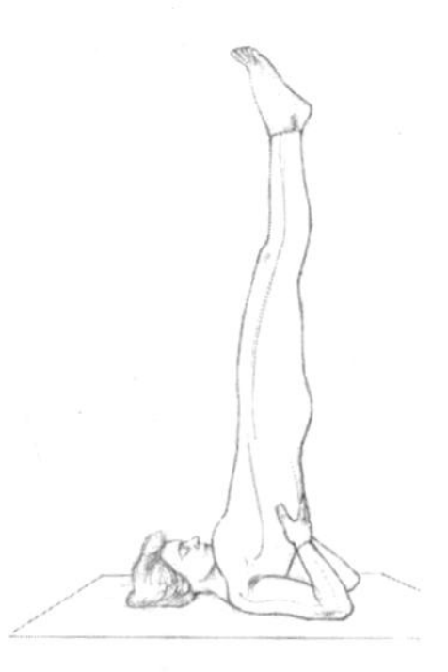

Shoulderstand

Deep Relaxation Pose

Suggested Reading

Asana & Pranayama

Iyengar, B. K. S. *Light on Yoga.* New York: Schocken Books, 1979.

Myers, Esther & Wylie, Lynn. *The Ground, the Breath & the Spine.* Toronto: self-published, 1992.

Myers, Esther. *Relaxation*, an audio tape (3 spoken guided relaxations, no music).

Ohlig, Adelheid. *Luna Yoga*. Woodstock, New York: Ash Tree Publishing, 1994.

Scaravelli, Vanda. *Awakening the Spine*. San Francisco: HarperCollins, 1991.

Stewart, Mary. *Yoga for Children*. New York: Simon & Schuster, 1992.

Stewart, Mary. *Yoga over 50*. New York: Simon & Schuster, 1994.

Vanda Scaravelli: *On Yoga.* A 35-minute video, including interviews with Vanda, as well as examples of her practice and her teaching.

Anatomy & Body Structure

Kapit, Wynn, & Elson, Lawrence M. *The Anatomy Coloring Book*. New York, San Francisco, London: HarperCollins, 1993.

Rolf, Ida. *Rolfing, The Integration of Human Structures*. New York: Harper & Row, 1977.

Yoga Philosophy & Psychology

Easwaran, Eknath, trans. *The Bhagavad Gita.* Berkeley: Nilgiri Press, 1985.

Hewitt, James. *The Complete Yoga Book.* New York: Schocken Books, 1977.

Mascaro, Juan, trans. *The Bhagavad Gita.* London: Penguin Books, 1988.

Prabhavananda, Swami and Isherwood, C. *How to Know God: The Yoga Aphorisms of Patanjali.* New York: New American Library, 1969.

Prabhavananda, Swami and Manchester, Frederick. *The Upanishads.* New York: Mentor, 1975.

Taimni, I. K. *The Science of Yoga.* Wheaton, Illinois; Madras, India; London, England: The Theosophical Publishing House, 1961, 1981.

Wilber, Ken. *No Boundary.* Boston & London: Shambhala, 1985.

Kundalini & Chakras

Judith, Anodea. *Wheels of Life: A User's Guide to the Chakra System.* St. Paul, Minn.: Llewellyn Publications, 1989.

Kason, Yvonne and Degler, Teri. *A Farther Shore.* Toronto: HarperCollins, 1994.

Selby, John. *Kundalini Awakening: A Gentle Guide to Chakra Activation and Spiritual Growth.* New York, Toronto, London, Sydney, Auckland: Bantam Books, 1992.

Meditation

Friedman, Lenore. *Meetings with Remarkable Women: Buddhist Teachers in America.* Boston & London: Shambhala, 1987.

Han, Thich Nhat. *Being Peace.* Berkeley: Parallax Press, 1987.
The Miracle of Mindfulness: A Manual on Meditation. Boston: Beacon Press, 1987.

Kabat-Zinn, Jon. *Full Catastrophe Living.* New York: Delta, 1990.

Kornfield, Jack. *A Path With Heart.* New York, Toronto, London, Sydney, Auckland: Bantam Books, 1993.

Rinpoche, Sogyal. The *Tibetan Book of Living & Dying.* San Francisco: HarperSanFrancisco, 1992.

Suzuki, Shunrya. *Zen Mind, Beginner's Mind.* New York & Tokyo: Weatherhill, 1986.

Friends of Peace Pilgrim. *Peace Pilgrim: Her Life and Work in Her Own Words*. 43480 Cedar Avenue, Hemet, California 92344. Write for a free copy.

Personal Growth

Baldwin, Christina. *Life's Companion*. New York, Toronto, London, Sydney, Auckland: Bantam Books, 1990.
Borysenko, Joan. *Guilt Is the Teacher, Love Is the Lesson*. New York: Warner Books, 1990.
Exeter, Nancy Rose. *Magic at our Hand*. 100 Mile House, B.C.: Foundation House Publications, 1988.
Goldberg, Natalie. *Writing Down the Bones*. Boston & London: Shambhala, 1986.
Keen, Sam. *Fire in the Belly: On Being a Man*. New York, Toronto, London, Sydney, Auckland: Bantam Books, 1991.
Laing, R.D. *The Politics of Experience*. Harmondsworth, Middlesex, England: Penguin Books, 1967.
Levine, Stephen. *Healing into Life & Death*. New York: Anchor Press/Doubleday, 1987.
Mallasz, Gita (transcription). *Talking with Angels*. Einsiedeln, Switzerland: Daimon Verlag, 1992.
Markova, Dawna. *No Enemies Within*. Berkeley: Conari Press, 1994.

Glossary of Sanskrit Terms

Ananta: In Hindu mythology, Ananta is the Chief of Serpents who upholds the globe of the earth and keeps it in orbit around the sun. He is the symbolic representation of the force of gravity.

Asana: In Patanjali, asana meant the place on which the yogi sits and the manner in which he sits there. It now refers to all the yoga postures.

Astanga: Eight-limbed. The eight limbs of yoga are described in Patanjali's *Yoga Sutras*.

Bhagavad Gita: Song of God, a classical yoga scripture, part of the epic poem, *The Mahabharata*.

Bhakti Yoga: The yoga of devotion.

Chakras: Energy centres. There are seven major centres of energy located on the spine: the base of the spine, the genitals, the solar plexus, the heart, throat, between the eyebrows and the crown of the head.

Dharana: Concentration, the sixth of Patanjali's eight limbs of yoga.

Dyana: Contemplation or absorption/meditation, the seventh of Patanjali's eight limbs of yoga.

Guru: Teacher.

Hatha Yoga: The practice of yoga postures. The word is derived from "Ha" meaning sun, and "Tha" meaning moon. It implies the integration and balancing of these two principles of energy.

Jnana Yoga: The yoga of study or self-knowledge.

Karma: Action, and the consequences of one's actions.

Karma Yoga: Selfless service.

Kriyas: Purification practices.

Kundalini: The energy of the spine. Kundalini is often described as a serpent, coiled at the base of the spine. Through practice, this energy is awakened and moves up through the spine.

Mahabharata: The great story of the Bharatas, a classical Indian epic poem.

Mandala: A circle, or a circular image that serves as a focus for concentration.

Mantra: A sacred syllable or phrase.

Mantra Yoga: The repetition of a sacred syllable or phrase, a form of meditation practice.

Nirvana: Literally, extinction. Nirvana refers to the cessation of all desire.

Niyamas: Disciplines which are concerned with the inner life, and relate to the committed practitioner. The second of Patanjali's eight limbs.

Prana: The universal life force.

Pranayama: Breathing practice, regulates and harmonizes the breath and its rhythm.

Pratyahara: Contemplation or absorption, the sixth of Patanjali's eight limbs of yoga.

Raja Yoga: The royal yoga. The method of practice and meditation described in Patanjali's *Yoga Sutras*.

Samadhi: Ecstatic union, the last of Patanjali's eight limbs of yoga.

Sutras: Threads. The name given to Patanjali's aphorisms on the meaning and practice of yoga.

Tapas: Heat. It implies both psychic heat in the form of anger and aggression, and a burning fervour or zeal.

Vedas: The earliest Indian scriptures (3000–1200 B.C.).

Vipassana: Insight.

Yamas: Universal ethical principles or disciplines. The first of Patanjali's eight limbs.

Yantra: A geometric form used as a focus for concentration.

Yoga: The joining or union of the individual self or soul with the higher Self — God. Yoga means mystical union *and* the disciplines or practices that lead toward this union.

Yuj: The root of the word yoga. To join, to yoke, to direct and concentrate one's attention on.

Index

The main listing for a pose or breathing technique is given in boldface.

A

Adho Mukha Svanasana **92**, 106
Adho Mukha Vrksasana **131**
Alignment 14, 16, 38-41, 48, 54, 84
Alternate Nostril Breathing **74-77**
  Alternate Nostril Exhalation **75**
  Alternate Nostril Inhalation **75**
  Full Alternate Nostril Breathing **77**
  Inhalation through the Left Nostril **76**
  Inhalation through the Right Nostril **76**
Ananta 14, 16
Anjaneyasana **94**, 104, 106
Anuloma Pranayama **75**
Ardha Baddha Padmottasana **111**
Ardha Chandrasana **121**
  Parivrtta Ardha Chandrasana **121**
Ardha Matsyendrasana **202-203**
Ardha Padma Paschimottanasana **193**
Ardha Padmasana **189**
Arm Balances 125, **155-157**,181
Asana 11, 14, 15, 16, 21, 45
Astanga
  Namaskar **105**
  Yoga 11, 107
Asthma 69
Aum **79**

B

Backbends 25, 32, 36, 37, 39, 43, 90, 97, 150, 155, **159-179**, 182
  Dropping into **169-175**
  Standing 104, 106, 113, **173-174**
  Other Advanced **176-179**
  Prone 95, **165-168**
Baddha Konasana **188**
Bakasana **156**
Balances
  Arm 125, **155-157**
  Standing 111, 114, **118-121**
Basic Sitting Forward Bend 54, 184, **190**, 191
Basic Standing Forward Bend 41, 50, 54, 99, 103, 104, 106, **111**, 133
Bee's Breath **78**
Bhagavad Gita 10, 24, 59, 195
Bhakti yoga 17
Bhramari **78**
Bhujangasana 105
Bladder 144, 188
Blood Pressure 69, 71, 125
Body Image 26-28
Bound Angle Pose 127, 139, 143, 182, 184, **188**, 189, 193
  Half 177, **191**, 193, 194
    Twist 187, **201**, 205
Bow Pose 165, **168**
Breathing **59-79**
  Alternate Nostril **74-77**

Other Breathing and
Sounding Techniques **78-79**
Practices **66-79**
Rapid Abdominal
Breathing 25, 34, 50, **68-69**, 78, 130, 182
Retention 71, **73**, 77
Rhythms and Timing **70-72**
Strong **68-69**
Bridge Pose **161**, 163
From Shoulderstand **169**
Single Leg **170**
Supported **144**, 145
Butterfly Pose **188**

C
Camel Pose **175**
Cancer 6-7, 19, 38
Cat Pose **90-91**, 101, 105, 127, 165
Chair Pose **84**
Chakra 16, 65, 159
Chandra Bhedana Pranayama **76**
Chaturanga Dandasana 105, **128**
Child's Pose 25, 36, 50, 54, 56, **89**, 100, 105, 165, 182
Circulation 126
Legs 55, 143, 144
Cobbler's Pose **188**
Cobra Pose 37, 95, 101, 105, 159, 165, **167**
Colds 144
Colitis 155, 199
Complete Yoga Breath **66**
Constipation 199
Cooling Breaths **78**
Corpse Pose 53, **54**
Cough 144
Cow's Head Pose 120, **186**, 202
Crow Pose 37, 47, 93, 155, **156-157**, **194**
Lotus in **157**
Cystitis 155, 199

D
Dancer Pose **179**
Simple 118
Deep Relaxation 36, 46, **53-57**, 60
Pose **54**
Dhanurasana **168**
Urdhva **163**
From Standing **173-174**
Diaphragm 61, 63, 65
Digestion 126, 199, 202
Dip Pose 50, 101, **105**
Disks, Herniated 159, 167, 182
Dog Pose 41, **92**, 127, 133
Head Down **92**, 102, 106
Head Up 101, 105, **165**, 167
Dwi Pada Viparita Dandasana **170**

E
Eagle Pose **120**, 139
Eight Parts Pose 50, **105**
Eight-fold Path 11-15
Eka Pada Raja Kapotasana **95**, **176-177**
Eka Pada Sirsasana **139, 196**
Eka Pada Sarvangasana **148**
Eka Pada Viparita Dandasana **172**
Elbow Balance 41, 127, 130, **132**
Emotions 12, 18-19, 23-25, 27, 48, 57, 59, 60, 65, 68
Emphysema 69
Extended Exhalation **66**

F
Feelings *See* Emotions
Fierce Pose **84**
Fight or Flight 22-23
Forward Bends
Advanced **195-196**
One Leg Straight, One Leg Bent **191-194**
Simple **184-190**
Sitting 25, 29, **181-197**
Standing 41, 50, 54 **111-112**

G
Garland Pose **93**, 156, 194, 196
Garudasana **120**
Gomukhasana **186**

H
Ha 15, 22, **68**, 69, 130
Halasana **150**
Parsva **152**
Half Bound Angle Pose 177, **191**, 193, 194
Twist 187, **201**, 205
Half Hero's Pose 177, **192**, 205
Half Lotus Pose 184, **189**, 194, 205
Forward Bend 189, **193**
In Standing Forward Bend **111**
In Tree Pose **119**
Lying down **141**
Half Moon Pose **121**
Twist **121**
Half Shoulderstand **145**
Handstand 25, 41, 126, **130-131**, 132, 155
Hanumanasana **178**
Hatha Yoga 4, 15-16
Head Balance Back Arch **171**
Single Leg Variation **172**
Head Down Tree Pose **131**

Head Down Dog Pose **92**, 102, 106
Headstand 25, 37, 39, 41, 47, 85, 120, 126-127, 130, 132, **133-142**, 171
  Cat Pose Preparation **135**
  Dog Pose Preparation **135**
  Dropping Back from **172**
    Single Leg Variation **172**
  Going Up **136**
  In the Pose **137**
  Lotus Pose in 140, **141**
  Lotus Forward Bend in **142**
  Preparation **134-135**
  Single Leg Variation **139**
  Tripod Headstand **142**, 156
  Twist **140**
  Variations **139-142**
Head Up Dog Pose 101, 105, **165**, 167
Hero's Pose 139, 140, **185**
  Half 177, **192**, 205
Heron Pose **192**
Humming Breath **78**

I
Illness 24, 36, 42, 57, 60
Imagery 48, 62, 83
Injury 11, 16, 21, 228, 38, 39, 40, 41-43, 48, 79, 126, 127
  Repetitive Stress 42-43, 181
Insomnia 74
Intense Spinal Twist **203**
Interval Breath **71**
Inverted Poses 25, 32-33, 39, 42, 48, **125-157**
Irritable Bowel 199
Iyengar, B. K. S. 4, 14, 45
  Yoga 4-5, 35, 107

J
Janu Sirsasana **191**
  Parivrtta **201**
Jnana Yoga 17

K
Kapalabhati Breathing **68-69**
Kapotasana **175**
  Eka Pada Raja **95**, **176-177**
Karma 9
  Yoga 17
Karna Pidasana **151**
  Parsva **152**
Knees
  Injuries 41, 42, 62, 89, 185, 187
  Torn Cartilage/Meniscus 185, 192
Krounchasana **192**
Kumbhaka **73**
Kundalini 16
Kurmasana **195**
  Supta **196**

L
Legs
  Circulation 55, 143, 144
  Resting on the Wall **143**, 182
  Single Leg Bridge Pose **170**
  Stretch in Headstand **139**
  Stretch in Head Balance Back Arch **172**
  Stretch in Shoulderstand **148**
Wide in Plough **152**
  Wide Standing Forward Bend **111**
Lion **68**
Little Boat Pose 36, 54, 56, **87**, 89, 162
  Twist **88**
Lotus Pose 11, 61, 188, **189**, 193, 196
  Forward Bend In Headstand **142**
  Half *See* Half Lotus
  In Crow Pose **157**
  In Headstand 140, **141**
  In Plough Pose **154**
  In Plough Twist **154**
  In Shoulderstand **153**
  In Shoulderstand Twist **154**
  Inverted 127
  Lying down **141**
  Variations in Headstand **141-142**
  Variations in Shoulderstand **153-154**
Lunge Pose **94**, 100, 102, 104, 106, 159, 176, 177
Lying Release Pose 54, **55**, 161

M
Malasana **93**
Mantra 14, 15, 79
  Yoga 15, 17
Marichyasana
  I, Forward Bend **194**
  I, Twist **204**
  III **205**
Marjarasana **90-91**, 105
Mastectomy 6, 25, 28, 34, 49
Matsyendrasana **202-203**
  Ardha **202-203**
  Paripurna **203**
Meditation 6, 14-15, 17, 18, 24, 32, 38, 65, 81, 184, 187
Men 18, 28, 29
Menopause 27
Menstruation 90, 125, 155, 188, 199
Mountain Pose 81, **83**, 85

N
Nadi Sodhana Pranayama **77**
Namaste 104, 106
Natarajasana **179**

O
Om **79**
One Leg Behind the Head Pose **196**
One Leg King Pigeon Pose **176-177**

P
Padmasana **189**
  Ardha **189**
Paripurna Matsyendrasana **203**
Parsva Halasana **152**
Parsva Karna Pidasana **152**
Parsvakonasana **116**
  Parivrtta **123**
Parsva Urdhva Padmasana Sarvangasana **154**
Parsva Pindasana in Sarvangasana **154**
Parsva Sarvangasana **149**
Parsva Sirsasana **140**
Parsvottanasana **112**
Pasasana **207**
Paschimottanasana **190**
  Ardha Padma **193**
  Triang Mukhaikapada **192**
  Urdhva Mukha **190**
Patanjali 10-15
Pavana Muktasana **87**
  Parsva **88**
Peacock Tail-Feather Pose **132**
Pelvic Tilt 37, **161**, 183
Perfect Posture **184**
Pigeon Pose **175**
  One Leg King Variations **176-177**
  Preparation Stretch **95**, 176, 189, 193
Pincha Mayurasana **132**
Pindasana
  In Sarvangasana **154**
    Parsva **154**
  In Sirsasana **142**
Plank Pose 100, 105, **128**
  Sideways Plank Pose **128**
Plough 127, 143, 147, **150**, 182
  Legs Wide in **152**
  Lotus in **152**
    Twist **152**
  Twist **152**
  Variations **151-152**
  With Knees Bent 127, **151**
    Twist **152**
Posture of the Adept **184**
Practice 31-43
  Finding the Time 33-34
  Finding Support 35-36
  Guidelines 32-33
  How to Structure 36-38
  Obstacles to 24-25
  Starting 34-35
Prana 14, 59
Pranatasana **89**, 105
Pranayama 10, 11, 14, 15, 17, 22, 57, **59-79**
Prasarita Padottanasana **111**
Pratiloma Pranayama **75**
Prayer Position 99, 103, 104, 106, 112, 174
Pregnancy 69, 71, 88, 90, 93, 122, 127, 144, 155, 182, 188, 199, 200
  Breech Position 144
  Post-Partum 155
Prstha Vakrasana 104, 106

R
Raja Yoga 10
Rapid Abdominal Breathing 25, 34, 50, **68-69**, 78, 130, 182
Reclining Forward Bend **190**
Relaxation 14, 21, 22, 25, 31, 36, 37, 47-48, 59
  Deep Relaxation 36, 46, **53-57**, 60
  Deep Relaxation Pose **54**
  Relaxation Response 22, 56
Repetitive Stress Injury 42-43, 181
Retention *See* Breathing

S
Sage's Forward Bend **194**
Sage's Twist 194, **204-205**
Sama Vrtti Pranayama **72**
Sarvangasana **143-154**
  Eka Pada **148**
  Parsva **149**
  Pindasana in **154**
    Parsva **154**
  Setu Bandha **161**
    Eka Pada **170**
  Setu Bandhasana from **169**
  Urdhva Padmasana Sarvangasana **154**
    Parsva **154**
Savasana **54**
Scaravelli, Vanda 4-5, 21, 27, 33, 45, 48, 50, 81, 109, 182
Scissors Twist In Headstand **140**
Setu Bandha Sarvangasana **161**
  Eka Pada **170**
  From Shoulderstand **169**
Sexuality 16, 28

Shoulderstand 37, 41, 43, 85, 97, 126-127, 130, 133, **143-154**, 171, 193
- Bridge Pose from **169**
- Half 143, **145**, 147
- Lotus in **154**
  - Twist **155**
- Preparation Poses **143-45**
- Single Leg Stretch in 127, **148**
- Supported Bridge Pose 143, **144**
- Supported Inverted Practice **144**
- Twist **149**
- Variations **148-154**

Siddhasana **184**
Side Angle Pose 109, 115, **116**, 121
- Twist 109, 121, 122, **123**

Side Angle Poses **116-117**
Sideways Plank Pose **129**
Simhasana **68**
Simple Crossed Legs **184**
Simple Sitting Poses 56, 61, **184-190**
  - Twisting in **200**

Simple Dancer Pose 118
Simple Stretches 31, **87-95**
Single Leg Bridge Pose **170**
Sirsasana **133-142**
- Sirsasana II **142**
- Eka Pada **139, 196**
- Parivrttaikapada **140**
- Parsva **140**
- Pindasana in **142**
- Urdhva Padmasana **141**

Sitakari **78**
Sitali **78**
Sitting 31, 32, 41, 47
- For Pranayama 61-64
- Poses 29, 41, 48, 95, 152, **181-197**, 200
- Forward Bends 25, 36
- Simple 56, 61, **184-190**
  - Twisting in 200

Sleeping Tortoise Pose **196**
Sleeping Yoga Pose **197**
Spinal Twist **202-203**
- Intense **203**

Spine 16, 27, 40, 41, 42, 49-51, 54, 61, 81, 87, 85, 97
Splits **178**
Square Breath 71, **72**
Squatting **93**
- Twist **207**

Standing 24, 26, 33, 31, 47, 49, **81-85**
- Back Bends 104, 106, 113, **173-174**
- Balances 111, 114, **118-121**, 179
- Basic Standing Forward Bend 41, 50, 54, 99, 103, 104, 106, **111**, 133
  - Basic Standing Forward Bend Balance **111**
- Forward Bends **111-112**, 182
- Poses 25, 32, 48, 50, **109-123**, 126, 163, 182
- Side Angle Poses **116-117**
- Straight 41, 81, **83**, 99, 103, 104, 106, 118, 173
- Twists **122-123**
- Wheel from **173**

Star Pose **187**
Stick Pose **128**
Stress 27, 39, 41, 46, 53, 56, 60, 67
- Stress Management 22-23
- Repetitive Stress Injury 42-43, 181

Supported Inverted Practice **144**
Supported Bridge Pose **144**
Sukhasana **184**
Sun Salutation 25, 31, 32, 50, 91, 94, **97-107**, 165
Supta Konasana **152**
Supta Kurmasana **196**
Surya Bhedana Pranayama **76**
Surya Namaskar **97**
Svanasana
- Adho Mukha **92**, 106
- Urdhva Mukha 105, **165**

T

Tadasana **83**, 104, 106
Throat 60, 68, 78, 125, 126, 169
Thunderbolt Pose **184**
- Toes Turned Under **185**

Tiredness 38, 57, 60, 144
Tortoise Pose **195**, 196
- Sleeping **196**

Tree Pose **119**
- Head Down **130-131**

Triang Mukhaikapada Paschimottanasana **192**
Triangle
- Forward Bend 109, **112**
- Pose 109, **117**
- Twist 109, **122**, 123

Trikonasana **117**
- Parivrtta **122**

Tripod Headstand **142**
Twists 37, 97, 160
- In Headstand **140**
  - Scissors **140**
- In Shoulderstand **149**
- Inverted 127
- Lotus in Shoulderstand **155**
- Sitting 43, **199-207**
- Standing **122-123**

U
Ujjayi **67**
Upavista Konasana **187**
Upright Forward Bend **190**
Urdhva Dhanurasana **163**
From standing
Urdhva Kukkutasana **157**
Urdhva Mukha Svanasana **165**
Urdhva Padmasana Sirsasana **141**
Urdhva Prasarita Ekapadasana **111**
Uterus, Prolapsed 152
Ustrasana **175**
Utkatasana **84**
Uttanasana 104, 106, **111**

V
Vajrasana **184**
Vasisthasana **129**
Viloma **71**
Viparita Dandasana
Eka Pada **172**
Dwi Pada **170**
Viparita Karani **144**
Virabhadrasana I **113**
Virabhadrasana II **115**
Virabhadrasana III **114**
Virasana **185**
Vrksasana **119**
Adho Mukha **131**

W
Warrior Poses **113-115**
Warrior I **113**, 159
Warrior II **115**
Warrior Balance **114**
Wheel Pose 132, 161, **163**, 171
From standing 163, **173**, 175, 179
Wide Angle Pose 62, 139, 152, 184, **187**, 189, 193, 195, 201
Women 17-18, 28, 130

Y
Yoga Sutras 10-15, 19
Yoga
Astanga 11, 107
Bhakti 17
Classes 35
Hatha 4, 15-16
Iyengar 4-5, 35, 107
Jnana 17
Karma 17
Mantra 15
Raja 10
Sutras 10-15, 19
Yoga Nidrasana **197**

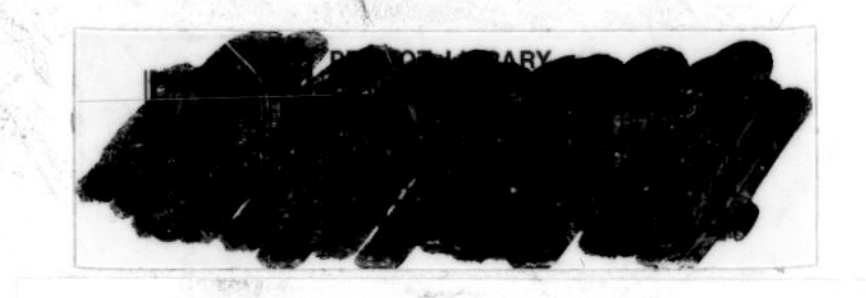

DATE DUE

FEB 1 4 1997	
APR 1 2 1997	
JUN 1 1 1997	
JUL 1 6 1997	
AUG 0 6 1997	
AUG 2 5 1997	
OCT 0 9 1997	
JUL 2 8 1998	
AUG 2 5 1998	